The AOTA Practice Guidelines Series

Occupational Therapy Practice Guidelines for Children and Adolescents With Challenges in Sensory Processing and Sensory Integration

Renee Watling, PhD, OTR/L, FAOTA
Visiting Assistant Professor
University of Puget Sound
School of Occupational Therapy
Tacoma, WA

Kristie Patten Koenig, PhD, OTR/L, FAOTA
Assistant Professor
New York University
Steinhardt School of Culture, Education, and Human Development
Department of Occupational Therapy
New York

Patricia L. Davies, PhD, OTR, FAOTA
Associate Professor
Colorado State University
Department of Occupational Therapy
Fort Collins

Roseann C. Schaaf, PhD, OTR/L, FAOTA
Professor and Vice Chairman
Department of Occupational Therapy
Faculty, Farber Institute for Neurosciences
Thomas Jefferson University
Philadelphia

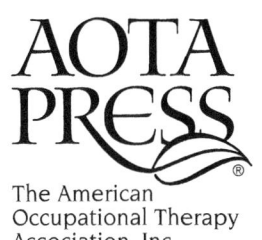

The American Occupational Therapy Association, Inc.

AOTA Centennial Vision

We envision that occupational therapy is a powerful, widely recognized, science-driven, and evidence-based profession with a globally connected and diverse workforce meeting society's occupational needs.

Mission Statement

The American Occupational Therapy Association advances the quality, availability, use, and support of occupational therapy through standard-setting, advocacy, education, and research on behalf of its members and the public.

AOTA Staff

Frederick P. Somers, *Executive Director*
Christopher M. Bluhm, *Chief Operating Officer*

Chris Davis, *Director, AOTA Press*
Ashley Hofmann, *Development/Production Editor*
Victoria Davis, *Production Editor/Editorial Assistant*

Beth Ledford, *Director, Marketing*
Emily Zhang, *Technology Marketing Specialist*
Jennifer Folden, *Marketing Specialist*

American Occupational Therapy Association, Inc.
4720 Montgomery Lane
Bethesda, MD 20814
Phone: 301-652-AOTA (2682)
TDD: 800-377-8555
Fax: 301-652-7711
www.aota.org

To order: 1-877-404-AOTA or http://store.aota.org

© 2011 by the American Occupational Therapy Association, Inc. All rights reserved.
No part of this publication may be reproduced in whole or in part by any means without permission.
Printed in the United States of America.

Disclaimers

This publication is designed to provide accurate and authoritative information in regard to the subject matter covered. It is sold or distributed with the understanding that the publisher is not engaged in rendering legal, accounting, or other professional service. If legal advice or other expert assistance is required, the services of a competent professional person should be sought.
—*From the Declaration of Principles jointly adopted by the American Bar Association and a Committee of Publishers and Associations*

It is the objective of the American Occupational Therapy Association to be a forum for free expression and interchange of ideas. The opinions expressed by the contributors to this work are their own and not necessarily those of the American Occupational Therapy Association.

ISBN: 978-1-56900-320-6
Library of Congress Control Number: 2011924389

Cover Design by Sarah Ely and Jennifer Farr
Composition by Maryland Composition, *Laurel, MD*
Printed by Automated Graphic Services, *White Plains, MD*

Citation: Watling, R., Koenig, K. P., Davies, P. L., & Schaaf, R. C. (2011). *Occupational therapy practice guidelines for children and adolescents with challenges in sensory processing and sensory integration.* Bethesda, MD: AOTA Press.

Contents

Acknowledgments vii

Introduction 1
    Purpose and Use of This Publication 1
    Domain and Process of Occupational Therapy 2

Overview of Children and Adolescents With Challenges in Processing and Integrating Sensory Information 5
    Sensory Integration Theory: Concepts, Neuroscience Underpinnings, Subtypes, and Prevalence 5
    A Word About Terminology 8

The Occupational Therapy Process for Children and Adolescents With Challenges in Sensory Processing and Sensory Integration 9
    Referral: Diagnostic vs. Intervention Planning Assessment 9
    Evaluation 10
    Evidence-Based Review of the Performance Challenges Related to Sensory Processing
        and Sensory Integration 25
    Intervention 27
    Evidence-Based Review of the Effectiveness of Occupational Therapy Intervention
        Using a Sensory Integration Approach 40
    Evidence-Based Review of the Effectiveness of Occupational Therapy Intervention
        Using Approaches Other Than Sensory Integration 47
    Foundations of Occupational Therapy Services for Children and Adolescents With Challenges
        in Sensory Processing and Sensory Integration 50
    Evidence-Based Review of the Neuroscience Literature 50
    Sensory Function and Dysfunction 54
    Evidence-Based Review of Subtypes of Children and Adolescents With Challenges in Processing
        and Integrating Sensory Information 60

Safety and Risk Issues 64
Mentorship and Training in Using a Sensory Integration Approach 65
Summary of the Evidence-Based Literature Reviews and Recommendations for
    Occupational Therapy Interventions. 66

Appendixes

Appendix A. Preparation and Qualifications of Occupational Therapists and
    Occupational Therapy Assistants 73
Appendix B. Evidence-Based Practice 75
Appendix C. Evidence Tables 81
Appendix D. History and Occupational Profile 189
Appendix E. Selected *CPT™* Coding for Occupational Therapy Evaluations and Interventions. 197
Appendix F. Data Collection Forms 199
Appendix G. Application to Adults With Mental Health Concerns 203
Appendix H. Glossary. 205

References 209

Figures, Boxes, and Tables Used in This Publication

Figure 1.   Occupational therapy's domain 3
Figure 2.   Aspects of occupational therapy's domain 3
Figure 3.   Occupational therapy's process of service delivery as applied within the
            profession's domain. 4

Box 1.   Questions to Aid Development of the Occupational Profile 11

Table 1.   Play Observations 15
Table 2.   Selected Evaluation Instruments of Occupational Performance for Children and
            Adolescents With Challenges Processing and Integrating Sensory Information. 17
Table 3.   Structured Observations of Fine Motor Performance 20
Table 4.   Observation of Social Skills. 23
Table 5.   Context Considerations and Activity Demands in Evaluation 24
Table 6.   Approaches and Sensory Strategies for Occupational Therapy Intervention in
            School-Based Practice 41

Table 7.	Recommendations for Occupational Therapy Interventions for Children and Adolescents With Challenges in Processing and Integrating Sensory Information	67
Table 8.	Application of Practice Guideline to Cases: Examples of Evaluation and Intervention	69
Table B1.	Levels of Evidence for Occupational Therapy Outcomes Research	75
Table B2.	Search Terms for Occupational Therapy Sensory Integration (SI) and Non-SI Intervention Systematic Reviews	79
Table B3.	Number and Levels of Evidence for Articles Included in Each Review Question	80
Table C1.	Neuroscience Evidence for the Effectiveness of Using a Sensory-Based Approach in Occupational Therapy With Children and Adolescents	83
Table C2.	Summary of the Evidence Supporting Subtypes of Children With Difficulty Processing and Integrating Sensory Information	107
Table C3.	Evidence for Functional Performance Difficulties in Children and Adolescents With Difficulty Processing and Integrating Sensory Information: Play–Leisure and Social Participation; ADLs and IADLs; Rest and Sleep; and Education and Work	146
Table C4.	Summary of the Evidence of the Effectiveness of Occupational Therapy Interventions Using a Sensory Integration Approach for Children and Adolescents	161
Table C5.	Summary of the Evidence of the Effectiveness of Occupational Therapy Interventions Other Than the Sensory Integration Approach for Children and Adolescents	180

■ ■ ■

Acknowledgments

The authors acknowledge the following individuals for their contributions to the evidence-based literature review:
Noemi Cantin, OT Reg. (Ont.)
Patricia L. Davies, PhD, OTR, FAOTA
Kristie Patten Koenig, PhD, OTR/L, FAOTA
Jane A. Koomar, PhD, OTR/L, FAOTA
Shelly J. Lane, PhD, OTR/L, FAOTA
Teresa A. May-Benson, ScD, OTR/L
Helene J. Polatajko, PhD, OT Reg. (Ont.), OT(C), FCAOT, FCAHS
Sarah G. Rudney, MS, OTR/L
Roseann C. Schaaf, PhD, OTR/L, FAOTA
Rebecca Tucker, MS, OTR/L

Issue Editor
Marian Arbesman, PhD, OTR/L
President, ArbesIdeas, Inc.
Consultant, AOTA Evidence-Based Practice Project
Adjunct Assistant Professor
University at Buffalo
Department of Rehabilitation Science
Buffalo, NY

Series Editor
Deborah Lieberman, MHSA, OTR/L FAOTA
Program Director, Evidence-Based Practice Project
Staff Liaison to the Commission on Practice
American Occupational Therapy Association
Bethesda, MD

The authors acknowledge and thank the following individuals for their participation in the content review and development of this publication:
Stefanie Bodison, OTD, OTR/L
Diana A. Henry, MS, OTR/L, FAOTA
Jane A. Koomar, PhD, OTR/L, FAOTA
Shelly J. Lane, PhD, OTR/L, FAOTA
Teresa A. May-Benson, ScD, OTR/L
Lucy J. Miller, PhD, OTR, FAOTA
Diane Parham, PhD, OTR/L, FAOTA
Sandra Schefkind, MS, OTR/L
Sarah A. Schoen, PhD, OTR
Susanne Smith Roley, MS, OTR/L, FAOTA
V. Judith Thomas, MGA

Introduction

Purpose and Use of This Publication

Practice guidelines have been widely developed in response to the health care reform movement in the United States. Such guidelines can be useful tools for improving the quality of health care, enhancing consumer satisfaction, promoting appropriate use of services, and reducing costs. The American Occupational Therapy Association (AOTA), which represents the interests of 140,000 occupational therapists, occupational therapy assistants (see Appendix A), and students of occupational therapy, is committed to providing information through relevant practice guidelines and other resources to support decision making that promotes high-quality health care and wellness and educational systems that are affordable and accessible to all.

Using an evidence-based perspective and key concepts from the *Occupational Therapy Practice Framework: Domain and Process* (2nd ed.; AOTA, 2008b), this guideline provides an overview of the occupational therapy process for children and adolescents with challenges in processing and integrating sensory information. It defines the occupational therapy domain, process, and intervention that occur within the boundaries of acceptable practice. This guideline does not discuss all possible methods of care, and although it does recommend some specific methods of care, the occupational therapist makes the ultimate judgment regarding the appropriateness of a given procedure in light of a specific client's circumstances and needs.

It is the intention of AOTA, through this publication, to help occupational therapists and occupational therapy assistants, as well as individuals who manage, reimburse, or set policy regarding occupational therapy services, understand the contribution of occupational therapy in evaluating and serving children and adolescents with challenges in processing sensory information. This guideline also can serve as a reference for parents; school administrators, educators, and other school staff; health care facility managers; education and health care regulators; third-party payers; and managed care organizations. This document may be used in any of the following ways:

- To assist occupational therapists and occupational therapy assistants in communicating about their services to external audiences
- To assist other health care practitioners, teachers, and program administrators in determining whether referral for occupational therapy services would be appropriate
- To assist third-party payers in understanding the therapeutic need for occupational therapy services for children and adolescents with challenges in processing and integrating sensory information
- To assist health and education planning teams in determining the developmental and educational need for occupational therapy
- To assist legislators, third-party payers, and administrators in understanding the professional education, training, and skills of occupational therapists and occupational therapy assistants
- To assist program developers, administrators, legislators, and third-party payers in understanding the scope of occupational therapy services
- To assist program evaluators and policy analysts in determining outcome measures for analyzing the effectiveness of occupational therapy intervention
- To assist policy, education, and health care benefit analysts in understanding the appropriateness of occupational therapy services for children and adolescents with challenges in processing sensory information
- To assist occupational therapy educators in designing appropriate curricula that incorporate the

role of occupational therapy with children and adolescents with challenges in processing sensory information.

The introduction to this guideline provides a brief discussion of the domain and process of occupational therapy. Next is an overview of sensory integration theory, including neuroscience underpinnings, subtypes, and prevalence of challenges in sensory processing and integration. This overview is followed by a detailed description of the occupational therapy process for children and adolescents with challenges in processing and integrating sensory information, including evaluation and intervention processes. Embedded within these descriptions are brief summaries of the results of systematic reviews of evidence from the scientific literature regarding performance challenges and best practices in occupational therapy intervention for this population. The guideline also includes a section on the foundations of occupational therapy services with this population, including history and theory development, and comprehensive summaries of the systematic review of the neuroscience literature and scientific literature supporting subtypes for children and adolescents with challenges in processing and integrating sensory information, as well as content addressing training and safety concerns. Finally, appendixes contain a description of the preparation and qualifications of occupational therapy practitioners, an outline of evidence-based practice and the methodology used in the literature review, evidence tables, a form for use in compiling a client history and occupational profile, guidelines related to use of *CPT*™ codes in billing, data collection forms, a review of application to adults with mental health concerns, and a glossary of related terms.

Domain and Process of Occupational Therapy

Occupational therapy practitioners'[1] expertise lies in their knowledge of occupation and how engaging in occupations can be used to improve human performance and ameliorate the effects of disease and disability (AOTA, 2008b).

In 2002, the AOTA Representative Assembly adopted the *Occupational Therapy Practice Framework: Domain and Process*. Informed by the previous *Uniform Terminology for Occupational Therapy* (AOTA, 1979, 1989, 1994) and the World Health Organization's (2001) *International Classification of Functioning, Disability and Health*, the *Framework* outlines the profession's domain and the process of service delivery within this domain. In 2008, the *Framework* was updated as part of the standard 5-year review cycle (AOTA, 2008b). The revisions included in the second edition focused on refining the document and updating it to reflect language and concepts relevant to current and emerging occupational therapy practice.

Domain

A profession's *domain* articulates its members' sphere of knowledge, societal contribution, and intellectual or scientific activity. The occupational therapy profession's domain centers on helping others participate in daily life activities. The broad term that the profession uses to describe daily life activities is *occupation*. As outlined in the *Framework*, occupational therapists and occupational therapy assistants[2] work collaboratively with clients to support health and participation through engagement in occupation (see Figure 1). This overarching mission circumscribes the profession's domain and emphasizes the important ways in

---

[1] When the term *occupational therapy practitioner* is used in this document, it refers to both occupational therapists and occupational therapy assistants (AOTA, 2006).

[2] Occupational therapists are responsible for all aspects of occupational therapy service delivery and are accountable for the safety and effectiveness of the occupational therapy service delivery process. Occupational therapy assistants deliver occupational therapy services under the supervision of and in partnership with an occupational therapist (AOTA, 2009a).

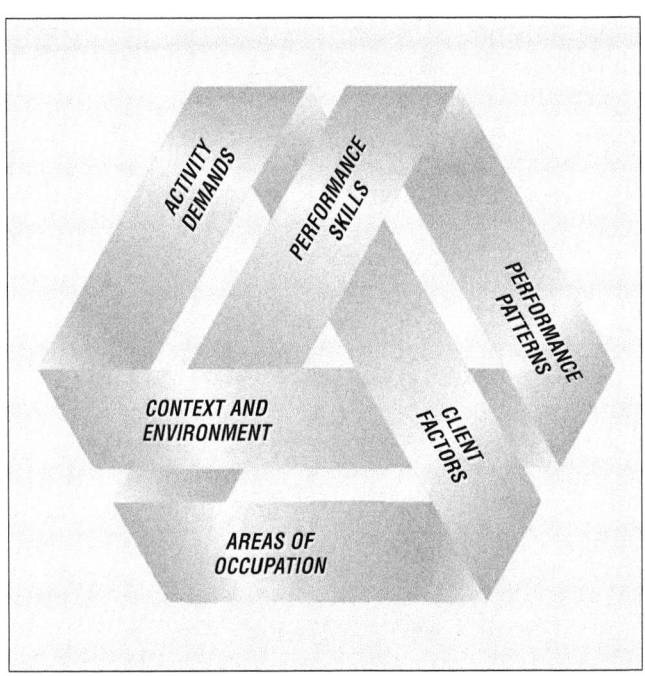

Figure 1. Occupational therapy's domain.

Reprinted from "Occupational Therapy Practice Framework: Domain and Process" (2nd ed., p. 627), by American Occupational Therapy Association, 2008, *American Journal of Occupational Therapy, 62,* 625–683. Used with permission.

AREAS OF OCCUPATION	CLIENT FACTORS	PERFORMANCE SKILLS	PERFORMANCE PATTERNS	CONTEXT AND ENVIRONMENT	ACTIVITY DEMANDS
Activities of Daily Living (ADL)*	Values, Beliefs, and Spirituality	Sensory Perceptual Skills	Habits	Cultural	Objects Used and Their Properties
Instrumental Activities of Daily Living (IADL)	Body Functions	Motor and Praxis Skills	Routines	Personal	Space Demands
Rest and Sleep	Body Structures	Emotional Regulation Skills	Roles	Physical	Social Demands
Education		Cognitive Skills	Rituals	Social	Sequencing and Timing
Work		Communication and Social Skills		Temporal	Required Actions
Play				Virtual	Required Body Functions
Leisure					Required Body Structures
Social Participation					
*Also referred to as *basic activities of daily living (BADL)* or *personal activities of daily living (PADL).*					

Figure 2. Aspects of occupational therapy's domain.

Reprinted from "Occupational Therapy Practice Framework: Domain and Process" (2nd ed., p. 628), by American Occupational Therapy Association, 2008, *American Journal of Occupational Therapy, 62,* 625–683. Used with permission.

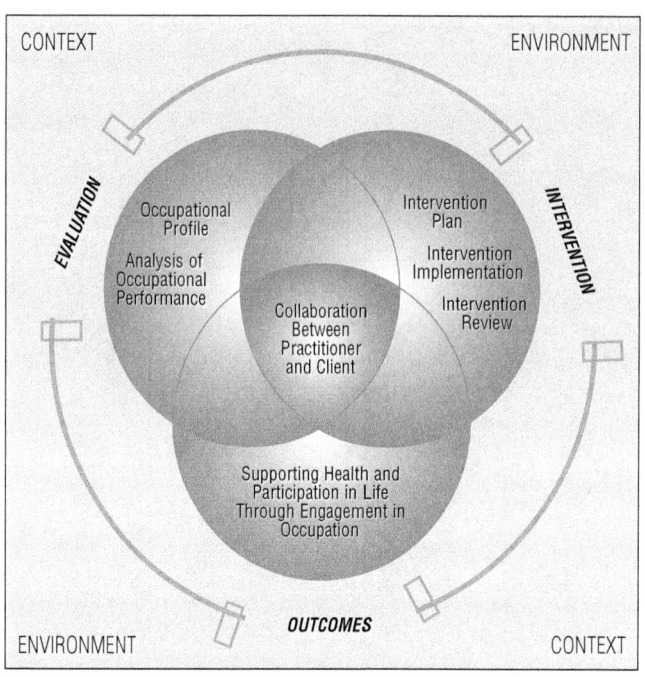

Figure 3. Occupational therapy's process of service delivery as applied within the profession's domain.

Reprinted from "Occupational Therapy Practice Framework: Domain and Process" (2nd ed., p. 627), by American Occupational Therapy Association, 2008, *American Journal of Occupational Therapy, 62*, 625–683. Used with permission.

which environmental and life circumstances influence the manner in which people carry out their occupations. Key aspects of the domain of occupational therapy are defined in Figure 2.

Process

Many professions use the process of evaluating, intervening, and targeting outcomes that is outlined in the *Framework*. Occupational therapy's application of this process is made unique, however, by its focus on occupation (see Figure 3). The process of occupational therapy service delivery includes an *occupational profile*; an assessment of the client's occupational needs, problems, and concerns; and the *analysis of occupational performance*, which includes the skills, patterns, contexts, activity demands, and client factors that contribute to or impede the client's satisfaction with his or her ability to engage in valued daily life activities. Therapists *plan and implement intervention* using a variety of approaches and methods in which occupation is both the means and the end (Trombly, 1995). Occupational therapists continually assess the effectiveness of the intervention they provide and the client's progress toward targeted outcomes. Ongoing *intervention review* informs decisions to continue or discontinue intervention and to make referrals to other agencies or professionals. Therapists select outcome measures that are valid, reliable, and appropriately sensitive to the client's occupational performance, adaptation, health and wellness, prevention, quality of life, role competence, self-advocacy, and occupational justice.

■ ■ ■

Overview of Children and Adolescents With Challenges in Processing and Integrating Sensory Information

Occupational therapy practitioners are concerned with an individual's ability to engage in and perform all activities that are required of him or her and any that he or she desires to do in the course of daily life (AOTA, 2008b). As a discipline, occupational therapy is steeped in the sciences that provide knowledge and understanding of human development and function and the many variables that influence these aspects of human life. Occupational therapy recognizes that the registration, processing, and integration of sensory information can both support and inhibit an individual's ability to function in context. It is the aim of this document to describe the relationship between sensory processing and participation in everyday activities, including development of sensory integration theory, concepts of function and dysfunction, approaches to evaluation, strategies for intervention, and elements of training and specialization. This section includes sensory integration concepts and the current evidence related to the neuroscience underpinnings, subtypes, and prevalence of challenges in sensory processing and integration.

Sensory Integration Theory: Concepts, Neuroscience Underpinnings, Subtypes, and Prevalence

Sensory Integration Concepts

Nearly 50 years ago, A. Jean Ayres introduced the idea that central nervous system processing and integration of sensation create a foundation upon which functional behavior develops. Ayres (1972b) posited that sensory information was nourishment for the nervous system and that the nervous system responded to sensory information with alterations in function, structure, and output. She used the term *sensory integration* to identify "the neurological process that organizes sensation from one's own body and from the environment and makes it possible to use the body effectively within the environment" (p. 11).

A primary principle upon which Ayres based her work is that of neuroplasticity (Jacobs & Schneider, 2001). Ayres consulted both human and animal neuroscience literature to ensure that her theory was grounded in empirical findings. Her work was based on the many animal studies examining the effects of sensory deprivation and of enriched environments, which provided evidence that organism–environment interaction could alter brain structure and function (e.g., Harlow, 1958; Harlow, Harlow, & Suomi, 1971).

Ayres generated postulates about the relationship between sensation and typical development, the manner in which sensory integrative dysfunction interferes with development, and the way in which sensation could be used to remediate dysfunction and support development. The first postulate of sensory integration theory purports that successful sensory integrative function creates a foundation for behavior and learning. Ayres hypothesized that integration of sensory information provides an individual with a reference for the body's relationship to itself, gravity, and people and objects in the environment and helps an individual perceive relationships between other people and objects in the environment. Sensory information arises from multiple sources, both within and outside the human body. All sensation is essential for the individual to develop an awareness of himself or herself as an integrated whole and helps to build a foundation for learning and skill development, including *praxis*, the ability to plan and organize motor behavior in time and space. As the child with typical development grows, sensory integrative functions become established, and the child gains in cognitive, psychosocial, and regulatory capacity and skill. The interaction of sensory integrative functions with these capacities supports the child in producing adaptive responses, a primary emphasis of sensory integration theory. Adaptive response and praxis are further discussed later in this document.

The second postulate of sensory integration theory describes the limitations in function that can occur when processing and integration of sensory information are inadequate. Ayres (1979) described dysfunction in sensory integration as a condition in which "the brain is not processing or organizing the flow of sensory impulses in a manner that gives the individual good, precise sensory input well. . . [and] is not directing behavior effectively" (p. 51). This ineffective sensory processing and behavioral organization interfere with the individual's ability to use sensation as a foundation for function. The manifestation of sensory integration dysfunction is multifaceted, with individuals displaying clusters of signs and symptoms in cognitive, motor, and emotional behavior, as well as dyspraxia. Thus, sensory integration dysfunction is seen not as an absence of function but as a malfunction in brain processing, with such dysfunction leading to impairments in occupational performance and participation in context.

The third major postulate of sensory integration theory expresses concepts related to therapeutic intervention aimed at improving nervous system processing and integrating sensory information. Ayres (1972b) proposed that sensation could be used intentionally and strategically to enhance the individual's ability to detect, register, perceive, and respond adaptively to stimuli in an organized and appropriate manner that is reflected in cognitive, motor, and emotional responses. Thus, sensory experiences could be used to create a foundation for successful occupational engagement and functional performance.

Neuroscience Underpinnings

Ayres's work was grounded in the neuroscience knowledge available to her from the 1950s through the 1980s. Since then, dramatic advances in neuroscience have led to a rapidly expanding body of literature that has bearing on both the distinct components and the totality of Ayres's theory. Lane and Schaaf (2010) conducted a systematic review of the neuroscience literature published between 1996 and 2006. Specifically, they addressed the question, What is the neuroscience evidence that occupational therapy using a sensory integration framework with children and adolescents will be effective? This question was designed to investigate the basic neural and developmental science literature that might support or refute the provision of occupational therapy using a sensory integration approach for intervention. The methodology for the review can be found in Appendix B.

Through the review, Lane and Schaaf (2010) found the literature investigating environmental enrichment to be relevant because it offers the participant (animal or human) control over activity, engagement, novelty, and challenge; a "playful" environment; and a more lifelike context (Bennett, Diamond, Krech, & Rosenzweig, 1964; Rosenzweig & Bennett, 1972), thus most closely resembling occupational therapy using a sensory integration approach. In general, this body of work shows that environmental enrichment can enhance neural plasticity. In addition, studies of specific sensory systems, sensory–motor activities, and multisensory integration also demonstrate that sensation and/or sensory–motor activity serves as a catalyst for neuroplasticity. Finally, several of the specific principles that Ayres (1972b) identified as key components of the sensory integration approach are at least indirectly supported. For example, the idea that intervention is best delivered in a child-directed, playful manner that allows for flexible adaptations to achievable challenges is supported in the human data demonstrating that brain processing of sensory input is flexible and dynamic and that the greatest changes come when interaction with the environment is self-initiated rather than forced (van Praag, Kempermann, & Gage, 1999). The idea that enriched sensory–motor experience enhances the brain's processing of information and provides a foundation for learning is demonstrated in Level I animal studies and human studies showing that enriched conditions (sensory, motor, and problem-solving opportunities) produced neuroplastic changes in areas of the brain related to learning and memory and that these changes were concurrent with behavioral improvements in learning (Kempermann & Gage, 1999). Thus, it appears that as science advances our knowledge about brain–behavior interactions, Ayres's (1965) original ideas—that learning is a function of the brain and that sensation provides nourishment for brain development and function—are gaining support and validation. All studies identified by the review are summarized in Table C1 in Appendix C, and full reference citations are listed in the "References" section. A more in-depth analysis of this review can be found beginning on page 50.

Subtypes

Since the theory of sensory integration was first proposed in 1963, Ayres's work has been continued and expanded upon by many theorists, researchers, and clinicians. In addition, an increasing number of investigations of sensory integration theory and intervention and new empirical evidence have emerged, including new models of function and dysfunction. Each model has specific strengths and weaknesses, and further research is needed to validate these models and subtypes. The complexity of the role of sensation in function remains a challenge to developing an integrated model that addresses all aspects of this multifaceted area. Thus, current models often explicate only certain aspects of sensory function and dysfunction.

An evidence-based review of the literature examining subtypes of dysfunction in processing and integrating sensory input was conducted by Davies and Tucker (2010). Information about the methodology for the review is included in Appendix B, and a summary of the incorporated articles is presented in Table C2 in Appendix C. Highlights of that review are presented here, and a more in-depth summary is provided in the section "Evidence-Based Review of Subtypes of Children and Adolescents With Challenges in Processing and Integrating Sensory Information" beginning on page 60.

Four studies directly examining subtypes of sensory integration and processing were found in the literature and included in the review (Dunn & Bennett, 2002; Liss, Saulnier, & Kinsbourne, 2006; Mulligan, 1998, 2000). Since the review was completed, an additional study has been published that provides evidence for subtypes. Together, these studies suggest that subtypes exist. However, each study used a different assessment measure, which resulted in each study yielding different clusters or groupings. Two of the studies had clusters related to dyspraxia, one had clusters related to modulation and attention, and one had clusters related to modulation. This finding emphasizes the need for a comprehensive assessment of sensory function and sensory-based motor performance that includes sensory perception, discrimination, modulation, and praxis in a single study. In addition, studies that include multiple assessment items and tools also will increase their probability of capturing patterns of sensory processing abilities that lead to function or dysfunction in everyday activities, provided they are comprehensive in their scope. Finally, more studies using multivariate methods are needed to confirm or dispute the existence of subtypes of sensory integrative dysfunction or sensory processing disorder. Researchers should be attentive to the assessments used in future research aiming to identify or confirm subtypes.

Prevalence

Ayres (1972b) hypothesized that 5% to 15% of the population had some form of dysfunction in sensory integration that interfered with occupational performance. Recent work suggests that her hypothesis was accurate. For example, Ahn, Miller, Milberger, and McIntosh (2004) found that 5% to 15% of the general population of kindergarten-age children in the United States have difficulties with sensory modulation. Estimates are even higher among individuals with a clinical diagnosis. For children with an autism spectrum disorder, estimates range from 80% to 100% (Dawson & Watling, 2000; Tomchek & Dunn, 2007), and estimates of prevalence among individuals with developmental disabilities range from 40% to 80% (Baranek et al., 2002).

A Word About Terminology

When presenting the theory of sensory integration, Ayres used terminology that was not commonly understood within occupational therapy. Terms such as *registration, habituation, modulation,* and *integration* were used to describe key concepts in the theory and were defined according to the available neuroscience literature at the time. As familiarity with the theory of sensory integration has expanded, so has common understanding of the terms used by Ayres. However, these terms have been used differently in other fields. Advances in the neurosciences have led to a refinement of many of these terms. As a result, there is inconsistency in the literature, with the same terms meaning different things, and at times debate has occurred regarding which is the best or most appropriate term for conveying a given concept. Some of the inconsistency is reflective of the terminology in vogue at the time a paper was published, some reflects an inaccurate understanding of concepts by a paper's authors, and some reflects differences in philosophical positions. As the theory of sensory integration has evolved, the terminology also has shifted and evolved to reflect contemporary research and practice. At the present time, debate regarding terminology continues around some terms (Schaaf & Davies, 2010). A glossary for this text is provided to prevent misinterpretation or misrepresentation of terms and concepts as they are used in this document (Appendix H).

■ ■ ■

The Occupational Therapy Process for Children and Adolescents With Challenges in Sensory Processing and Sensory Integration

The process of occupational therapy for individuals with challenges in processing and integrating sensory information includes evaluation and intervention focused on salient outcomes that include but are not limited to the individual's occupational performance, adaptation, health and wellness, participation in the community, quality of life, role competence, self-advocacy, and occupational justice (AOTA, 2008b). The occupational therapy process aims to identify the individual's strengths and any areas of need related to occupational engagement and participation.

Services are initiated when an individual client demonstrates functional difficulties that impede engagement in occupations and participation in everyday life activities. The evaluation includes gathering, interpreting, and synthesizing information relevant to the client's past and current occupational engagement and performance as well as desired future participation and specific evaluation of current occupational performance.

Occupational therapy intervention is designed individually and is aimed at improving the client's desired and expected occupational engagement and participation through implementation of strategies and procedures directed at the client, the activity, and the environment. Occupational therapy services often build upon the client's demonstrated strengths and use them to support his or her success in additional areas of occupation.

When developing an intervention, occupational therapy practitioners always consider the dynamic nature of the context in which the client is expected to perform.

The occupational therapy process also includes monitoring the client's response to an intervention, reevaluating and modifying the intervention plan, and measuring intervention success through outcomes that are relevant and meaningful to the individual. The occupational therapy process is client- and family-centered and considers the dynamic interaction of the individual and the internal neurophysiological and external physical, social, and cultural contexts of function. Occupational therapy is fluid, dynamic, and interactive, using engagement in occupations as both the method and desired outcome of the process.

Referral: Diagnostic vs. Intervention Planning Assessment

The occupational therapy process usually begins with a referral initiated by a parent or caregiver, physician, or school personnel. Occupational therapy services are requested when performance limitations are suspected or limitations in adaptive behaviors are observed (e.g., in movement, play skills, self-regulation, fine motor function). In most cases, the evaluation is requested to document the individual's strengths and weaknesses and determine whether intervention is needed to assist the individual in improving engagement in needed and desired activities.

Occupational therapy evaluation may be requested for diagnostic and/or intervention planning purposes. In either case, the evaluation process should include measurement of the individual's abilities across the domain of occupational therapy with specific examination of sensory processing and integration patterns and careful assessment to determine which sensory systems support or inhibit the individual's occupational performance.

Occupational therapy evaluation should include an assessment of sensory processing and integration when referral concerns, report of individuals familiar with the client, results of other evaluations, or clinical observations suggest that dysfunction in sensory processing may be present. Assessment of sensory processing and integration should be conducted whenever conditions in which sensory processing and integration dysfunction are known to coexist or are diagnosed or suspected. These include autism spectrum disorders, fragile X syndrome, attention deficit hyperactivity disorder, developmental disability, postinstitutionalized children, low-birthweight infants, and some mental health disorders (Cermak, 2009; Mulligan, 2003a; Smith Roley, Blanche, & Schaaf, 2001; Watling, Bodison, Henry, & Miller Kuhaneck, 2006). Because dysfunction in sensory processing and integration also can play a role in regulatory disorders in young children (DeGangi, 2000; Williamson, Anzalone, & Hanft, 2000), these functions should be evaluated in children ages 0 to 3 years when self-regulation is a concern. When sensory processing and integration deficits are identified, they should be reported to all other members involved in the diagnostic process and to the client and his or her caregivers.

Although the methods used by occupational therapists are the same whether conducting evaluation to aid in diagnosis or treatment planning, interpretation of the evaluation results has a different focus for each of these distinct purposes. When the identified purpose of the occupational therapy evaluation is to assist in making a diagnosis, special attention is given to overall test scores and performance profiles. Results are interpreted with emphasis placed on identifying whether sensory processing and integration dysfunction exists, and if so, whether the dysfunction occurs in a pattern or profile consistent with that seen among children and youths with specific diagnostic classifications. This information is provided to the team for consideration in the diagnostic process.

When the stated purpose of the evaluation is to determine the most appropriate course of intervention services, scores on measures of sensory processing and integration are carefully analyzed for patterns and profiles. This analysis of test scores is complemented by careful consideration of the child's approach to tasks, self-organizational abilities and preferences, caregiver report about sensory reactivity and behavioral patterns, and observations of sensory responsiveness, among other factors. When patterns are found, the occupational therapist carefully reviews them to determine which areas of sensory processing and function are implicated. This information is then used to plan the intervention approach to be used in the initial course of intervention services.

Evaluation

Evaluation occurs formally and informally during all interactions and observations of the client. The evaluation process relies heavily on *clinical reasoning*, in which the occupational therapist synthesizes knowledge of human development and clinical conditions with the information gathered through interaction with the client to gain a greater understanding of the client's occupational performance. This process guides the therapist in analyzing observations, considering historical information about the client, and applying constructs of sensory integration theory. Clinical reasoning is a systematic process that aids in informed decision making about intervention context, activities, and appropriate outcomes.

Occupational therapists perform evaluations in collaboration with the client when possible, the client's family, and school staff when appropriate. The two elements of the occupational therapy evaluation are (a) the occupational profile and (b) the analysis of occupational performance (AOTA, 2008b). Occupational therapists may use standardized and nonstandardized assessments that are specifically designed for use with children and adolescents with challenges in processing and integrating sensory information, as well as other evaluation tools and methods. Occupational therapists should validate clinical observations with data from standardized assessments.

Occupational Profile

The purpose of the occupational profile is to allow the occupational therapist to gain an understanding of who the client or clients are, identify their needs or concerns, and determine how these concerns affect engagement in occupational performance. In addition, the occupational profile aims to help the therapist understand what is important to the client and what the client finds meaningful. Information for the occupational profile is gathered through formal and informal interviews with the client and significant others. When working with children, the client includes the child as well as significant family members and other care providers. Interviews explore the client's history and experiences; patterns of daily living; and interests, values, and needs.

Development of the occupational profile varies somewhat according to the context of service provision and can be influenced by availability of persons needed to participate in the process. Generally, the occupational profile is developed at the outset of services through a process of inquiry involving all persons who comprise the client. Inquiry focuses on what the client needs and wants to do, his or her interests and motivations, typical routines, past experiences, and current occupations in various contexts. With the client's help, the occupational therapist gains perspective of how the client spends his or her time and how the contexts and environments in which the client lives, learns, and plays support or hinder occupational engagement. An example of a history and occupational profile (Schaaf & Smith Roley, 2006) is included in Appendix D.

Issues of sensory processing and integration can influence the manner and nature of an individual's engagement in performance skills and patterns. It is important to investigate the nature of the client's choices and preferences for engagement as well as whether special accommodations are made by the family (and school or other agencies or programs when appropriate) for the client. Some questions that may be helpful in addressing these issues and that can be incorporated into the occupational profile are listed in Box 1.

The occupational profile identifies the child's occupational history and current occupations in various contexts and discusses typical routines and the child's interests and motivations. Additionally, the profile explores problematic daily routines. The current social supports (e.g., family and friend membership,

---

Box 1. Questions to Aid Development of the Occupational Profile

1. How does the child's response to sensation affect the engagement of the family in daily activities, particularly social activities like birthday parties; daily routines such as mealtimes, bedtime, and getting out of the house in the morning; and necessary activities such as errands?
2. Does the child seem to avoid or seek sensory-rich activities (e.g., frequently seeks out rough or intense physical play opportunities such as wrestling, swinging, spinning, or inversion; often initiates physical touch with people and objects and seeks out opportunities for messy play; refuses or resists participation in movement-based activities, messy arts and crafts, cooking projects, or activities with large groups of people)?
3. How do the individual's sensory processing and praxis skills affect his or her co-occupations with significant others such as family members and classmates (e.g., does the child avoid interaction with certain people because of a loud voice, boisterous or unpredictable behavior, tendency to touch or hug)?
4. Are special accommodations related to sensory processing regularly used with the child (e.g., time of day activities occur, changes to environmental stimuli, declining invitations to crowded or noisy places or events)?
5. How has the family been affected by the child's needs? Have significant changes been made to accommodate the child's needs, such as a parent quitting work in order to care for the child?

peer relationships, community resources, intervention programs) are identified to guide information gathering related to functioning and engagement in childhood occupations. The profile also includes concerns, questions, and priorities of the client. To develop the occupational profile for a child with concerns related to sensory processing and integration, interviewing the family using the Canadian Occupational Performance Measure (COPM; Law et al., 2005) can yield information about how and when the sensory processing challenges affect the child and family during daily life. The COPM can be administered to the child and/or a family member to gain insight into the respondent's perspective regarding occupational performance challenges. Additional instruments that may be useful include the Perceived Efficacy and Goal Setting System (PEGS; Missiuna, Pollock, & Law, 2004) and Children's Assessment of Participation and Enjoyment and Preferences for Activities of Children (CAPE/PAC; King et al., 2005). These instruments provide information about a child's participation in activities outside of school along the dimensions of diversity, intensity, physical and social context, and enjoyment. Results can help the occupational therapist understand how sensory processing and integration challenges may be affecting the child's activity preferences.

Information gathered in the occupational profile is used to guide the family-centered evaluation and intervention process. Using this information, the occupational therapist can identify the strengths and limitations of the child and family and, in turn, identify relevant evaluation methods to assess the underlying components of the identified impairments. The evaluation findings are used to establish goals and guide intervention planning.

Evaluation Considerations

Occupational therapy practitioners work in many settings (e.g., schools, clinics, homes) and with a variety of other professionals (e.g., educators, speech–language pathologists, physical therapists, psychologists) and paraprofessionals (e.g., instructional assistants, bus drivers, lunchroom personnel) when providing services for children and adolescents with challenges in processing and integrating sensory information. Factors that influence the evaluation process are briefly described in the following sections.

Setting and context considerations. The setting in which the occupational therapist works influences the focus of the evaluation. Services provided within a child's school are governed by federal and state legislation and must address the child's performance and participation in academic and nonacademic activities at school. Evaluation of sensory processing and integration in the school setting includes measurement of the child's ability to adapt, organize, and integrate sensory information in the many different school environments, such as the lunchroom, art class, and playground, and during varied school tasks and activities. An occupational therapist working in other settings, such as hospitals or community-based practices, may focus more broadly during the evaluation on the child's ability to adapt, organize, and integrate sensory information during tasks and activities related to engagement and participation in multiple settings and contexts.

Standardized vs. nonstandardized assessments. Assessment typically involves the use of multiple measures, including both standardized and nonstandardized instruments. Standardized assessments have fixed protocols for administering test items and specific guidelines for scoring and interpreting the client's performance (Kielhofner, 2006; Urbina, 2004). Such instruments offer in-depth measurement of the client's performance in the area evaluated by the test and can aid in determining whether delays or deficits in performance are significant enough to warrant intervention. Standardized instruments must be administered under controlled conditions for results to be valid; however, the standardized testing conditions rarely represent the conditions in which the client is expected to perform on an everyday basis, so performance on standardized tests may not be representative of the client's daily performance in other contexts. In addition, some individuals with challenges in sensory processing and sensory integration cannot conform to the specific procedures and protocols required during administration, precluding the use of these tools for these clients. Nonstandardized measures are more flexible in that they do not require adherence to a specified protocol for administration and may be used to supplement standardized test results. However, these tools do not yield standard scores and therefore are generally not sufficient for determining eligibility for services (Richardson, 2010). A few standardized and norm-referenced rating instruments are now available (e.g., Sensory Processing Measure and Sensory Processing Measure–Preschool; Miller Kuhaneck, Henry, & Glennon, 2007, 2010) that may be sufficient alternatives for qualifying children for services in some settings without need of scores on a performance-based measure.

Regardless of whether one uses standardized or nonstandardized instruments, the focus of the assessment process should be on obtaining accurate information about the individual's occupational performance. A variety of strategies, including direct assessment, naturalistic observation, and structured interview, should be used to obtain the most accurate and representative results.

Reliability and validity issues. When measuring a child's abilities, it is important to determine whether the measurements obtained are reliable and valid. *Reliability* is measured in various ways to determine the extent to which the scores obtained from a given measure can be expected to be consistent and stable when the individual is tested over time, with different sets of test items, or under different contextual conditions (Kielhofner & Fossey, 2006). *Validity* informs test users whether a given test measures the construct it intends to measure (Kielhofner & Fossey, 2006). Test validity is determined by comparing the test to other established tests measuring the same construct, expert review of the test items, and careful and specific analysis of the items included on the test. The reliability and validity of evaluation results depend on the appropriate and accurate use of the assessment tools and methods. Manuals include specific instructions for administering tests according to standardized procedures. Any deviations from the standard procedures must be documented in the evaluation report, and the impact on performance must be described. Deviation from standard administration procedures invalidates test scores, so therapists should refrain from calculating and reporting scores when standard procedures are not used. Specific reliability and validity of assessment tools typically are reported in the manual for each test, with additional data sometimes available in the professional literature. Occupational therapists should be familiar with the reliability and validity values of the assessment tools they use and be able to interpret test scores in accordance with these parameters.

Analysis of Occupational Performance

Evaluation of individuals with challenges in processing and integrating sensory information addresses components of sensory processing (e.g., registration, modulation, discrimination), as well as praxis, functional skills, and organization of behavior (Smith Roley, 2006a). Participation of the child in family, school, and community roles also is addressed in this process. Information from the occupational profile is used by the occupational therapist to determine the specific areas of occupation and contexts to address. Analysis of occupational performance includes the following steps:

- Observe the client performing activities in the natural or least restrictive environment, and note the effectiveness of the client's performance skills (e.g., motor, praxis, sensory–perceptual, emotional regulation, social) and performance patterns (e.g., habits, routines, rituals, roles).
- Select specific assessment tools and methods that will identify and measure factors related to sensory processing and integration that may be influencing the client's performance.
- Interpret the assessment data to identify which aspects of sensory processing and integration support and which hinder performance.
- Develop or refine a hypothesis regarding the client's performance.

Analysis of occupational performance culminates in a collaborative process of developing goals that address the desired outcome for the client. With consideration for the evaluation results, desired outcomes, and scientific evidence, the occupational therapist then identifies potential intervention approaches and discusses them with the client. Finally, the evaluation process and results are documented and communicated to the family, appropriate team members, and community agencies.

Participation in areas of occupation. Individuals with challenges in processing and integrating sensory information often have performance limitations in one or more areas of occupation. Depending on the concerns identified for the individual being assessed, play performance, school-related occupations, leisure and social participation, and adaptive behavior and activities of daily living may be evaluated. In addition to these everyday occupations, it is important to note that children with challenges processing and integrating sensory information frequently choose their occupational engagement according to their sensory responding patterns (Dunn, 2001). Thus, in addition to measuring performance in these areas, it is important to determine the influence of the individual's sensory processing and integration patterns on his or her preferences and choices for activity engagement.

Play. Play is a child's main occupation and therefore requires special attention in the evaluation. Children with challenges in processing and integrating sensory information often have difficulty with play. A limited play repertoire due to a lack of ideation, avoidance of certain play experiences due to overresponsiveness, inappropriate intensity or aggression during play, clumsiness, and ineffective use of the body to interact with play materials due to dyspraxia are some behaviors that may be present. Assessment of play skills occurs through both formal and informal methods. The Knox Preschool Play Scale (Knox, 2008) can be used to gather information about the types of play a child demonstrates. The Test of Playfulness (Skard & Bundy, 2008) examines a child's playfulness and motivation for play in an unstructured play situation. When conducting assessments of play, it is important for the occupational therapist to focus not only on what the child does and does not do in a play scenario, but also on *how* the child plays, *what* motivates him or her in play, and what is going on *around* the child while a certain type of play is demonstrated. In order to understand the way in which sensory processing and integration may be supporting or hindering a child's ability to play, assessment of play should be supplemented by skilled observation of the manner in which the child plays. Assessment of play should describe a child's level of play skills and take into account the qualitative and contextual aspects of the play. Some key features to incorporate into observations of play are provided in Table 1. These may be especially useful when time or contextual factors preclude structured evaluation of play skills.

School occupations. Analysis of the child's school-related occupations helps the therapist develop an understanding of how the sensory aspects of the classroom, playground, auditorium, cafeteria, library, and other school environments support or inhibit the child's ability to be successful as a learner, peer, and participant in school and extracurricular activities. Initial information is gathered from the family and school personnel regarding their concerns about the child's strengths and areas of challenge within the school context. Evaluation of school-based performance can be accomplished through use of the School Function Assessment (Coster, Deeney, Haltiwanger, & Haley, 1998). This tool yields data about the child's performance of functional tasks within the school context and identifies supports needed for successful participation in the academic and social contexts of elementary school. The School Version of the Assessment of Motor and Process Skills (School AMPS; Fisher, Bryze, Hume, & Griswold, 2005) is available for use with children ages 3 to 12 years. The School AMPS is an observation-based assessment that measures motor and process skills during performance of schoolwork in the child's typical classroom setting. These performance-based measures can be supplemented by administration of the Main Classroom and School Environment Forms of the Sensory Processing Measure (Miller Kuhaneck et al., 2007), the School Forms of the Sensory Processing Measure–Preschool (Miller Kuhaneck et al., 2010), or the Sensory Profile School Companion (Dunn, 2006). These tools yield information about the impact of sensory processing challenges on the child's function in

Table 1. Play Observations

Area	Observation
Toy Use	• Is the child able to select and engage with a toy independently? • Does the child have ideas about what to do with objects? • Does the child use toys creatively? • Does the child use the toy as it is intended? • Is the child able to expand a play activity independently? With suggestions from others? • How does the child interact with toys? Are interactions limited, repetitive, or stereotypic? • Does the child share toys with others? • Do the child and family members engage together in toy play?
Developmental	• What forms of play are observed? Parallel, cooperative, pretend, symbolic? • How long does the child persist in a play activity? • Does the child demonstrate emotions during play? Humor? Mischief? Frustration? • Is the child able to transition between play activities? • Is the child able to conclude play activities?
Context	• Is the child able to engage in play when the surrounding environment is noisy? Quiet? • Is the child able to engage in play when the surrounding environment contains moving objects or people? When the environment is still? • Does the child have regular opportunities to engage in a variety of play experiences, including indoor, outdoor, home-based, community-based, play group experiences?
Family Observations	• Do the child and family members regularly spend time playing together? • Who typically initiates family play? Child? Parent? Sibling? • Does the child seek out participation of other family members in his or her play episodes? If so, which family members? • How does the child respond when a family member attempts to participate in the child's play? • For how long is the child able to persist in play with other family members? • What is the usual reason that family play time concludes? Natural end to the activity? Family member chooses to stop playing? Child chooses to stop playing? Child's behavior interferes with play episode?
Play Preferences	• Is the child attracted to or does the child avoid toys with certain sensory qualities? • Does the child seek out sedentary play? • Does the child seek out movement-based play? • Does the child engage in antigravity play (e.g., jumping, climbing)? • Does the child invert his or her head during play? • Are the child's play preferences age-appropriate?

the school and preschool environments. Evaluation is supplemented by observations of the child participating in context to identify any performance limitations present and the types of supports needed for success.

Adaptive behavior and activities of daily living. Measurement of performance in activities of daily living (ADLs) is important for understanding the affect of sensory processing and integration on daily life skills. Evaluation of ADLs can be accomplished using both observation and formal assessments. Formal assessments such as the Pediatric Evaluation of Disability Inventory (Haley, Coster, Ludlow, Haltiwanger, & Andrellos, 1992), Adaptive Behavior Assessment System II (Harrison & Oakland, 2003), and Vineland Adaptive Behavior Scales, 2nd Edition (Sparrow, Cicchetti, & Balla, 2005) can be helpful because they can be completed through caregiver interview. In addition to determining the child's strengths and areas of concern, it is important to determine whether special accommodations have been made previously, such as only using clothing that does not require the use of fasteners or allowing extra time to complete tasks to account for distractibility. Supplemental interviews with the child's caregivers also can be used to gather information about their concerns and priorities for their child's adaptive behavior and performance of ADLs.

Leisure and social participation. Sensory processing patterns can influence an individual's leisure choices and social participation behaviors. Information about these areas of occupation can be gathered through interview (using questions about choices and preferences), formal assessment (see Table 2), and informal methods such as interest checklists and observations such as the Sensory Processing Measure (Parham, Ecker, Miller Kuhaneck, Henry, & Glennon, 2007) and Social Responsiveness Scale (Constantino & Gruber, 2005). Just as with other areas of occupation, it is important to determine whether and to what degree sensory processing and integration influence the individual's performance in these areas.

Analysis of performance skills and performance patterns. *Performance skills* are the observable, goal-directed actions by which an individual engages in an occupation. These can be subdivided into motor and praxis, sensory–perceptual, cognitive processing, emotional regulatory, and communication and social skills (AOTA, 2008b). *Performance patterns* are the habits, routines, rituals, and roles a person performs while engaging in activities or occupations. Performance skills and patterns can influence and be influenced by sensory processing and integration. For the purpose of this section, assessment of performance skills is divided into the broad areas of gross motor and praxis skills, fine/visual–motor development, sensory–perceptual skills, emotional regulation, cognitive skills, and communication and social skills. Each section will address formal and informal measurement methods.

Motor and praxis skills. Assessment of motor performance involves evaluation of foundations for movement such as postural stability and neurodevelopment, including muscle tone. A child's readiness to move is affected by the status of his or her muscles. A child with abnormal muscle tone has greater difficulty activating muscles to move the body in a desired manner against the force of gravity. Assessment of muscle tone is best accomplished through clinical observations of posture and movement (e.g., Blanche, 2010) and palpation of the muscle belly.

Gross motor skills typically are evaluated through administration of developmental tests to measure achievement of motor milestones and the characteristics and quality of movements. Commonly used standardized measures of motor performance for children include the Bayley Scales of Infant and Toddler Development, 3rd Edition (Bayley, 2005), the Peabody Developmental Motor Scales, 2nd Edition (Folio & Fewell, 2000), and the Bruininks–Oseretsky Test of Motor Proficiency, 2nd Edition (Bruininks & Bruininks, 2005). In addition to measuring the child's performance on specific gross motor test items, the occupational therapist observes the child during standardized test activities and documents the quality of the child's performance, noting aspects such as organization, initiation, termination, and fluidity of movement, as well as overall coordination. Information about the consistency with which gross motor skills are demonstrated across environments and settings can be obtained through interview with the child's caregiver.

The client's skill in integrating cognition, sensation, and motor skills for praxis is challenging to measure. A few formal assessments are available that specifically evaluate this complex skill. The Sensory Integration and Praxis Tests (Ayres, 1989) include four specific tests of *practic* abilities and can be used with children ages 4 to 8 years, 11 months. The Test of Ideational Praxis (TIP; May-Benson & Cermak, 2007) specifically evaluates the ideation component of praxis by examining a child's ability to use and manipulate simple objects in novel ways. The TIP is still in development, but preliminary data suggest that this tool shows promise as an objective and reliable measure for examining ideational abilities of children ages 5 to 8 years (May-Benson & Cermak, 2007). The motor planning aspect of praxis often is evaluated through a child's ability to imitate movements such as gestures or postures (May-Benson, 2010). Motor execution is evaluated as the child uses his or her body to engage with the environment, especially when encountering a novel task or challenge. Observations of the child's ability to initiate motor action, learn from mistakes in order to modify subsequent attempts, and fine tune

Table 2. Selected Evaluation Instruments of Occupational Performance for Children and Adolescents With Challenges Processing and Integrating Sensory Information

Domain of Occupational Therapy	Sample Assessments Used in Occupational Therapy Practice
Areas of Occupation • Activities of daily living • Instrumental activities of daily living • Rest and sleep • Education • Work • Play • Leisure • Social participation	• Achenbach System of Empirically Based Assessment (ASEBA; Achenbach, 2009) • Adaptive Behavior Assessment System, 2nd ed. (Harrison & Oakland, 2003) • Adaptive Behavior Assessment System–School, 2nd ed. (Harrison & Oakland, 2003) • Behavior Assessment System for Children, 2nd ed. (C. R. Reynolds & Kamphaus, 2006) • Canadian Occupational Performance Measure (Law, Baptiste, Carswell, McColl, Polatajko, & Pollock, 2005) • Children's Assessment of Participation and Enjoyment and Preferences for Activities of Children (King et al., 2005) • Children's Engagement Questionnaire (McWilliam, 1991) • Communication and Symbolic Behavior Scales–Developmental Profile (Wetherby & Prizant, 2002) • Evaluation Tool of Children's Handwriting (Amundson, 1995) • Knox Preschool Play Scale (Knox, 2008) • Miller Function and Participation Scales (L.J. Miller, 2006) • Minnesota Handwriting Assessment (Reisman, 1999) • Pediatric Evaluation of Disability Inventory (Haley, Coster, Ludlow, Haltiwanger, & Andrellos, 1992) • Perceived Efficacy and Goal Setting System (Missiuna, Pollock, & Law, 2004) • Play Preference Inventory (Wolfberg, 1995) • Preschool Activity Card Sort (Berg & LaVesser, 2006) • Scales of Independent Behavior–Revised (Bruininks, Woodcock, Weatherman, & Hill, 1997) • School Assessment of Motor and Process Skills (Fisher, Bryze, Hume, & Griswold, 2005) • School Function Assessment (Coster, Deeney, Haltiwanger, & Haley, 1998) • Test of Handwriting Skills (Gardner, 1998) • Test of Playfulness (Skard & Bundy, 2008) • Transdisciplinary Play-Based Assessment, 2nd ed. (Linder, 2008) • Vineland Adaptive Behavior Scales, 2nd ed. (Sparrow, Cicchetti, & Balla, 2005)
Performance Skills • Sensory–perceptual skills • Motor and praxis skills • Emotional regulation skills • Cognitive skills • Communication and social skills	• Adaptive Behavior Assessment System, 2nd ed. (Harrison & Oakland, 2003) • Battelle Developmental Inventory, 2nd ed. (Newborg, 2004) • Bayley Scales of Infant and Toddler Development, 3rd ed. (Bayley, 2005) • Behavior Assessment System for Children–II (BASC–II; C. R. Reynolds & Kamphaus, 2006) • Behavior Rating Inventory (Gioia, Isquith, Guy, & Kenworthy, 2000) • Bruininks–Oseretsky Test of Motor Proficiency, 2nd ed. (Bruininks & Bruininks, 2005) • DeGangi–Berk Test of Sensory Integration (Berk & DeGangi, 1983) • Developmental Test of Visual–Motor Integration, 5th ed (Beery, Buktenica, & Beery, 2004) • Developmental Test of Visual Perception (Hammill, Pearson, & Voress, 1993) • Developmental Test of Visual Perception—Adolescent and Adult (C.R. Reynolds, Pearson, & Voress, 2002) • Infant/Toddler Sensory Profile (Dunn, 2002) • Miller Assessment for Preschoolers (L. J. Miller, 1988) • Miller Function and Participation Scales (L. J. Miller, 2006) • Motor-Free Visual Perception Test, 3rd ed. (Colarusso & Hammill, 2003) • Peabody Developmental Motor Scales, 2nd ed. (Folio & Fewell, 2000) • Sensory Integration Inventory–Revised (Reisman & Hanschu, 1992) • Sensory Integration and Praxis Tests (Ayres, 1989) • Sensory Processing Measure: Home (Parham & Ecker, 2007); Main Classroom and School Environment Forms (Miller Kuhaneck, Henry, & Glennon, 2007) • Sensory Processing Measure–Preschool (SPM–P): Home (Ecker & Parham, 2010); SPM–P: School (Miller Kuhaneck, Henry, & Glennon, 2010)

(Continued)

Table 2. Selected Evaluation Instruments of Occupational Performance for Children and Adolescents With Challenges Processing and Integrating Sensory Information *(cont.)*

Domain of Occupational Therapy	Sample Assessments Used in Occupational Therapy Practice
Performance Skills *(cont.)*	• Sensory Profile (Dunn, 1999) • Sensory Profile School Companion (Dunn, 2006) • Social Responsiveness Scale (Constantino & Gruber, 2005) • Social Skills Improvement System (Gresham & Elliott, 2008) • Test of Sensory Functions in Infants (DeGangi & Greenspan, 1989) • Test of Visual–Motor Skills–Revised (TVMS–R; Gardner, 1995) • Test of Visual–Motor Skills–3 (TVMS–3; Martin, 2010) • Test of Visual–Motor Skills Upper Level (Gardner, 1992) • Test of Visual–Perceptual Skills–3 (TVPS–3; Martin, 2006) • Test of Visual–Perceptual Skills Upper Level (Gardner, 1997) • Touch Inventory for Elementary-School-Aged Children (Royeen & Fortune, 1990) • Touch Inventory for Preschoolers (Royeen, 1987)
Performance Patterns • Habits • Routines • Roles • Rituals	• Activity Card Sort, 2nd ed. (Baum & Edwards 2008) • Canadian Occupational Performance Measure (Law et al., 2005) • Children's Assessment of Participation and Enjoyment and Preferences for Activities of Children (King et al., 2005) • Perceived Efficacy and Goal Setting System (Missiuna et al., 2004)
Context • Cultural • Physical • Social • Personal • Temporal • Virtual	• Canadian Occupational Performance Measure (Law et al., 2005) • Children's Assessment of Participation and Enjoyment and Preferences for Activities of Children (King et al., 2005) • Perceived Efficacy and Goal Setting System (Missiuna et al., 2004)

Adapted from *Occupational Therapy Practice Guidelines for Children and Adolescents With Autism*, by S. D. Tomchek and J. Case-Smith, 2009, p. 22. Copyright © 2009 by the American Occupational Therapy Association. Adapted with permission.

movements to achieve the desired outcome are important to document.

Additional information about a child's practic abilities can be obtained through structured and unstructured clinical observations. Blanche's (2010) *Observations Based on Sensory Integration Theory* provides a format for analyzing and interpreting the practic components of behaviors when standardized assessments are not appropriate and when supplemental information is desired. These observations can be conducted via structured or unstructured activities.

Fine/visual–motor development. Skilled fine motor performance is dependent on sufficient registration and discrimination of tactile, proprioceptive, and visual stimuli in conjunction with development of age-appropriate motor control of the upper extremity and intrinsic hand musculature. Foundations for fine motor control include proximal stability of the shoulder musculature, establishment of a hand preference or dominance, and development of grasp and prehension patterns and manipulative skills. Sensory processing and integration can affect fine motor development when tactile and kinesthetic awareness are limited, coordination of visual and tactile inputs are insufficient, dyspraxia is present, and neuromotor development is delayed. Occupational therapy assessment of fine motor skill typically occurs through administration of standardized tests in conjunction with observations of engagement in purposeful fine motor tasks. Standardized tests of fine motor skill include performance-based measures of manipulation, prehension patterns, isolation of finger movements, dexterity, bilateral hand use, and tool use (Mulligan, 2003b). Tests of visual–motor integration reflect the manner in which a child relates to visual stimuli by way of his or her motor response. Related functions include visual localization of stimuli, scanning, visual tracking, and somatosensory abilities. These skills are essential for success in activities such as writing, drawing, catching a ball, completing puzzles, copying from the board, and locating materials needed for a task. Observation of fine and visual–motor skills should supplement formal assessment and should include subskills or other aspects of performance that are not directly measured by formal tests, such as direction of eye gaze during fine motor performance, the ability to efficiently coordinate eyes and hands together in space to reach for objects, and motor control and coordination of hands and fingers. Qualitative observations should address specifically whether tactile, proprioceptive, and visual input support or inhibit fine and visual motor performance. Suggested questions to guide observations are provided in Table 3.

Sensory–perceptual skills. Sensory–perceptual skills are those "actions or behaviors a client uses to locate, identify, and respond to sensations and to select, interpret, associate, organize, and remember sensory events via sensation" (AOTA, 2008b, p. 640). Sensory perception includes visual, auditory, tactile, vestibular, proprioceptive, gustatory, and olfactory sensations. Perception of sensation creates a critical foundation for development of body image, relation of the body to the social and physical world, movement through space, and interaction with others. Deficiencies in one or more sensory systems can lead to deficiencies in occupational performance. Evaluation of sensory–perceptual skills in occupational therapy is guided by an understanding of the relationship between sensation and functional behavior and as such occurs within the context of occupational performance. This section addresses evaluation of visual perception and overall sensory processing and integration.

Visual perception functions such as visual discrimination, visual form constancy, visual memory, visual–spatial relations, visual–sequential memory, visual figure ground, and visual closure are all dependent on registration and integration of visual information for perception. These perceptual skills allow an individual to receive, interpret, and recognize visual stimuli in order to attach meaning to what is seen and understand the spatial relationship of self in the physical world. Visual perception is integrated with sensory input from many other systems to support optimal functioning of the individual.

A variety of formal visual–perceptual tests are available for use by occupational therapists (see Table 2). Some measures of visual perception (e.g., Motor-

Table 3. Structured Observations of Fine Motor Performance

Foundation Area	Example Observations

Hand Preference	• Does the child demonstrate use of a preferred hand, mixed dominance, or ambiguous handedness for skilled tasks?
	• If the child has mixed or no preference,
	  ○ Does he or she avoid crossing midline?
	  ○ Does he or she consistently accomplish certain tasks (e.g., self-feeding, coloring) with one hand?

Grasp and Prehension Patterns	• Does the child have adequate hand strength to hold onto objects? • Does the child have difficulty grading pressure (too much or too little) when holding objects? • Can the child isolate finger motions to pick up smaller objects? • Does the quality of the child's grasp and prehension abilities differ when he or she is grasping or manipulating an object versus using the object in a functional task? • When the child is grasping and manipulating objects, are there compensatory movements in the arms, shoulders, or trunk (e.g., shoulder elevation or associated reactions)?
Manipulation Skill	• What is the quality of the child's in-hand manipulation skill? • Can the child transition objects in his or her hand using transverse palmar (palm-to-finger and finger-to-palm) motions, or does he or she stabilize the object against the table or him- or herself and regrasp? • Does the child demonstrate different manipulation abilities when he or she is grasping, carrying, or manipulating an object versus using the object in a functional task?
Purposes and Quality of a Child's Interactions With Objects	• Does the child manipulate objects primarily for sensory gratification or for purposeful toy play? • Are tremors present, or do the child's movements appear ataxic? • Does the child have a hard time damping his or her reach? • Does the child frequently shift his or her position while interacting with an object, or does he or she frequently turn or reposition a task? • If so, is he or she doing so to avoid midline crossing or for visual inspection? • Does the child use peripheral vision or central vision, or does he or she accomplish tasks "by feel"?
Cooperative Hand Use	• Does the child transfer objects between hands? • Does the child stabilize objects with one hand while manipulating with the other? • Does the child bring both hands to midline to enable better visual or tactile exploration? • Do the two hands work together with symmetry and strength for efficient and skilled function? • Does the child recognize his or her hands as useful in enabling accomplishment of his or her objectives?

Reprinted from *Occupational Therapy Practice Guidelines for Children and Adolescents With Autism*, by S. D. Tomchek and J. Case-Smith, 2009, p. 25. Copyright © 2009 by the American Occupational Therapy Association. Used with permission.

Free Visual Perception Test, 3rd Edition [Colarusso & Hammill, 2003]; Test of Visual–Perceptual Skills (non-motor), 3rd Edition [Martin, 2006]) are motor-free, allowing the child to respond to test stimuli by indicating his or her answer choice from available options using gestural or verbal responses. Other tools (e.g., Developmental Test of Visual Perception, 2nd Edition [Hammill, Pearson, & Voress, 1993]) incorporate both nonmotor visual–perceptual tasks with visual–motor integration tasks for a more comprehensive assessment of how visual skills affect the child's function. In addition, the Sensory Integration and Praxis Tests (SIPT; Ayres, 1989) have several subtests that assess visual perception (Space Visualization, Figure Ground, Manual Form Perception, and Design Copying).

Specific evaluation of *sensory processing and integration* includes both formal and informal methods. Table 2 includes selected assessments that may be used when evaluating sensory processing and integration in children. The SIPT (Ayres, 1989) are often referred to as the "gold standard" for comprehensive evaluation of sensory integration and praxis (Smith Roley, 2006a, p. 25; Windsor, Smith Roley, & Szklut, 2001, p. 218). This test battery requires advanced training to administer and interpret and includes 17 subtests that measure vestibular processing, visual and tactile processing, kinesthetic awareness, and praxis.

The test involves direct administration of test items and provides scoring norms for children ages 4 years to 8 years, 11 months. Each of the 17 subtests yields specific data about the individual's sensory processing abilities, and computerized interpretation of the entire test battery produces information about how the individual integrates multisensory information for functional engagement.

Other formal measures can be used to gather information about certain aspects of the individual's sensory processing or integration. Many of these are limited in range (i.e., measure only one aspect of sensory processing), basis of measurement (i.e., based on assessment of general rather than specific sensory functions), or elements of test construction (e.g., lacking psychometrics or standardization). However, these measures are useful in developing an understanding of the client and his or her ability to use sensory information for occupational performance. Used in the context of a comprehensive evaluation, each measure contributes to the sum total of data about the client and his or her strengths and areas of concern.

In addition to performance-based measures, caregiver report measures can be used to gather data about the child's typical functioning in home and school environments. The Sensory Profile series of tests (Dunn, 1999, 2002, 2006) consists of questionnaires completed by the caregiver, school personnel, or the client. The rater records the frequency with which specific behaviors are demonstrated by the client. Results yield information about the client's typical sensory-processing patterns and their possible contributions to daily occupational performance. The Sensory Processing Measure: Home and School Forms (Miller Kuhaneck et al., 2007; Parham & Ecker, 2007) and the Sensory Processing Measure–Preschool Home and School Forms for 2- to 5-year-olds (Ecker & Parham, 2010; Miller Kuhaneck et al., 2010) use standardized normed rating questionnaires to examine the child's sensory processing. The various forms include questions specific to the respective environments within which the child functions and allow for identification of differences in sensory-based behaviors across settings.

As with all other areas evaluated by occupational therapists, assessment of sensory processing that is completed with standardized and nonstandardized tools is complemented with observations. Observations of sensory processing and integration can occur through structured and unstructured methods, depending on what questions the therapist seeks to answer and the capacity of the child to comply with structure and engage in directed activities. Observations should include sensory qualities of the testing environment (e.g., ambient noise, visual stimuli such as pictures on walls, quality and type of lighting, size of space, openness of space, smells) and the type, frequency, and intensity of the child's responses to these aspects of the evaluation situation. Specific observations of sensory processing and practic functions can be guided by use of the *Observations Based on Sensory Integration Theory* (Blanche, 2010).

Emotion regulation. Emotion regulation has been described as "a complex process involving physiological, cognitive, and behavioral responses to internal and external factors in an attempt to maintain homeostasis of the body and engage effectively in context" (Watling & Miller Kuhaneck, 2010, p. 116). Because of the multiple neuropsychophysiological mechanisms involved, evaluation of specific emotion regulation is complex. Observation of behaviors such as emotional reactivity to stimuli, intensity of response, ability to calm or recover following an intense response, latency and duration of response, and match between emotional response and contextual factors are important aspects of emotion regulation assessment. Current tools that may be used when measuring emotion regulation are those questionnaires designed to measure sensory processing that include subsets of questions addressing this area, such as the Sensory Processing Measure: Home (Parham & Ecker, 2007), Sensory Processing Measure: Main Classroom and School Environments Forms (Miller Kuhaneck et al., 2007), Sensory Processing Measure–Preschool: Home (Ecker & Parham, 2010); Sensory Processing Measure–Preschool: School (Miller Kuhaneck et al., 2010), and Sensory Profile (Dunn, 1999). Other tools that may be useful include the Coping Inventory (Zeitlin, 1985) and Early Coping Inventory

(Zeitlin, Williamson, & Szczepanski, 1988). These tools measure behavior patterns and skills used by children to meet personal regulatory needs and the contextual demands of the environment.

Cognitive skills. Occupational therapists recognize that the ability to plan and manage the performance of activity depends on cognition. Although specific and thorough measurement of cognitive skills typically is performed by a psychologist, occupational therapists intentionally consider the impact of cognitive abilities on the child's occupational performance. Some aspects of cognition that may be considered specifically during evaluation by an occupational therapist include the child's ability to select appropriate materials for a task, sequence steps within a task or activity, organize activities in time and space, plan what to do, and generate new ideas. These abilities can be observed while conducting standardized tests of the child's performance skills and during skilled clinical observations in which the occupational therapist creates scenarios that challenge the child to demonstrate these cognitive skills. Information from measures such as the Behavior Rating Inventory of Executive Function (Gioia, Isquith, Guy, & Kenworthy, 2000) informs the therapist about the child's cognitive skills.

Communication and social skills. The ability to interact with others forms the basis for social relationships and participation. Challenges in processing or interpreting auditory information may impair an individual's ability to develop effective communication and social skills. Formal evaluation of communicative abilities usually is performed by a speech–language pathologist; however, occupational therapists, through their interaction with the client, become aware of any communicative difficulties and seek to understand how they influence the client's performance and social interaction. Challenges with communication can result in frustration and cause children to withdraw from social interaction, have low self-confidence, experience anxiety or tension, or easily become upset in unfamiliar situations. Due to the interactive nature of the evaluation process, a child experiencing any of these may be uncomfortable or uncooperative. This should be noted and accommodations made in order to obtain meaningful evaluation data. Children and adolescents who demonstrate significant communication challenges should be referred to a speech–language pathologist for evaluation if one has not yet been conducted.

Assessment of social skills includes measurement of skills necessary for interacting with others, such as using gestures or interpreting the gestures of others, initiating interaction, taking turns, and maintaining appropriate physical space in relation to others. Social skills assessment is conducted through both formal and observational measures. Formal measures include standardized test instruments that rely on reports of the caregiver or other adults who know the child well or tools that use self-report by the child (see Table 2). Observations of social interactions with peers can be conducted in natural settings, whereas social interactions with adults can occur through natural observations as well as during the evaluation process. Suggested observations of social skills are identified in Table 4.

Performance patterns. Examination of the daily routine of the client within the family, school, and community provides information about the client's patterns of engagement and participation. Questions about whether the client has established habits, routines, or rituals should be incorporated into interviews, as should inquiry about the usual role the client fills in each of the groups and contexts in which he or she regularly participates. The COPM (Law et al., 2005) can be used to guide incorporation of such questions into interviews with caregivers and other informants. When informant responses suggest that a sensory base may be influencing habits, routines, or rituals of the client, further questioning or assessment examining this possibility should be incorporated. If possible, the client should be evaluated while engaged in the habits, rituals, or routines to gain information about the nature of these performance patterns and their relationship to the client's functioning in daily life activities.

Contexts and environments. Occupational therapists acknowledge that occupational performance is characterized by dynamic interaction between an individual and the contexts and environments within

Table 4. Observation of Social Skills

Area	Observation
Physical Space	• Does the child maintain appropriate body space when interacting with others (e.g., positions own body too close or too far away from social partner)? • Does the child orient his or her body toward the social partner?
Nonverbal Cues	• Does the child direct eye gaze at the social partner when talking, if culturally appropriate? • Can the child interpret body language? • Does the child respond to gestures and nonverbal communication? • Do the child's facial expression and tone match the content of the interaction?
Social Interaction	• Does the child approach and interact with adults? In what way? • Does the child approach and interact with peers? In what way? • How does the child respond when approached by others? • Does the child take turns appropriately during conversation? • Does the child take turns appropriately during physical interactions such as when playing a board game, participating in a physical game, or playing on the playground? • Does the child share materials and toys spontaneously? • Does the child notice when another person is sad or hurt? • Does the child understand or participate in joking? • Does the child participate appropriately during family mealtimes, family gatherings, or family outings?

which the person engages and participates. *Contexts* are identified as the cultural, personal, temporal, and virtual factors that exist within and around a person. *Environments* are those external physical and social factors that surround the client (AOTA, 2008b). Because challenges in processing and integrating sensation are a function of the individual's interaction with the environment, the presentation of an individual's sensory processing and integration patterns can vary according to features of the contexts and environments within which the person lives and functions. For example, a child with heightened sensory sensitivities may perform well in the typical standardized testing environment, which consists of a private room with bare walls and the absence of ambient noise. However, the same child may have considerable difficulty focusing attention on a task in a typical elementary school classroom when other children cough, fidget, talk, turn pages of a book, or move about the room. Thus, evaluation of performance and behaviors across various settings is important, and the contextual and environmental factors that support or inhibit performance should be identified during the evaluation process.

Consideration of the physical and social contextual features that affect performance also can have implications for planning intervention. Information on the pattern of engagement in various contexts allows the therapist to evaluate the contributions of different conditions to the individual's performance and can help the therapist begin devising a plan for how to structure the environment during intervention activities. Consideration should be given the sensory aspects of both human and nonhuman facets of the environment. Elements of context that should be considered during evaluation are listed in Table 5.

Activity demands. Determining whether a child may be able to complete an activity depends not only on the performance skills, performance patterns, and client factors but also on the demands of the activity itself. The *demands* of an activity are aspects of the activity that include the tools needed to carry it out; the space and social demands required by the activity; and the skills, body functions, and body structures needed to take part in the activity (AOTA, 2008b). During evaluation, the occupational therapist observes the child's performance and the impact of the activity demands, including any supports or modifications that the child relies on to increase success. The therapist may provide varying forms and levels of assistance to determine whether a change in activity demands alters the child's occupational performance. The therapist

Table 5. Context Considerations and Activity Demands in Evaluation

	Context Considerations

Cultural	• Cultural beliefs about
	  ○ Diagnosis and labeling
	  ○ How to care for those with limitations in participation
	  ○ Who in a family takes on the role supporting participation

Personal	• Age of client and family members • Awareness of personal space • Preferred or nonpreferred activity • Pleasure and motivation (natural and/or secondary) to engage present in the activity
Physical	• Size of space • Lighting • Noise level of the environment • Pleasure and motivation (natural and/or secondary) to engage present in the activity
Social	• Number of people in the environment (peers and adults) • Presence of parents • Level of initiation and response to people • Response of others to the individual • Individual or group activity • Level of support to facilitate participation and the child's response to that support • Social communication during the activity • Awareness of interpersonal space
Temporal	• Time of day • Open-ended activity or one with a clear ending point • Activity duration
	Activity Demands
	• Activity type • Sensory aspects of activity (auditory, tactile, visual, olfactory, gustatory, vestibular, proprioceptive) • Preferred or nonpreferred activity • Activities by choice or scheduled • Visual supports used (e.g., schedules, activity progression indicators, visual indicator of completion of an activity/finish box) • Pleasure and motivation to engage in the activity • Materials concrete and meaningful • Facilitation of transitions within an activity and between activities

Adapted from *Occupational Therapy Practice Guidelines for Children and Adolescents With Autism*, by S. D. Tomchek and J. Case-Smith, 2009, p. 15. Copyright © 2009 by the American Occupational Therapy Association. Adapted with permission.

aims to balance the level of assistance offered to create the "just-right challenge" with regard to activity demands. The just-right challenge is evidenced when the demands of the activity (including therapist support) and the client's abilities are matched in such a way that the child is successful in adaptively accomplishing something more difficult than he or she was able to do before (Smith Roley, 2006b). In addition, the therapist carefully analyzes the sensory features of the activity and materials used in order to assess the manner in which they contribute to the child's success or challenge. Table 5 identifies aspects of activity demands that should be addressed during evaluation.

Client factors. Client factors include the values, beliefs, and spirituality; body functions; and body structures that affect the individual's occupational performance (AOTA, 2008b). In order to successfully meet the activity demands common to childhood occupations, a child must have adequate cognitive, sensory, and motor functioning. Evaluation of these client factors (e.g., body functions) includes measuring the function of specific sensory systems as well as the detection/registration, modulation, and integration of sensation.

Interpretation of Evaluation Results

Determining the meaning of the evaluation results requires synthesis of all evaluation data from multiple sources to identify the client's strengths and any areas of engagement, participation, and performance for which the client needs intervention. The occupational therapist synthesizes all assessment data and looks for patterns and convergence in the data to form a cohesive image of the child's participation in daily activities and the ways the child's sensory processing and integration patterns affect engagement and participation. Evaluation data are interpreted with consideration of the child's ability to register and discriminate sensory information, self-regulate behavioral responses to sensory stimuli, and integrate sensory information with cognitive and motor functions to demonstrate effective practic abilities. The occupational therapy evaluation results are integrated with those of other professionals, if available, to gain a more comprehensive understanding of the effect of sensory processing and integration on various aspects of function, including strengths and limitations in performance. This information guides development of the intervention plan, including which combinations of sensations provided during meaningful activities can be used to support performance.

Evidence-Based Review of the Performance Challenges Related to Sensory Processing and Sensory Integration

Children and adolescents with challenges processing and integrating sensory information may display a wide range of performance challenges, some sensory-based. Identification of the particularly challenging performance areas will help guide occupational therapy assessment and intervention for these children. Identification of these performance challenges is particularly important because occupational therapy services emphasize improving performance in areas that restrict full participation in daily life tasks. Koenig and Rudney (2010) conducted an evidence-based review of the literature spanning 1996 to 2008 to explore the evidence regarding performance difficulties in the areas of activities of daily living (ADLs), instrumental activities of daily living (IADLs), rest and sleep, education, work, play, leisure, and social participation for children and adolescents with challenges in processing and integrating sensory information. See Table C3 in Appendix C for details about each study.

Daily Living Skills

In the area of ADLs and IADLs, evidence suggests that children and adolescents with challenges processing and integrating sensory information demonstrate difficulty with functional performance, especially as related to the motor aspects of these activities. Nine studies addressed performance in ADLs and IADLs, including eating, dressing, grooming, and hygiene. Of these 9, 2 were Level II studies, 4 were Level III studies, 2 were Level IV studies, and 1 was a qualitative study. Several studies revealed that children with challenges processing and integrating sensory information demonstrated difficulties with fine motor skills that affected performance on tasks involving skills such as using a mature grasp to hold a pencil and a pair of scissors (Case-Smith, 1995; Rodger et al., 2003). Another study found that children with atypical scores on the Sensory Profile (Dunn, 1999) displayed more problems with motor aspects of ADLs compared to children developing typically (B. P. White, Mulligan, Merrill, & Wright, 2007). In a qualitative study based on parent interviews, children with developmental coordination disorder (DCD) performed in the average range on visual–motor integration, mobility, and social function but below average in self-care functions for their age (Rodger et al., 2003). In 2 case study design articles, participants who had challenges processing and integrating sensory information were shown to have deficits in feeding and other functional ADL behaviors (Linderman & Stewart, 1999; Reeves, 1998). In a case study description of 3 children with sensory overresponsiveness, S. Reynolds and Lane (2008) reported that sensitivities, especially in the tactile area, were related to disruption of family routines and self-care performance, such as tooth brushing, hair and face washing, hair combing, eating (restricted food preferences), and dressing.

Rest and Sleep

One Level III study associated sensory hypersensitivity with sleep disturbances (Shochat, Tzischinsky, & Engel-Yeger, 2009). In this study, tactile sensitivity accounted for 25% of the variance in sleep disturbances. Underresponsive and sensation-seeking attributes also related to day and night sleep and behavior.

Education and Work

Seven articles addressing education and work occupations in children with challenges processing and integrating sensory information were reviewed. These articles included 5 Level II studies, 1 Level III study, and 1 Level V study. Evidence from several of these indicated that children with challenges processing and integrating sensory information demonstrated decreased academic achievement and attention, were at a higher risk for learning difficulties, and showed lower participation in school activities (Baranek et al., 2002; Dewey, Kaplan, Crawford, & Wilson, 2002; Parham, 1998).

Play, Leisure, and Social Participation

Seventeen articles were found examining the occupations of play, leisure, and social participation; 13 were Level II studies and 4 were Level III studies. Overall, these studies revealed decreased quality and quantity of social participation and play skills. One study of 36 children with autism spectrum disorders found a significant correlation between sensory processing as measured by the Sensory Profile (Dunn, 1999) and social competence (Hilton, Graver, & LaVesser, 2007). In another study, neuromotor coordination scores were found to be related to social problems in children with DCD (Cummins, Piek, & Dyck, 2005). The children with DCD spent more time alone and were more often onlookers in social play compared to their typically developing peers, indicating that poor motor coordination was related to decreased involvement in play (Smyth & Anderson, 2000). However, no difference was found between children with and without DCD in social fantasy play. Physical social play and variance in physical activity were decreased in children with DCD (Cairney et al., 2005; Smyth & Anderson, 2000). Boys with DCD were found to participate less in structured and unstructured physical activities than boys without DCD (Poulsen, Ziviani, Cuskelly, & Smith, 2007). These researchers also found a relationship between motor coordination and loneliness that was mediated by participation in team sports, suggesting that social participation was a protective factor for boys with DCD who participated in team sports as compared to boys with DCD who did not participate in team sports.

Implications for Clinical Practice and Research

This review found evidence supporting the assumption that children and adolescents with challenges processing and integrating sensory information display performance deficits in occupations such as social participation, play, ADLs, IADLs, and school function (Koenig & Rudney, 2010). This evidence-based review highlights the importance of occupational therapists including performance-based assessments when evaluating performance in everyday occupations in the home and at school for children with sensory-based difficulties. Assessments should include evaluation of both motor and sensory functions to understand the relationship between sensory function and motor performance so that intervention can be individualized to achieve successful participation in occupations that are meaningful to the child.

Koenig and Rudney (2010) encouraged occupational therapy practitioners working with children with challenges in processing and integrating sensory information to include intervention strategies that promote social skill development and community participation in natural settings. Social competence, social participation, and participation in school and play activities all have been shown to be compromised in children with challenges in processing and integrating sensory information, especially for children with deficits in motor planning and coordination. These vulnerabilities have great implications for social and emotional well-being. Occupational therapy practitioners should not only intervene at the sensory function and motor performance level but also keep participation in home, school, and community activities as a central theme.

This evidence-based review exposed a paucity of studies that directly examined and described the relationships between sensory processing and integration and everyday performance of occupation in the areas of education, play, ADLs, IADLs, leisure, work, and social participation. Because this relationship will likely differ across clinical conditions, it is important for studies to be conducted within and among various diagnostic groups. As our understanding of subtypes of dysfunction in sensory processing and integration becomes more established, it will be important to study occupational performance within and across the subtypes. For example, if research demonstrates that children with sensory overresponsive patterns and sensory-related motor disorders have more difficulty with social participation and ADL performance than children with underresponsive patterns, occupational therapists can target these areas of occupation during assessment and intervention for children who exhibit these specific subtypes. Research in the area of occupational performance in children with sensory-based difficulties is essential to guide occupational therapy intervention to successfully engage children in social participation and everyday activities in the home, at school, and other environments.

Intervention

Occupational therapy practitioners use the information about the child or adolescent and his or her family gathered during the evaluation to direct client-centered and occupation-based interventions. The intervention process consists of the skilled actions taken by occupational therapy practitioners in collaboration with the child and other service providers and the family to facilitate engagement in occupation related to health and participation (AOTA, 2008b). This intervention process is divided into three steps: (1) planning, (2) implementation, and (3) review. During the intervention process, information from the evaluation is integrated with theory, practice, frames of reference, intervention methods, and evidence from the literature. This information guides the clinical reasoning of the occupational therapist in the development, implementation, and review of the intervention plan.

Clinical Reasoning

Clinical reasoning is a complex and multifaceted process in which the practitioner dynamically uses a variety of metacognitive processes to consider scientific knowledge of the client's condition, the meaning of the condition to the client, the practical issues that might affect delivery of services to the client, moral issues that may affect therapeutic choices or actions, and knowledge and skills related to interpersonal relationships and interactions (Schell, 2009). This process, which the occupational therapy practitioner uses to "plan, direct, perform, and reflect on intervention" (Schell, 2009, p. 314), is central to occupational therapy intervention addressing sensory needs. The clinical reasoning process begins when the occupational therapy practitioner first reviews the request for services for the client, and it continues throughout the process of preparing for, conducting, and reflecting on the evaluation and intervention sessions.

When providing intervention to address challenges in sensory processing and integration, occupational therapy practitioners consider the client and his or her family, the contexts in which the client needs to function, the client's desired outcomes, knowledge of sensory processing, the theory and intervention principles associated with occupational therapy using a sensory integration approach, the *Occupational Therapy Practice Framework* (AOTA, 2008b), and the evidence base for the interventions being considered. The clinical reasoning process assists the practitioner in thinking and making decisions about those occupations the client needs and wants to engage in and the manner in which sensation can be used to support the client's function in areas that are challenging. For example, the occupational therapist asks himself or herself, How do deficits in sensory registration and discrimination affect this client's ability to maintain balance while standing on one foot, use arms together to swing a baseball bat to hit a balloon, maneuver through an obstacle course, and attend to instructions provided in a noisy classroom? How do challenges in self-regulation affect the client's ability to recover when distressed, focus attention to a task, and negotiate different ideas while playing with a peer? What sort of sensory experiences, including the type, intensity, rate, duration, and frequency of sensation, should I offer to this client to help support his or her success in desired occupations? By continuously and dynamically engaging in the clinical reasoning process, the occupational therapy practitioner is able to provide occupational therapy services that are consistent with the intervention approach, relevant to the client's occupational needs, and responsive to the client's ongoing sensory integration and processing.

Intervention Plan and Intervention Implementation

The occupational therapist develops the intervention plan collaboratively with the client, basing it on the client's goals and priorities. Depending on whether the client is a person, organization, or population, others, such as family members, significant others, board members, service providers, and community groups, also may collaborate in the development of the plan. The selection and design of the intervention plan and goals are directed toward addressing the client's current and potential problems related to engagement in occupations and/or activities. The design of the intervention plan is directed by the following: (1) client's goals, values, and beliefs; (2) client's health and well-being; (3) client's performance skills and performance patterns; (4) collective influence of activity demands, client factors, and the context, which includes the environment; (5) context of service delivery in which the intervention is provided; and (6) best available evidence. Several of these considerations are highlighted specifically in this discussion of intervention planning.

The goal of intervention for children and adolescents with challenges in sensory processing and sensory integration is to promote successful engagement in areas of occupation by addressing performance limitations in key areas such as play and leisure, social participation, education, rest and sleep, and ADLs (AOTA, 2008b; Koenig & Rudney, 2010). Occupational therapists provide intervention using sensory integration and sensory-based approaches to address difficulties across all areas of occupation. The specific emphasis is on sensory modulation disorders linked to emotion regulation difficulties, deficits related to motor and praxis skills, and sensory–perceptual skills (Ayres, 1979; Bundy, Lane, & Murray, 2002; Schaaf & Smith Roley, 2006; Smith Roley et al., 2001).

Collaboration. Throughout the assessment and intervention process, the occupational therapy practitioner collaborates with the family, child, and team members to establish meaningful goals and identify relevant outcomes. Because the overall goal of intervention is to improve participation in home, school, and community environments, collaboration is essential. The occupational therapist communicates with parents and teachers and other relevant people who are involved with the ongoing development of the child or adolescent. Initial collaboration involves gathering data and discussing the child's strengths and reactions to sensory stimuli, for example, and how those reactions may affect school performance and behavior at home. After the evaluation, collaboration continues to delineate goals and objectives that are identified as meaningful by the child, and particularly the adolescent, relevant to family priorities and, if collaboration is occurring within the context of a school system, in conjunction with improving participation in the educational setting. Ongoing discussions and communications should occur throughout the course of intervention to identify how the child's sensory systems and motor-planning efforts are affecting his or her ability to participate in home, school, and the community, as well as track improvements and outcomes. Often, children and adolescents with challenges in sensory processing and sensory integration receive services from both community- and school-based therapists, and it is essential that the roles of each practitioner be defined and close collaboration between them occur in order to meet the needs of the child or adolescent.

Intervention Review and Outcome Monitoring

Intervention review is a continuous process of reevaluating and reviewing the intervention plan, the effectiveness of its delivery, and the progress toward targeted outcomes (AOTA, 2008b). This regular monitoring of the results of occupational therapy intervention determines the need to continue or modify the intervention plan, discontinue intervention, provide follow-up, or refer the client to other agencies or professionals. Reevaluation may involve readministering assessments used at the time of initial evaluation, parent or client completion of a satisfaction questionnaire, or practitioner–client interview using individually developed questions that evaluate the status of each client goal. Reevaluation normally substantiates progress toward goal attainment, indicates any change in functional status, and directs modification to the intervention plan, if necessary (Moyers & Dale, 2007). Additionally, this review of intervention may require revisiting available literature if occupational performance of the individual has changed.

Intervention review for children and adolescents with challenges in processing and integrating sensory information is an ongoing process, with the setting and context again playing a significant role. For example, practitioners working in natural environments in early intervention programs conduct ongoing assessment as part of the intervention process and as members of the interdisciplinary team. Here, family outcomes written on the individualized family service plan are monitored. In addition to these child-specific outcomes, the occupational therapist also contributes developmental reassessment components to the state-level child outcome reporting system for indicators within the State Performance Plan and Annual Performance Report required by the U.S. Office of Special Education Programs (U.S. OSEP, 2006).

Intervention review and outcome monitoring in the public schools for children receiving occupational therapy services under the Individuals with Disabilities Education Improvement Act (IDEA) are completed formally on an annual basis when goals on an individualized education program (IEP) are reevaluated. Each year, the IEP team reevaluates the goals, establishes eligibility for continued special education and related services, establishes new goals, and outlines changes to specially designed instruction to address these goals. Children and adolescents with challenges processing and integrating sensory information also may receive private services from occupational therapy practitioners with expertise in sensory integration theory and practice. Intervention review and outcome monitoring are determined by the practitioner and may or may not occur in conjunction with annual school reviews.

Monitoring progress. Progress is monitored both formally and informally through standardized assessments; clinical observations; and contextual data from families, teachers, and related personnel and is related directly to the functional outcomes. As Coster (1998) stated, "the measure of successful outcome of intervention . . . is not whether there is a change in sensory processing but whether there has been a change in his or her occupational engagement into a pattern that is more personally satisfying and more growth supporting" (p. 340). When a child can adequately modulate, discriminate, and process sensory information, the result is a child or adolescent who can self-regulate his or her behavior with adequate attention, arousal, and activity level (Schaaf et al., 2010), which will support learning and social participation. Motor outcomes include improved praxis and motor organization, including use of both sides of the body in a coordinated manner, postural and ocular control, and sequencing of motor tasks, which will support engagement in ADLs, play, and leisure pursuits, as well as participation in play contexts (e.g., recess) within the educational setting. Standardized tests and clinical observations can be used to monitor progress as well as determine attainment of goals. Goal attainment scaling (GAS) has been used effectively to track progress of occupational therapy interventions using sensory integration and sensory-based approaches (Mailloux et al., 2007; L. J. Miller, Anzalone, Lane, Cermak, & Osten, 2007; Schaaf & Nightlinger, 2007). GAS is used to measure the attainment of intervention goals, producing a goal attainment score that allows the occupational therapy practitioner to track progress as a promising outcome measure.

Transition

Children transition throughout their schooling to different settings, grades, and situations. Under IDEA, children with disabilities are entitled to transition planning and services at two points in time: when the child moves from early intervention (Part C) into preschool and kindergarten (Part B) and when the student moves from high school to postsecondary education and community living. As part of the transition team, occupational therapy practitioners support positive transition outcomes to prepare the family and child for changes in roles and routines; facilitate academic and functional living skills for school participation; and facilitate community integration, including skills for employment, further education, and adult living. The occupational therapy practitioner also provides extensive information to the family about the new setting and program, explains how expectations for the child will change, and facilitates communication with the providers of the child's future program. Interventions are reviewed and outcomes are monitored to develop new IEP goals and specially designed services for the child that are appropriate to the new setting and staff within that setting.

Transition planning may include postsecondary education, vocational training, integrated employment (including supported employment), continuing and adult education, adult services, independent living, and community participation. Development of social participation skills, self-regulation, and self-advocacy remains an important goal for the adolescent; however, the focus may change from the social performance needed in play interactions to that needed for dating or vocational tasks. To negotiate with employers for accommodations requires self-knowledge and self-advocacy skills; therefore, the adolescent's independence in self-advocacy is an important outcome for services in secondary education (Graetz & Spampinato, 2008) and is essential to success whether the adolescent plans to enter college, employment, or supported employment. Because services change dramatically after high school, both the adolescent and his or her family should be well-informed about the differences in services when exiting the public education system. As part of the transition planning, IDEA requires that the school develop a summary of performance to help with planning. This summary includes recommendations specific to the adolescent's plans for continuing on to higher education, seeking employment, and living in the community. This summary may identify the coping skills, resources, and supports needed for successful transition to the community (Graetz & Spampinato, 2008).

Discontinuation, Discharge Planning, and Follow-Up

Like transition, discontinuing and discharging from services requires planning and should begin at the time services are initiated. During the annual review of services provided under IDEA, a practitioner, as part of the IEP team, may recommend discontinuation of services when the student either has met goals requiring occupational therapy collaboration and no additional goals are appropriate or when the student has achieved maximal benefit from occupational therapy services (AOTA, 2008a). In addition, services may be discontinued if they no longer are needed; at the request of the family; or if the child is unable to participate because of extenuating medical, financial, social, or psychological challenges. As part of the discharge process, occupational therapists document the plan for discontinuing services, including a summary of progress and recommended follow-up, if any.

Occupational therapy services may be requested and required at different points in the development of children and adolescents with challenges in sensory processing and sensory integration. Therefore, additional intervention may be needed following discharge from services if the child's developmental profile and/or the contexts (e.g., home and community; day care; classroom; or other school environments such as art, music, PE, playground, cafeteria, or bus) that affect occupational performance are changed. In addition to a formal request, routine follow-up may be conducted within various settings. In a school setting, routine follow-ups may be done as part of ongoing educational screening efforts. Private clinics and diagnostic centers may conduct follow-up services to monitor developmental progress and provide program planning recommendations. Additionally, practitioners in some settings may follow up with a client via phone, letter, or questionnaire as part of ongoing quality assurance measures. In any case, follow-up is an important component of the occupational therapy process.

Documentation, Billing, and Reimbursement

Occupational therapists and occupational therapy assistants regularly and routinely document their services and outcomes (AOTA, 2010). This documentation should be completed "within the time frames, format, and standards established by the practice settings, agencies, external accreditation programs, payers, and AOTA documents" (AOTA, 2010, p. S109). Occupational therapy documentation meets four purposes:

1. Articulating the rationale for the provision of services and their relationship to the client's outcomes
2. Reflecting the therapist's clinical reasoning and professional judgment
3. Communicating information about the client from an occupational therapy perspective
4. Creating a chronological record of client status, occupational therapy services provided, and client outcomes (AOTA, 2008a).

The following types of documentation may be completed for each client, as required by law, the practice setting, third-party payers, or some combination of these:

- Occupational therapy evaluation, including history and results of special testing or assessments
- Occupational therapy intervention plan, including goals and objectives
- Progress reports
- Prescription/recommendation for adaptive equipment
- Reevaluation reports
- Discharge or discontinuation report (AOTA, 2008a).

Readers should refer to the *Guidelines for Documentation of Occupational Therapy* (AOTA, 2008a) for specific report contents and fundamental elements of documentation.

It is essential that occupational therapy practitioners document how the problems in sensory processing and integration affect functional behaviors and engagement in daily occupations in their clients and write intervention plans with clear long- and short-term goals that are objective, functional, and measurable (Hinojosa & Foto, 2004). Such documentation can aid in obtaining reimbursement for occupational therapy services provided. Appendix E provides guidelines for occupational therapy evaluation and intervention billing using *CPT*™ codes (American Medical Association, 2010). Occupational therapy practitioners should use the most relevant *CPT* code based on the specific services provided, patient goals, and payer coding policy.

Interventions

The following section provides an overview of common occupational therapy interventions for children and adolescents with challenges in sensory processing and sensory integration. This overview is organized into three broad categories: (1) Occupational therapy using a sensory integration approach, (2) occupational therapy using sensory-based interventions, and (3) other occupational therapy interventions used with children and adolescents who have challenges in processing and integrating sensory information. The section concludes with a summary of the systematic reviews of occupational therapy using a sensory integration approach; sensory-based approaches; and other, nonsensory strategies.

Occupational therapy using a sensory integration approach. Sensory integration intervention has been well-described in the occupational therapy literature (e.g., Ayres, 1979; Bundy et al., 2002). The aim of occupational therapy intervention using a sensory integration approach is to improve the efficiency of the nervous system in interpreting sensory information for functional use (Parham & Mailloux, 2010). Bundy et al. (2002) define *sensory integration intervention* as an approach "involving meaningful therapeutic activities characterized by enhanced sensation, especially tactile, vestibular, and proprioceptive (inputs), active participation, and adaptive interaction" (p. 479). An important emphasis of occupational therapy using a sensory integration approach is the adaptive response. Ayres (1972b) defined *adaptive response* as "purposeful, goal-directed actions" that are "more effective than that which [an individual] has been able to demonstrate previously" (p. 126). Ayres explained that when an individual demonstrates the ability to engage effectively in context to meet a demand, that is, adapt and succeed, the individual gains mastery over the situation rather than the situation having mastery over the individual. The ability of an individual to demonstrate an adaptive response is considered during occupational therapy evaluation, and strategies to support and enhance the individual's capacities in this area are emphasized in intervention.

Ayres also gave special attention to the relationship among cognition, sensation, and movement, describing these as critical elements of *praxis*, which she defined as "the ability to plan and carry out an unfamiliar action" (Ayres, 1979, p. 87). In the current literature, praxis is described as a three-part process in which the individual conceptualizes, plans, and executes a motor act (May-Benson & Cermak, 2007). The process involves cognitive functions, referred to as *ideation*, for creating ideas about how to act and interact with the environment and motor functions for skilled execution of the necessary movements.

Praxis is dependent upon integration of tactile, vestibular, and proprioceptive input; an organized body concept; and recognition of self as an agent of action and interaction. Practic abilities allow an individual to organize behavior in time and space in a manner that is fairly automatic and effective in achieving a desired outcome. When practic abilities are well-developed, the individual is able to develop an idea for action, create a plan, and carry out the plan, including actively adjusting his or her actions so that the motor activity is matched to the environmental challenge, resulting in an adaptive response (Smith Roley, 2006a).

When Ayres first introduced the sensory integration theory and began using sensory integration principles in her practice, her therapeutic strategies were very distinct from previous and concurrent approaches. Since that time, a range of methods and approaches using sensation in various ways has emerged both within and outside of occupational therapy, raising concerns about issues of fidelity to treatment. To address this problem, scholars, scientists, and researchers with expertise in sensory integration used systematic procedures to identify the core elements of the sensory integration intervention process (see Parham, Ecker, et al., 2007, for a description of the process used). Ten core elements were identified and defined that address both the structural and procedural elements of sensory integration intervention. The consistent provision of these core elements within occupational therapy intervention is referred to as *Ayres Sensory Integration*™ (ASI) intervention (Smith Roley, Mailloux, Miller Kuhaneck, & Glennon, 2007). The broader phrase of *occupational therapy utilizing a sensory integration approach* is used in this document to describe intervention that follows the 10 key principles of sensory integration intervention to address deficits in modulating responses to sensory input, poor sensory discrimination, and sensory-based motor deficits.

The 10 core elements of ASI intervention are (1) ensuring physical safety; (2) presenting a range of sensory opportunities (specifically, tactile, proprioceptive, and vestibular); (3) using activity and environmental factors to help the child maintain self-regulation and alertness; (4) challenging postural, oral, ocular, or bilateral motor control; (5) challenging praxis and organization of behavior; (6) collaborating with the child on activity choices; (7) tailoring activities to present the just-right challenge; (8) ensuring that activities are successful; (9) supporting the child's intrinsic motivation to play; and (10) establishing a therapeutic alliance with the child (Parham, Ecker, et al., 2007; Parham et al., 2011). These 10 elements are outlined more extensively in the Ayres Sensory Integration Fidelity Measure (Parham, Ecker, et al., 2007), which serves to assess the integrity with which the intervention is implemented (Parham, Ecker, et al., 2007; Parham et al., 2011).

When using a sensory integration approach to occupational therapy intervention, the therapist provides an environment rich in sensory experiences and offers activities that challenge the child to gradually engage in more difficult tasks and produce more complex responses (Parham et al., 2007, 2011). Selection of intervention activities is guided by the 10 core elements of ASI, and each is designed carefully according to the individual needs of the child (Parham et al., 2011). The activities created by the therapist are developmentally appropriate, offer a just-right challenge to the child, and are designed to engage the child in activities that will evoke an adaptive response. The adaptive response helps the child organize the sensory information and produce a functionally appropriate response (Ayres, 1972b). The therapist supports the child's adaptive responses by monitoring the child's interests and responses; giving verbal cues or physical support during the activity; or modifying the activity if the child becomes frustrated, overstimulated, or unsuccessful (Ayres, 1972b, 1972c; Tomchek & Case-Smith, 2009). The therapist's skill at eliciting an adaptive response by determining a just-right challenge is essential in improving functional outcomes throughout the course of therapeutic intervention. Sensory integration intervention is aimed at addressing the underlying deficits experienced by children and adolescents with challenges in sensory processing and sensory integration, including deficits in modulating sensory input; discrimination; postural control, bilateral integration, and sequencing; and praxis.

Challenges in modulating sensory input. One of the aims of occupational therapy using a sensory integration approach is to address deficits in modulation of sensory input that lead to poor self-regulation of behavior and may interfere with the child or adolescent's ability to participate in home, school, and community occupations. Addressing sensory modulation difficulties often is the initial focus of intervention, because atypical responses to sensory information make it difficult for the child or adolescent to cope with various intensities and types of environments adaptively. The occupational therapy practitioner uses the clinical reasoning process to construct activities that offer vestibular, proprioceptive, and tactile sensations to increase the child's organization using either a facilitatory (for a child who is underresponsive) or inhibitory (for a child who is overresponsive) manner, adjusting the intensity, duration, quality, and predictability of the sensory experience in accordance with the child's response. For example, vestibular input can be primarily inhibitory if it occurs in a slow, rhythmical, sustained fashion and alternatively, can be very alerting if it occurs quickly, with sudden changes in direction and incorporates the use of rotation. If the child demonstrates a low level of arousal or is slow to respond to sensations, the practitioner may use activities that offer quick and irregular movements to alert the child and facilitate more rapid responses. Proprioceptive sensations (i.e., exerting physical effort against resistance, such as pulling on elastic roping while swinging or pushing off of a surface while on a scooter board) often are combined with vestibular activities to help the child modulate arousal and organize an adaptive behavioral and emotional response. Anecdotal evidence suggests that proprioceptive input has an influence on arousal levels in general and can help regulate overresponsiveness to tactile and vestibular input (Blanche & Schaaf, 2001; Shoener, Kinnealey, & Koenig, 2008). It is important for the occupational therapist to use clinical reasoning to consider the child's optimal level of responsiveness, which is closely tied to arousal level, and the type, intensity, and combination of sensations within an activity the child or adolescent needs in order to achieve the optimal level of responsiveness. Schaaf and colleagues (2010) discussed how difficult it is for a child or adolescent with challenges in processing and integrating sensory information to self-regulate arousal level and described how the child may become easily overaroused during sensory play. The therapist must be able to "(1) recognize the signs of overarousal, (2) try to modify the environment or the activities to decrease the likelihood of an overaroused response, and (3) utilize strategies to help the child maintain or regain self-regulation in the face of potentially disorganizing activities" (p. 162). When a child is at the optimal level of arousal, learning can occur, focus and attention will improve, and the child can begin to self-regulate the response to sensory stimuli. The types of input used to facilitate optimal levels of arousal vary depending on the individual child's initial state of arousal and response pattern, the environment(s) the child is in, and daily life activities and routines in which the child engages. The occupational therapist can play a key role in integrating sensory activities throughout the child's day and modifying the environment to assist the child in maintaining a calm, steady state in response to the disorganizing sensory aspects of the environment.

Overresponsiveness to vestibular and proprioceptive input may manifest as gravitational insecurity or aversion to movement. *Gravitational insecurity* is described as a primal fear response to changes in head position or base of support (Koomar & Bundy, 2002). This fear of movement is "out of proportion to that which could be accounted for by poor posture or ocular movements alone" (Koomar & Bundy, 2002, p. 272). Aversion to movement is characterized by autonomic responses, including nausea, dizziness, and general feelings of discomfort that lead the individual to avoid movement experiences such as long rides in a car. Interventions for overresponsiveness to vestibular and proprioceptive input require the practitioner to have advanced knowledge of neurophysiology and mastery of the principles guiding sensory integration intervention. The occupational therapy practitioner uses this knowledge in conjunction with the clinical reasoning process to devise intervention activities that help the child develop adaptive responses to the vestibular and proprioceptive input associated with movement. The overarching goal is to increase awareness of the body's speed and direction of movement through space and help the client tolerate everyday movement experiences (e.g., riding on an escalator) in order to extend active engagement in meaningful daily activities.

Intervention for deficits in sensory modulation centers around providing graded sensation both directly (e.g., deep pressure touch by the occupational therapist) and indirectly (e.g., crawling over textured surfaces) in order to help the child achieve and maintain an optimal level of arousal. The occupational therapy practitioner again uses clinical reasoning and sensory integration theory to design and implement therapeutic intervention activities that provide input that either facilitates an adaptive response or inhibits a maladaptive response pattern. Strategies for supporting modulation often include balancing excitatory and inhibitory movement and tactile experiences with the deep input of proprioception. As the child and adolescent matures, it is important for the occupational therapy practitioner to give them knowledge, tools, and strategies that can help them address their modulation needs independently and in the most natural environment possible. This may include constructing their own activity routines that provide graded sensations throughout typical experiences in natural environments and developing methods for manipulating sensory aspects of play and work to be comfortable and successful. An adolescent who seeks out increased proprioceptive input to help maintain an optimal level of arousal can be taught a gym routine with weights or enrolled in a yoga or Pilates class, which supports not only his or her sensory needs but general health and fitness as well. Development of independent strategies to support improved sensory responsiveness is important because sensory modulation patterns and individual differences appear to be lifelong tendencies (Dunn, 2001). The occupational therapist can be an advocate to support and identify choices and activities that help the child or adolescent engage and participate in meaningful roles.

Challenges in sensory discrimination. Children who are able to discriminate sensory information can develop and use that information to build accurate perceptions of the world and events that help guide a variety of planned movements. This includes being able to discriminate between various stimuli by touch alone; localize and visually track objects in the environment; grade the force, timing, and distance of movements to develop advanced motor skills; and possess good sensory awareness of the body and use it in a coordinated manner. Intervention for children with difficulty discriminating sensory information is addressed in occupational therapy using a sensory integration approach by providing opportunities for the child to develop tactile, proprioceptive, and vestibular discrimination to increase accurate body awareness to guide more accurate planned movements. Feedback is essential to developing improved sensory discrimination and body awareness. The occupational therapy practitioner devises activities that provide the child with increased sensory feedback through multiple sensory systems to enhance awareness of the body in space and in relation to other objects in the environment. In addition, the therapist offers verbal feedback to the child regarding position and relationship of the body to the environment and objects within the environment. To enhance tactile discrimination, the occupational therapist works to engage the child in a variety of experiences to improve manual use of the hands in skilled activities and overall body awareness.

Challenges in postural control, bilateral integration, and sequencing. Sensory integration theory and subsequent analysis of subtypes or clusters of dysfunction have consistently identified deficits in bilateral integration and sequencing as having a vestibular and proprioceptive base. The occupational therapist uses the clinical reasoning process to identify deficits in bilateral integration and sequencing and then provide rich vestibular and proprioceptive activities along with visual information to improve balance, antigravity control, prone extension, core stability, and ability to cross the midline and use two sides of the body together in a coordinated manner. In addition to balance and bilateral skill deficits, children also tend to have difficulty with timing and sequencing of activities. Attention to timing and sequencing of activities includes offering graded opportunities for projecting these actions in future time and space while coordinating postural control, including balancing and segmenting movements. Often, visual targets are used during movement activities to develop timing and visual–spatial skills and specific activities emphasizing sequencing (beginning, middle, and end) are planned, with the child articulating the sequence and developing self-organization (Schaaf et al., 2010, p. 155).

Challenges in praxis. According to sensory integration theory, *praxis deficits* encompass difficulties conceptualizing, planning, or carrying out motor plans. The sensory supports for praxis can be auditory, visual, or somatosensory, and a core difficulty may be poor somatosensory integration, challenges in processing and organizing auditory language to plan actions, and difficulty using vision to guide and monitor new and novel actions. Children and adolescents with deficits in praxis frequently have difficulty developing an adequate body scheme to support novel motor plans and actions. They also may have difficulty either drawing on motor memory and previous plans to problem solve or being able to represent a plan with good ideation. Intervention strategies specific to deficits in motor function and praxis include

> (1) utilization of activities that have high levels of somatosensory input in order to help the child develop a better body scheme; (2) provision of environments that are novel, with a variety of shapes, sizes, and planes of movement, in order to challenge the child's ability to plan in space; (3) encouraging the child to imitate and then expand on the therapist's idea; (4) having the child engage in problem-solving in order to assist in the self-generation of motor plans; and (5) increasing and varying the motor demands faced by the

child, with particular attention to repetitive practice in order to master the motor plan and skill. (Schaaf et al., 2010, p. 154)

In addition to sensory integration theory, concepts in motor control and motor learning emphasize the task demands and motor skills in context. So the type of strategies used, the type of feedback the therapist gives, and the optimal forms of practice to plan novel motor tasks are critical to having an understanding of skill development.

Occupational therapy using sensory-based interventions. In addition to occupational therapy using a sensory integration approach, which is typically a one-to-one direct intervention in a specific environment, children and adolescents with challenges in sensory processing and integration may receive occupational therapy interventions that emphasize the provision of sensory input and its effect on behavior but that do not strictly follow the principles of occupational therapy with a sensory integration approach. Sensory-based interventions are used to address specific issues in sensory modulation or sensory discrimination and may involve providing enhanced vestibular and proprioceptive sensation throughout daily routines to prepare the child for engagement, support his or her ability to focus on learning activities, and regulate his or her behavior as task demands change (Tomchek & Case-Smith, 2009). Sensory-based interventions are often an integral part of occupational therapy in early intervention and school-based practices, in which the occupational therapist can contribute his or her knowledge base of sensory processing and integration to an interdisciplinary team in an effort to improve engagement and participation. Specific aspects of addressing a student's sensory needs in the school setting are discussed in the section "Occupational Therapy Using a Sensory Integration Approach and Sensory-Based Interventions in School-Based Practice."

A common sensory-based intervention used in conjunction with clinic-based activities, as well as in school systems, is the development and utilization of a sensory diet (Wilbarger & Wilbarger, 2002). Sensory diets are daily programs implemented in the child's routines at home and school. Each sensory diet is individually designed for the child by the therapist but may be monitored and reinforced by parents and teachers. Although unique to the child or adolescent, there are some common elements of sensory diets. The sensory diet is designed to help the child use sensory strategies to regulate his or her arousal level and behavioral responses to sensation throughout the day. This program enables the child to participate in activities throughout the day by helping him or her maintain optimal arousal and avoid disorganized behaviors from overstimulation or lack of involvement due to understimulation. Sensory diets most often involve specific calming or alerting activities or a retreat from sensory stimulation at regular intervals throughout the day (Tomchek & Case-Smith, 2009). A sensory diet is designed to present these sensory experiences in natural environments, with increased frequency during normal routines.

The type and duration of the activity differ depending on the age of the child or adolescent and the presenting problems. For example, a sensory diet for a young child who demonstrates sensory overresponsiveness will emphasize sensory elements that include providing deep-pressure input with towels after his bath, playing calming music, and rocking slowly prior to bedtime. Similarly, a sensory diet for an adolescent who displays sensory underresponsive patterns and seeks tactile, proprioceptive, and vestibular input might include an intensive aerobic workout in the morning; chewy foods that provide increased proprioceptive input throughout the day (e.g., bagels); seated arm push-ups while at the desk in school; and opportunities for more proprioceptive and vestibular input after school, including weight lifting, swimming, swinging on a rotary swing, and so on. In general, the goal is to help optimize the child's arousal, attention, and focus and promote organized, appropriate behavior. However, it is important that the child or adolescent is taught ways to access, alter, and adapt his or her unique sensory diets in ways that are age-appropriate and support self-efficacy. Sensory diets must be assessed continually to gauge the child's response to the intervention and revisions made to promote attention and focus throughout the day (Tomchek & Case-Smith, 2009).

Sensory-based interventions can have a multisensory approach (e.g., sensory diet) or focus on one sensory system to effect change. It is important to recognize that, although occupational therapists may use a variety of sensory-based interventions in practice, there is weak evidence to suggest that such interventions can improve outcomes, and investigations of these interventions are of poor quality and include poorly designed studies that lack protocols, large enough sample sizes, to control groups. Among these are listening programs and brushing programs, which are briefly described below. Until empirical evidence emerges to support or refute the use of these sensory-based interventions, they should be considered only as a supplement to occupational therapy, and the emphasis should remain on an occupation-based program that encourages a child's successful participation in daily life activities.

Sound-based interventions have been suggested as a supplement to occupational therapy. For example, Therapeutic Listening® (Frick & Hacker, 2001) is a home-based, therapist-directed program in which children listen to modulated music while wearing headphones for 20-minute sessions several times a day. This method was reported to reduce sensory-based behaviors (temper tantrums) when used in conjunction with a sensory diet, but these results were mixed and inconclusive (Hall & Case-Smith, 2007). Sound-based interventions often are used as part of a sensory diet with stated goals to improve arousal, attention, focus, and organization (Frick & Hacker, 2001).

The Wilbarger Deep Pressure and Proprioceptive Technique (Wilbarger & Wilbarger, 1991), a program involving a prescribed schedule of brushing the skin and compressing joints, also has been recommended as a supplement to occupational therapy. However, there are no empirical studies that have demonstrated the effectiveness of the Wilbarger brushing protocol, and therapists are cautioned about using or recommending any specific protocol without strong evidence. Therapists considering an intervention that involves passively applied stimulation should bear in mind that the neuroscience evidence indicates that greater changes occur when interaction with the environment is self-initiated, actively engaged in, and meaningful to the individual.

Therapists choosing to use an unproven intervention should specify an occupation-based rationale for selecting the intervention, outcomes the intervention is intended to address, and a valid and reliable method for measuring the intervention's effect on the identified outcomes.

Reframing a child or adolescent's behavior in terms of sensory integration and sensory processing is often a successful strategy to address sensory-based issues. Once the child, parents, and teachers learn to reinterpret difficult child behaviors in light of sensory differences, strategies can be developed to support success and reduce stress. For example, the Alert Program for Self-Regulation: How Does Your Engine Run? by M. S. Williams and Shellenberger (1994) can be used to increase awareness of sensory processing and to identify strategies that the child and teacher can use to support behavioral regulation in daily routines. This program views a child's arousal levels as fluctuating throughout the day at optimal and non-optimal levels for learning. Teachers and other adults are trained in the key concepts so that they can help their students identify and recognize their levels of alertness and use sensorimotor experiences throughout the day to increase or decrease alertness as needed. These strategies have been applied successfully for individuals and large group settings. Empirical research on the efficacy of the Alert Program for Self-Regulation, including How Does Your Engine Run? has not been conducted to date. However, research on the use of visual aids and prompts, a strategy that the Alert Program uses for the child to self-identify arousal state, is abundant in the special education literature (e.g., Bryan & Gast, 2000; Dettmer, Simpson, Myles, & Ganz, 2000; Dooley, Wilczenski, & Torem, 2001).

In occupational therapy intervention, occupational therapy using a sensory integration approach or sensory-based strategies is paired with play-based or functional activities. Often, the sensory intervention is viewed as preparation for the child to participate in an activity designed to enhance specific skills (e.g., social interaction, pretend play, visual–motor performance). These skill-building activities are woven into the treatment session or are implemented immediately following the sensory input (e.g., spinning or swinging, massage, brushing). This sequence allows the child to learn or practice an activity when arousal and attention are optimal. Sometimes, occupational therapists collaborate with other professionals (e.g., speech–language pathologists) to sequence sensory-intensive experiences with skill-focused interventions, priming the nervous system for learning (Tomchek & Case-Smith, 2009). These collaborations are often very productive and occur in clinic and school-based settings, and they are the framework for early intervention services.

Other occupational therapy interventions. There are many other occupational therapy interventions that are not sensory-based that are used with children and adolescents who have challenges in processing and integrating sensory information. Through the evaluation process, deficits may be identified in fine and visual–motor skills, visual–perceptual skills, and social skills that do not have a sensory basis and thus can be addressed via non-sensory-based intervention. In addition, methods such as direct instruction and cognitive-based approaches recognize the interplay between cognition and sensory–motor performance and have been shown to be successful in addressing coordination and motor skill deficits. These approaches are discussed briefly below.

Fine motor and visual–motor interventions. Challenges in processing and integrating sensory information can affect the development of fine and visual–motor skills and can be seen in decreased tactile discrimination, motor praxis deficits, and lack of coordination between visual and tactile inputs that affect such activities as writing, drawing, ball skills, puzzles, copying from a board, and organizing materials. Fine and visual–motor interventions focus on activities that target improving in-hand object manipulation, prehension patterns, isolation of finger movements, bilateral hand use, and tool use (scissors, crayons, pencils, eating utensils). Fine and visual–motor tabletop activities often are done after sensory input is given and may include hand-strengthening exercises with resistive materials, prewriting and handwriting activities, keyboarding, scissor and cutting activities, and functional ADLs that require fine motor skills for fastening clothing (e.g., buttons, shoe tying, zippers).

Occupational therapy practitioners also work on functional visual skills that support fine and visual–motor development. If the child or adolescent has weak oculomotor skills, the occupational therapy practitioner works on activities that require disassociation of the head and eyes, visual regard and focus, visual scanning, and visual tracking in order to improve functional vision that will support visual–motor development. In addition to working on foundational fine and visual–motor skills, many occupational therapy practitioners use available handwriting programs (e.g., Handwriting Without Tears) that have a multisensory base, often combining tactile, kinesthetic, and visual input to reinforce letter formation. These programs also emphasize directionality of letter and number formation, which is often helpful to children with challenges in processing and integrating sensory information. Use of multiple sensory systems and direct instruction of directional concepts appear to support the acquisition of writing skills, and school-based occupational therapy practitioners have been instrumental in increasing the use of such programs classroom-wide for all students.

Visual–perceptual interventions. Visual–perceptual skills (e.g., visual memory, visual figure ground) allow an individual to interpret and attach meaning to sensory input. Visual–perceptual skills are integrated with sensory input from many systems to support functional tasks such as reading, completing puzzles, building or construction activities, and writing. Children and adolescents with challenges in processing and integrating sensory information may have visual–perceptual deficits that interfere with optimal functioning. Occupational therapy practitioners often adapt materials to compensate for visual–perceptual deficits or use task-specific interventions that target deficient visual–perceptual skills. Common adaptations include using reading windows that block out extraneous text, highlighted papers that draw the eye to selected areas, and raised-line paper that provides a tactile stimulus to assist the client in knowing where to write. Task-specific interventions may include providing gradually increasing challenges with visual figure ground tasks, visual memory activities, or visual tracking.

Social skills interventions. Social skills are necessary for interacting with others both verbally and nonverbally, using and interpreting gestures, maintaining appropriate personal space, initiating interaction, taking turns, and engaging in play activities. Children and adolescents who have challenges in sensory processing and integration may misread subtle social cues, have difficulty planning and using gestures and imitation, and have secondary social skill deficits. Social skills interventions may take place individually but are more frequently done in groups to develop necessary skills to build and sustain interactions. Activities are aimed at group behavior skills (turn taking, voice modulation, give-and-take in conversation) and emotion regulation skills such as impulse control, recognizing emotional states, coping with frustration, and calming techniques. Social Stories™ (Gray Center for Social Learning and Understanding, n.d.), custom-written stories that describe the expected behavior in a social situation (e.g., expected voice modulation in the library, sharing a toy) may be written to outline the expected social behaviors in situations that may be overwhelming to the child. Sensory Stories (Marr & Nackley, 2009) are also custom-written to meet individual needs but address expected behaviors and potential coping strategies in distressing sensory situations (e.g., getting a haircut, brushing teeth). Social skills group activities often are developed around common interests (e.g., Lego® groups, computers) with older children in order to motivate participants to increase interactions and build foundational social skills.

Direct instruction and cognitive-based interventions. Occupational therapists recognize that the ability to plan and manage the performance of activity is dependent upon cognition. Interventions that provide direct instruction or target the cognitive aspects of skills such as motor planning, for example, rely on the child's ability to generate an idea, problem solve, sequence, organize, and use feedback and memory to enhance performance via repetitive practice. The Cognitive Orientation to Occupational Performance, or CO-OP, approach (Polatakjo, Mandich, Miller, & Macnab, 2001) is one such intervention that provides direct instruction using cognitive strategies to teach motor skills for children with mild coordination deficits and typically normal intelligence. Children self-identify a motor goal that they want to accomplish (jumping rope, riding a bike), and then a thorough comprehensive assessment and task analysis break down the performance to identify errors. The child is then taught a global problem-solving strategy (e.g., Goal/Plan/Do/Check) and then task-specific strategy (e.g., to ride a bike, you must pedal fast). The steps are cognitively driven versus working on foundational skills (e.g., processing visual and vestibular input) in order to acquire the new motor skill. "I want to jump rope" (Goal); "I am stopping my arms after one revolution with the rope, and I need to keep my hands moving in circles" (Plan); practice frequently with the plan (Do); and finally see if the plan worked—"Am I better at the skill?" (Check). The task-specific strategy would be unique to the jump-rope activity, such as hand placement on the rope.

Occupational therapy using a sensory integration approach and sensory-based interventions in school-based practice. Occupational therapy services in school systems include consultation (see Bundy, 2002) and direct intervention to support learning and educational goals of individual students, as well as system-wide interventions that can support the success of all children in the school context. Sensory-based interventions for an individual student may include educating school personnel to reframe student concerns from a sensory processing and integration perspective; providing recommendations for incorporation of specific sensory–motor activities throughout the day such as before, during, and after school; and making environmental modifications such as decreasing ambient visual and auditory stimuli in a classroom to support the student's school-related performance. In addition, direct intervention to address underlying sensory, motor, and praxis concerns may be provided (AOTA, 2009b). System-wide interventions that occupational therapists may coordinate include adoption of a handwriting curriculum that uses continuous strokes to support children with motor planning problems and those who are beginning to write, incorporation of physical activity at the beginning of the school day to help with self-regulation of all students, and designing and installing a playground designed for universal access (Case-Smith, 2010). The sensory integration and processing needs of all students can be addressed in schools with flexible models of service delivery in order to meet educational needs. Ideas and strategies for using sensory-based interventions in school-based practice are presented in Table 6.

Occupational therapists work with teachers and staff (paraprofessionals; gym, art, music teachers) to infuse sensory experiences into the classroom to promote learning and self-regulation (Polcyn & Bissell, 2005). Occupational therapy practitioners also propose classroom modifications, such as seating options, and use of play and learning materials that provide sensory input throughout the day, as well as environmental modifications that easily can be implemented in school settings. Examples include activities on the playground that provide heavy proprioception, such as climbing, tug of war, or holding the heavy door open as a line leader; messy play in art class; visual models of motor directions in gym class; or use of soft foam earplugs in a noisy lunchroom. There are many ways to enhance participation and provide a wide range of individualized sensory strategies that are embedded throughout the child's schoolday in the natural classroom environment. Occupational therapists are being called upon to provide "push in" services in the classroom, that is, to share their knowledge of sensory integration and sensory processing with teachers, versus the traditional "pull out" model in schools. This requires the occupational therapist to think creatively how to provide sensory-rich activities that support the classroom curriculum and may include large group and whole class interventions.

It is important to consider outcomes when modifying the environment and using sensory-based occupational therapy strategies in school-based practice. Outcome data should be logged regarding the type of input, activity or modification used, target behavior, and any observations related to whether or not the child appeared more or less organized and focused (e.g., improved time on task, decrease in verbal outbursts) after the strategy was implemented (Polcyn & Bissell, 2005). Appendix F provides examples of data collection forms that can be used in classrooms when assessing the effectiveness of classroom-based interventions. Demonstrating effectiveness of occupational therapy using a sensory integration approach and sensory-based interventions is critical, and payers and legislation require accountability and evidence of scientifically driven practice.

Evidence-Based Review of the Effectiveness of Occupational Therapy Intervention Using a Sensory Integration Approach

A systematic review of the literature addressing interventions for children and adolescents with challenges in processing and integrating sensory information published between 1996 and 2008 was conducted to examine the evidence for effectiveness of intervention. The methodology for the review can be found in Appendix B. All studies identified by the review are summarized in the evidence tables in Appendix C, and full references are provided in the "References" section. Separate reviews were conducted to examine the literature addressing occupational therapy using a sensory integration approach and sensory-based interventions. Summaries of those reviews are presented here.

This Practice Guideline specifically addresses children and adolescents with challenges in processing and integrating sensory information, but there is a growing body of knowledge related to the use of sensory integration and sensory-based interventions with other populations. Appendix G presents some information about the application to adults with mental health concerns.

This section of the evidence-based review of sensory integration addresses the question, What is the effective-

Table 6. Approaches and Sensory Strategies for Occupational Therapy Intervention in School-Based Practice

Occupational Therapy Approaches	Examples of Sensory-Related Strategies
Create, promote health and participation	• Conduct an in-service session or other education program for parents and/or educational staff to teach the relationships among sensory processing, learning, and behavior. • Promote increased physical activity for students to improve physical and mental health and cognitive and social performance. • Support installment of a variety of equipment at schools and public playgrounds to promote a diversity of sensory play experiences. • Design sensory-enriched classrooms with a variety of seating options to provide opportunity for tactile, movement, and proprioceptive experiences throughout the day.
Establish/restore performance skills and performance patterns	• Design activities rich in tactile, vestibular, and proprioceptive information that increase body awareness needed during activities of daily living. • Facilitate the development of appropriate sensory integration and motor-planning skills needed for organizing materials, completing tasks within an appropriate time frame, and adapting to transitions. • Establish/restore mobility needed for social and object play. • Provide controlled sensory input through activities that require increasingly more complex adaptive responses to novel activity to support ability to engage in group activities with peers.
Maintain student ability to engage and participate in academic and extracurricular activities to promote academic success and social participation	• Structure sensory environment to meet the student's needs, such as reducing distractions and improving attention to salient auditory and visual information. • Teach sensory strategies for emotional, physiological, behavioral, motor, and social self-regulation. • Maintain ability to organize behavior by providing scheduled sensory breaks and sensory accommodations, such as changing the size, texture, and location of the desk. • Maintain peer relationships by supporting and compensating for motor-planning needs in age-appropriate games and sports. • Maintain student productivity by providing compensation techniques for sensory and motor-planning deficits using study carrels, visual timers, weighted vests, alternate seating arrangements, modified writing tools, paper, and other assistive technology.
Modify activity to help student compensate for sensory, motor, and praxis deficits	• Through collaborative consultation with education staff and parents, using a team empowerment approach, develop strategies for modifying the sensory, motor, or praxis demands of assignments to increase student productivity. • Support student participation in general curriculum by modifying sensory and motor-planning (praxis) demands of activity. • Structure or modify the environment to support the student's sensory, motor, motor-planning, and self-regulatory capacities and needs.
Prevent barriers to participation and improve safety	• Prevent inattention, poor posture, and restlessness when sitting for prolonged periods by modifying seating options, allowing sensory breaks, and allowing student to work in various positions. • Prevent social isolation by providing motor-planning and social strategies to participate with peers. • Prevent socially inappropriate behaviors and behavioral distress or disruption by detecting and meeting sensory and self-regulatory needs. • Prevent injury by providing ergonomic seating and safety strategies for students whose nervous systems fail to register sensory information. • Prevent barriers to child participation by increasing the understanding of school district staff regarding the role that sensory integration and praxis play in influencing learning and behavior.

Adapted from "Providing Occupational Therapy Using Sensory Integration Theory in School-Based Practice," by the American Occupational Therapy Association, 2009, *American Journal of Occupational Therapy, 63*, p. 827. Copyright © 2009 by the American Occupational Therapy Association. Adapted with permission.

ness of interventions using the SI approach (including the effect of context [cultural, physical, social, personal, spiritual, temporal, and visual]) to create, promote, establish, restore, maintain, modify, and prevent future limitations in ADLs, IADLs, education/transition, play/leisure, and social participation in children and adolescents whose sensory integration and processing patterns are interfering with everyday life participation? (May-Benson & Koomar, 2010, p. 404). Studies included were those in which the authors reported the intervention to be based on the sensory integration approach as outlined by A. Jean Ayres. However, various authors appeared to interpret these principles in somewhat different ways.

Challenges of Conducting an Evidence-Based Review of the Sensory Integration Literature

The evidence for interventions using the sensory integration approach spans a period of more than 37 years, during which expectations for scientific rigor and detail of reporting have evolved. Thus, many studies reviewed have methodological problems, although more recent studies (L. J. Miller, Coll, & Schoen, 2007; L. J. Miller, Schoen, et al., 2007; Roberts, King-Thomas, & Boccia, 2007) demonstrated good scientific rigor. Some of the methodological issues of this literature include failure to use independent or well-qualified evaluators (e.g., Bullock & Watter, 1978; Polatajko, Law, Miller, Schaffer, & MacNab, 1991; Werry, Scaletti, & Mills, 1990) or to report on the qualifications of the evaluators or the treating therapists (e.g., Morrison & Sublett, 1986; Schroeder, 1982). In addition, it is often unclear whether the examiners administered standardized tests of sensory integration or only educational tests. On average, however, all studies reviewed demonstrated at least a moderate degree of scientific rigor according to the 24 components identified by MacDermid (2004) for rating the quality of research studies. In addition to these common methodological problems, major limitations are evident in six facets of this literature: (1) control for developmental maturation effects, (2) characteristics of the sample population, (3) statistical power and effect sizes, (4) dosing of intervention, (5) selection of outcome measures, and (6) lack of manualization and fidelity to intervention. These methodological problems limit the ability to adequately interpret the data and draw strong conclusions; nonetheless, the data point to promising evidence for the SI intervention approach and an urgent need for rigorous, methodologically sound investigations.

A second challenge to interpretation is that a number of systematic reviews of this literature have been conducted, but the findings are mixed. For example, Ottenbacher (1982b) reviewed 8 studies and concluded that the sensory integration approach demonstrated a large, significant, positive treatment effect in the area of motor outcomes in children of diverse ages with learning disabilities and mental retardation as compared with no-intervention control participants. This finding has not been replicated in subsequent reviews. A later meta-analysis by Vargas and Camilli (1999) found moderate effects in the areas of motor performance and psychosocial outcomes for the sensory integration approach compared with no treatment, although they found no difference in effectiveness of the sensory integration approach compared with other approaches, such as perceptual–motor. A systematic review by Polatajko, Kaplan, and Wilson (1992) of 10 intervention studies for children with learning disabilities concluded that the sensory integration approach was effective, but no more so than other interventions, and that the best gains were made in the areas of motor performance; however, a later systematic review by Hoehn and Baumeister (1994) that reexamined 7 of these 10 studies as well as 1 additional study (Ottenbacher, 1982a) found that although there were positive outcomes for some variables in some studies, they did not consistently demonstrate greater effects for the sensory integration approach over alternate treatments such as the perceptual–motor approach or tutoring. Thus, the authors concluded that the gains made were caused by maturation, not the sensory integration intervention. They did not, however, address the issue of small sample size and low power in regard to the lack of significant findings as an alternative explanation for their finding. More recently, a systematic review by Baranek (2002) of sensory-based interventions for children with autism concluded that although the limited studies available specifically addressing the sensory integration approach with this population suggest positive outcomes, the studies suffered from small samples (most were single-case designs) and weak individual study designs.

To address the limitations of the systematic reviews in the literature, May-Benson and Koomar (2010) conducted a recent review of original studies (i.e., systematic reviews were excluded) that examined the sensory integration intervention approach and did not rely on interpretations by previous reviewers. They included 27 individual studies, including 13 Level I randomized trials, 5 Level II studies, 3 Level III studies, and 6 Level IV studies. See Table C4 in Appendix C for details about each study. Findings are summarized below and presented by outcome area: motor performance, sensory processing, behavioral outcomes, academic and psychoeducational outcomes, and occupational performance.

Motor Performance

Fourteen articles examined motor outcomes of the sensory integration approach, including component skills such as fine and gross motor skills, general motor-planning skills, and more functional measures of motor performance and praxis, such as participation in gross and fine motor play. There were 6 studies evaluated as Level I (3 on children with learning disabilities and an additional 3 on other clinical populations), 3 Level II studies, and 2 Level IV studies (all detailed on Table C4 in Appendix C). Overall, some positive gains were found in several studies, suggesting that the sensory integration approach is better than no treatment and at least as effective as, and sometimes more effective than, perceptual–motor treatment in improving aspects of motor performance. The studies also suggested that these gains were maintained after the cessation of intervention. There was considerable variability across studies in the measures used and the type of results found; it appears that gains in praxis and overall motor skills most consistently may be found to occur with the sensory integration approach. However, findings are not conclusive, and ability to generalize is limited until further research occurs.

Level I studies. Three studies on children with learning disabilities—Humphries, Wright, McDougall, and Vertes (1990); Humphries, Wright, Snider, and McDougall (1992); and Humphries, Snider, and McDougall (1993)—found that both the sensory integration and perceptual–motor approaches improved motor performance skills better than no intervention. Humphries and colleagues (1990) found the sensory integration approach produced greater gains than both the perceptual–motor approach and no treatment in overall gross motor skills, bilateral coordination, strength, and motor accuracy and that the sensory integration approach was superior in improving the number of areas of sensory and motor dysfunction. Humphries and colleagues (1992) documented that the sensory integration approach was more effective than perceptual–motor and no treatment, specifically in motor-planning skills but not in other motor skills. On measures of visual–motor skills and balance, the perceptual–motor approach was more effective than the sensory integration approach, but no better than no treatment on measures of visual–motor skill and balance. On a measure of bilateral coordination, the perceptual–motor and sensory integration approaches were both more effective than no treatment, but Humphries and colleagues (1993) concluded that although the group receiving the sensory integration approach demonstrated improvement in twice as many ratings of severity of dysfunction as the perceptual–motor group, the sensory integration approach was only as effective as the perceptual–motor approach in decreasing the severity and number of symptoms of motor and sensory integrative dysfunction (e.g., bilateral coordination, praxis). Ziviani, Poulsen, and O'Brien (1982) found the sensory integration approach to be more effective than remedial classroom activities in improving fine motor performance, whereas Werry et al. (1990) found that both the sensory integration approach and the no-treatment group improved significantly on motor performance measures. Finally, Wilson and Kaplan (1994) conducted a follow-up study on children with learning disabilities and found that children who received 6 months of intervention using the sensory integration approach maintained the gains in their gross motor skills 6 months after the end of intervention.

Level II studies. Ayres (1977) found no significant difference on a fine motor test of motor accuracy between a small sample of no-treatment control participants and children with learning disabilities who had received the sensory integration approach. Similar to Humphries and colleagues (1993), Bullock and Watter (1978) found that the incidence of symptoms of sensory integration dysfunction (e.g., praxis, crossing the midline, skilled activities) and the level of severity of dysfunction of gross motor abilities decreased markedly after 6 months of intervention using the sensory integration approach. In this study, 86% of school-age children and 75% of preschool children in the sensory integration approach group demonstrated a decrease in the total number of symptoms of sensory integration dysfunction, compared with 7% of school-age and 14% of preschool-age children in the control group.

Bundy, Shia, Qi, and Miller (2007) examined motor performance and praxis in terms of playfulness. Although they initially anticipated that there would be a significant difference in playfulness scores between children with problems in sensory processing and typically developing no-treatment control participants, initial overall playfulness scores in the treatment group were relatively typical before therapy, suggesting little room for change. However, the study found that the children with problems in sensory processing were more likely to engage in sedentary play before intervention and showed increased levels of active play after intervention using the sensory integration approach. Similar pattern changes did not occur in the control group.

Level IV studies. Two single-case studies of children with motor coordination problems found positive results in improved motor performance (Allen & Donald, 1995; Leemrijse, Meijer, Vermeer, Adèr, & Diemel, 2000) and rhythm (Leemrijse et al., 2000). In addition, 1 study suggested that the sensory integration approach improved play skills in children with autism (Case-Smith & Bryan, 1999).

Sensory Processing

Thirteen Level I studies of intervention using the sensory integration approach examined outcomes thought to be indicators of improved sensory processing. Seven studies showed positive outcomes, including changes in duration of nystagmus, improvements in tactile function (e.g., tactile discrimination), reports of overall changes in sensory processing (e.g., electrodermal responsivity), and decreases in sensory defensiveness. These studies are detailed in Table C4 in Appendix C. May-Benson and Koomar's (2010) review suggests that positive outcomes in sensory processing abilities related to intervention using a sensory integration approach are found in these areas; however, the conclusiveness of results is hampered by the small sample sizes (e.g., groups of 5–18) in all studies except Ottenbacher, Short, and Watson (1979), resulting in possible underreporting of positive findings.

Level I studies. Ottenbacher and colleagues (1979) examined the effect of length of intervention on changes in nystagmus. Although a causal relationship could not be confirmed, they concluded that longer duration of therapy (e.g., 6 months vs. 3 months) was significantly related to increased duration of nystagmus in children with hyponystagmus, thereby suggesting more normalized processing of vestibular stimuli. Further, they ruled out maturation as a factor in the increased nystagmus: Older children were not found to have longer nystagmus than younger children at pretest. Carte, Morrison, Sublett, Uemura, and Setrakian (1984) examined changes in nystagmus in children with learning disabilities and found that the intervention that used an sensory integration approach resulted in significant increases in nystagmus duration in children with depressed nystagmus compared to a no-treatment condition. Morrison and Sublett (1986) examined changes in nystagmus in children with reading delays and problems in sensory integration and found no significant changes as a result of intervention using the sensory integration approach. More recently, L. J. Miller, Coll, and Schoen (2007) found that occupational therapy using a sensory integration approach for children with problems in sensory modulation resulted in a greater reduction in the amplitude of electrodermal responses compared with no-treatment and activity groups, indicating a decreased stress response to repetitive and potentially noxious sensory stimuli.

Level II studies. Schroeder (1982) found tactile discrimination gains, as measured by improved performance on the Manual Form Perception Test (Ayres, 1980), in children receiving intervention using the sensory integration approach. Children who received a combined approach of sensory integration and a perceptual–motor curriculum improved in visual, auditory, and tactile areas. Children who received only the perceptual–motor intervention demonstrated only auditory gains.

Level III studies. L. J. Miller, Schoen, and colleagues (2007) found significant gains on a parent-reported measure of sensory processing skills following occupational therapy using a sensory integration approach for children with problems in sensory processing.

Level IV studies. Ottenbacher (1982a) found that intervention using the sensory integration approach resulted in increased duration of nystagmus in 3 children with learning disabilities, whereas Leemrijse and colleagues (2000) found that using the sensory integration approach improved visual perception in children with developmental coordination disorder.

Behavioral Outcomes

Seven studies were identified that examined the effects of occupational therapy using a sensory integration approach on various behaviors. These studies showed improvements in areas such as self-esteem, attention, socialization, and cognitive skills and decreases in maladaptive behaviors. Application and interpretation of these studies is limited by methodological issues and failure to include a follow-up measure. It is promising, however, that the studies completed by L. J. Miller and colleagues used more rigorous methodologies and found improvements in several areas of behavior. These are summarized below.

Level I studies. In the area of behavior, attention, and self-esteem outcomes, Polatajko and colleagues (1991) found the sensory integration approach resulted in gains in self-esteem after 6 months of intervention. These gains were sustained at 3 months after discontinuation of therapy. However, the gains were not significantly greater than those demonstrated by children receiving a perceptual–motor treatment. B. N. Wilson, Kaplan, Fellowes, Gruchy, and Faris (1992) compared the effect of the sensory integration approach with tutoring and found no differences between interventions, except that the sensory integration group also improved on a measure of attention and maladaptive behaviors, with scores improving from dysfunctional levels to within normal limits after 6 months of intervention. More recently, L. J. Miller, Coll, and Schoen (2007) found that occupational therapists using the sensory integration approach saw significant gains in attention and cognitive and social skills among children with problems in sensory processing compared with children who received no treatment and an alternate activity-based treatment group.

Level III studies. L. J. Miller, Schoen, and colleagues (2007) found significant gains in socialization and a decrease in internalizing and externalizing behaviors after occupational therapy using the sensory integration approach with children with problems in sensory processing.

Level IV studies. Case-Smith and Bryan (1999) and Linderman and Stewart (1999) found that the sensory integration approach improved social interaction and decreased disruptive behaviors in children with autism. Roberts and colleagues (2007) found increased engagement and decreased aggression following treatment with an sensory integration approach in a child with sensory modulation disorder.

Academic and Psychoeducational Outcomes

Twelve studies examined academic and psychoeducational outcomes (e.g., math, reading, visual targeting, cognitive functions, language). Six of these studies suggested some positive results, particularly that reading skills improved with the sensory integration approach and were maintained at follow-up; however, it is unclear whether these effects were greater than gains achieved by alternate interventions. For example, Level I studies by M. White (1979) and Grimwood and Rutherford (1980) found that the sensory integration approach significantly increased reading skills in children at risk for reading failure and problems in sensory integration. Specifically, reading performance improved from dysfunctional levels to at or near the level of peers developing typically, and gains in reading accuracy were sustained over a 2-year follow-up period. Similarly, Carte and colleagues' (1984) Level 1 study found reading, math, and visual performance on a targeting test improved for children in both the sensory integration approach and the no-intervention groups. They suggested gains may have been caused by maturation but did not account for the poor power of their study caused by small sample size (i.e., groups of 7–15). Alternately, other Level 1 studies (Humphries et al., 1990, 1993) found no significant gains on a variety of psychoeducational variables reflecting higher cognitive functions, language, and academic skills for any group, and Polatajko and colleagues (1991) found that both sensory integration and perceptual–motor approaches were associated with significant gains in the reading, math, and written language outcomes of children with learning disabilities compared with typical norms and that these changes were sustained at the 9-month follow-up. There was no significant difference between children who received sensory integration and perceptual–motor approaches, except that math scores were maintained significantly better in the sensory integration group at the 9-month follow-up. In Level II studies, Ayres (1972a) found that intervention using the sensory integration approach produced significant gains in reading and auditory-language skills in children with learning disabilities compared with a no-treatment control group matched for type and severity of sensory integration problems, and Schroeder (1982) found all groups improved similarly in reading and spelling after intervention using the sensory integration approach, a perceptual skills curriculum, and a combination of both approaches. Of note, children who received the sensory integration approach improved more in math skills.

Occupational Performance

Three recent studies (1 Level I and 2 Level II) examined changes in individualized goals measuring functional occupational performance changes (e.g., goal attainment scaling), such as improved sleep patterns, increased repertoire of foods eaten, improved ability to participate in mealtime and homework activities, improved ability to manipulate fasteners, or improved ability to pump a swing. All studies demonstrated significant gains in self-identified tasks and activities, and positive changes were reported in both the performance of tasks and the satisfaction of performance of tasks.

Level I studies. L. J. Miller, Coll, and Schoen (2007) reported that occupational therapy using the sensory integration approach resulted in significantly greater improvements in individual functional goals than no treatment or an alternate activity-based intervention in children with problems in sensory processing.

Level III studies. Candler (2003) documented significant improvement in performance or satisfaction on individualized family-developed functional goals after an sensory integration–based summer program for children with problems in sensory modulation. L. J. Miller, Schoen, and colleagues (2007) also found significant gains on functional, parent-developed goals after occupational therapy using the sensory integration approach with these children.

Level IV studies. Roberts and colleagues (2007) documented gains in individualized functional, behavioral, and attention goals in a child with problems in sensory modulation.

Conclusions and Implications for Practice

May-Benson and Koomar (2010) provided a comprehensive review of original studies of the sensory integration approach. This synthesis of the evidence suggests that the sensory integration approach may result in positive outcomes in the areas of sensorimotor skills/motor planning; socialization, attention, and behavioral regulation; reading and reading-related skills; and individualized goals for the study participants. Various outcomes related to the sensory integration approach were better than the outcomes associated with the no-treatment control condition in more than half of the studies reviewed and were just as effective (although not better) than alternative treatments, including perceptual–motor-based therapies and tutoring/academic-based interventions, for some outcomes in some studies. Although limited, only the sensory integration approach, compared with perceptual–motor treatment and tutoring, showed any sustainable gains after intervention in the studies within this review. Results for specific outcomes varied among studies, and intervention effects also varied from small to large. Recent studies show positive trends supporting the effectiveness of the sensory integration approach, especially when measuring goals customized for the client. Overall, this review suggests that despite low power in most studies, there is a trend toward positive evidence to support the sensory integration approach.

Further research is needed to support the conclusiveness of these results, including more qualitative studies that examine the occupational performance and participation outcomes valued by the client's family (Cohn & Cermak, 1998). For clinicians, intervention planning for individual clients requires the review of both quantitative and qualitative study results and the integration of that information with specific knowledge of the client's needs, expert consensus within the field, and professional judgment. Occupational therapy practitioners, researchers, and educators can best help clients and their families when all levels of evidence are considered in evidence-based practice.

Evidence-Based Review of the Effectiveness of Occupational Therapy Intervention Using Approaches Other Than Sensory Integration

Occupational therapists have a variety of intervention approaches to choose from when working with children and adolescents experiencing challenges in processing and integrating sensory information. Accordingly, Polatajko and Cantin (2010) conducted an evidence-based review on occupational therapy interventions, other than the sensory integration approach, that would be appropriate for this population of children and adolescents. Challenges in processing and integrating sensory information are found in a variety of diagnoses; therefore, Polatajko and Cantin's review included children with sensory integration disorder, learning disabilities, attention deficit hyperactivity disorder (ADHD), developmental delays, pervasive developmental disorder (PDD), and developmental coordination disorder (DCD). They reviewed 20 articles, including 3 articles addressing the effectiveness of consultation, 13 articles addressing the effectiveness of direct service, and 4 review articles (i.e., systematic reviews and meta-analysis). See Table C5 in Appendix C for details about each of the studies.

Consultation

The 3 studies addressing consultation as an intervention strategy were positive, suggesting that consultation is an effective model of service delivery for children with challenges in processing and integrating sensory information (Dunn, 1990 [Level IV]; Kemmis & Dunn, 1996 [Level III]; Sugden & Chambers, 2003 [Level II]). Although Polatajko and Cantin (2010) cautioned that due to the small number of participants and weak study designs, conclusive recommendations could not be derived, they concluded that the results of the studies using a consultation approach were "particularly promising" (p. 431).

Direct Service

Thirteen articles examined direct service interventions and were organized by the review authors (Polatajko & Cantin, 2010) into four categories: sensory-based, sensorimotor, direct skills teaching, and cognitive-based approaches (see Polatajko & Cantin, 2010, for details about the types of interventions that fell into these categories).

Sensory-based. Three articles examined sensory-based approaches: wearing a weighted vest (Fertel-Daly, Bedell, & Hinojosa, 2001 [Level IV]; VandenBerg, 2001 [Level IV]) and using a sensory diet in combination with therapeutic listening (Hall & Case-Smith, 2007 [Level III]). Both of the single-case design studies examining the effectiveness of wearing a weighted vest demonstrated increased on-task behaviors in children with PDD (Fertel-Daly et al., 2001) and ADHD (VandenBerg, 2001). However, due to the studies' designs, it was not possible to determine whether the weighted vests or some other factors were responsible for the positive outcomes (Polatajko & Cantin, 2010). In a one-group pretest–posttest design study, a sensory diet in combination with a therapeutic listening program for children with ADHD facilitated considerable improvement in the children's behavior; however, the authors reported mixed results on the outcome measures (Hall & Case-Smith, 2007). Children who received the sound-based intervention and sensory diet showed improvements in sensory-related behaviors (decreased temper tantrums, reduced hyperactivity), but did not improve in any of the visual–motor or handwriting measures. No studies meeting the criteria for inclusion in the review were found that examined the effectiveness of the Wilbarger Deep Pressure and Proprioceptive Technique. Due to the heterogeneity of these studies with regard to both the type of children studied and the type of interventions used, it is difficult to reach conclusive recommendations regarding the effectiveness of sensory-based approaches. Some of the results were positive, but others were not.

Sensorimotor. Five studies examined the effectiveness of sensorimotor interventions, including a combination of sensory integration techniques, sensory diets, and therapeutic riding (Candler, 2003 [Level III]); movement therapy (Hartshorn et al., 2001 [Level I]); use of therapy balls as seating (Schilling & Schwartz, 2004 [Level IV]); physiotherapy (Chia & Chua, 2002 [Level I]); and educational kinesiology techniques (Inder & Sullivan, 2005 [Level IV]). The variety of designs and outcome measures used in these studies make it difficult to reach conclusions regarding the effectiveness of sensorimotor interventions. However, all 5 studies reported some positive behavioral outcomes related to the intervention, suggesting that sensorimotor interventions demonstrate some promise for children with challenges in processing and integrating sensory information.

Direct skills teaching. Direct skills teaching approaches were examined in 2 randomized controlled trial studies, each with three groups. Hodge, Murata, and Porretta's (1999) Level I study evaluated motor skills in children with learning and attention problems under three conditions. One group received mental preparation (MP), which included a practice period involving mental imagery and verbal directions after a demonstration of the target motor skill prior to the motor skill performance test. Another group received a task-specific warm-up period involving practice of the target motor skills prior to the test. The control group received no activities prior to the motor skill performance test. The MP group performed significantly better on a throwing accuracy item than the other groups. There were no other significant differences in motor performance between the groups. P. H. Wilson, Thomas, and Maruff's (2002) Level I study examined motor performance in children with motor coordination difficulties in three conditions. One group received motor imagery techniques that involved visual imagery, visual modeling of motor skills, mental rehearsal, and practice. A second group received a perceptual–motor program that involved gross, fine, and perceptual–motor activities. The control group received no intervention. The two groups that received the motor imagery and the perceptual–motor interventions demonstrated improvement in motor performance and performance that was superior to that of the control group. Although positive results were found in both of these studies, limitations in the number of studies and the heterogeneity of populations and interventions examined prevented decisive recommendations (Polatajko & Cantin, 2010).

Cognitive-based. Three articles described 4 studies (1 article reported 2 studies) examining the use of a cognitive-based approach, the Cognitive Orientation to Daily Occupational Performance (CO-OP) for children with DCD (Martini & Polatajko, 1998; L. T. Miller, Polatajko, Missiuna, Mandich, & Macnab, 2001; Polatajko et al., 2001). These studies included a 2-group randomized controlled trial (Level I), several single-case studies (Level IV), and a retrospective chart audit (Level IV). Collectively, the results of these studies provide evidence for the effectiveness of the CO-OP cognitive-based approach for children with DCD. However, limitations include limited generalizability of the case studies, lack of control group in the chart audit, and relatively small sample in the randomized controlled trial (Polatajko & Cantin, 2010).

The authors concluded that although this approach is promising, further study is needed.

Review articles.
Sensory-based and sensorimotor approaches. Two systematic reviews examined the effectiveness of sensory-based and sensorimotor interventions for children with autism. Baranek (2002) reviewed 29 studies that examined a variety of interventions, including sensory integration–like approaches, sensory stimulation techniques, auditory integration training, visual therapies, sensorimotor handling techniques, and physical exercise. Findings from these studies are mixed; however, several studies yielded some positive outcomes (Baranek, 2002). Unfortunately, methodological limitations restrict conclusive recommendations and generalizability of much of this research (Baranek, 2002). Sinha, Silove, Wheeler, and Williams (2006) reviewed randomized controlled trials investigating the effectiveness of sound therapy in autism. The results were mixed for the 6 studies that met the inclusion criteria; 3 studies reported improvement, and 3 studies failed to demonstrate positive effects, so no conclusions about this approach could be drawn.

Perceptual–Motor Interventions

One meta-analysis study was conducted on perceptual–motor interventions with a variety of children with learning problems (Kavale & Mattson, 1983). The results from the 180 studies that met the inclusion criteria indicated that the effect size for perceptual–motor intervention was no better than no intervention. However, Nolan (2004) more recently reviewed all 180 articles that were included in the Kavale and Mattson meta-analysis and found major methodological flaws in study selection, completeness of data, and analysis of outcomes. As a result of these methodological limitations, Nolan questioned the strong claims made by Kavale and Mattson that perceptual–motor training is not an effective intervention.

A final study that combined a systematic review and meta-analysis on the effectiveness of a variety of interventions for children with DCD included 21 studies in the systematic review and 13 studies in the meta-analysis (Pless & Carlsson, 2000). Pless and Carlsson divided the studies into three categories based on their interpretation of theoretical foundations of interventions used in each study. Those categories were general ability, sensory integration, and specific skills. All categories of intervention were found to have positive effects, with specific skills intervention having the largest effect, followed by general ability intervention and sensory integration. The authors concluded that their results support the use of specific skill approaches in the treatment of children with DCD (Pless & Carlsson, 2000).

Implications for Clinical Practice and Research

Due to the great heterogeneity of the articles reviewed, both in the variety of populations (9) included and the variety of interventions (10), Polatajko and Cantin (2010) were unable to formulate an overall conclusion for occupational therapy practitioners regarding which interventions may be most effective for children and adolescents experiencing challenges in processing and integrating sensory information. Notwithstanding the heterogeneity issues that permeate this area of research, Polatajko and Cantin stated that based on the articles reviewed, the consultation service delivery model with this population was particularly promising. The results for the direct service models were more mixed, with some direct service interventions demonstrating positive outcomes and other direct service interventions demonstrating mixed results. Polatajko and Cantin classified the interventions into sensory-based, sensorimotor, direct skills training, and cognitive-based approaches. Some studies in all four of the categories resulted in some positive outcomes. However, depending on the intervention, population, and outcome measures, many of the results were mixed, meaning that only some of the outcomes showed positive effects. In conclusion of their review, Polatajko and Cantin stated that support for the effectiveness of sensory-based and sensorimotor approaches is inconclusive, and support for the effectiveness of direct skills training and cognitive-based approaches is very encouraging but may be limited to children with normal intelligence and motor coordination.

The heterogeneity issues in this research area accentuate the urgent need for well-designed studies on the effectiveness of precise interventions in a well-defined homogeneous population. Studies need to use designs that provide a strong link between specific interventions and outcomes. Studies that use outcomes targeting participation in everyday activities are essential for helping to elucidate interventions that have positive outcomes for children and adolescents experiencing challenges in processing and integrating sensory information.

Foundations of Occupational Therapy Services for Children and Adolescents With Challenges in Sensory Processing and Sensory Integration

History and Theory Development in Sensory Processing and Integration

In her seminal work, A. J. Ayres, an occupational therapist, educational psychologist, and researcher, proposed that sensory information, as it was processed and utilized by the nervous system, affected behavior and learning (Ayres, 1972b). Ayres emphasized the contributions of sensation to the development of an individual's concept of self and environment. She recognized the five basic senses—taste, touch, sight, smell, and hearing—but highlighted the key importance of the body-centered senses of proprioception and vestibular input for helping an individual develop a body schema. She also promoted the importance of what she termed *interoception*, those sensations that arise from within the body, and the way in which such sensations interact with those that arise from outside the body *(exteroception)*. She conceptualized the interaction among interoception, proprioception, and exteroception as critical for an individual to interact meaningfully and functionally with the world (Smith Roley, 2006b).

Ayres hypothesized that a relationship between sensation and behavior existed in which neurological processing of sensation could support or inhibit function (Bundy et al., 2002). She also proposed that because of this brain–behavior relationship, sensation could be used strategically as an intervention to affect nervous system functions and, ultimately, behavior and learning (Ayres, 1972b). As part of Ayres's first description of sensory integration intervention, the following three major postulates of the theory emerged:

1. Learning is dependent on the ability to take in and process sensation from movement and the environment and use it to plan and organize behavior.
2. Individuals who have a decreased ability to process sensation may also have difficulty producing appropriate actions which, in turn, may interfere with learning and behavior.
3. Enhanced sensation, as a part of meaningful activity that yields an adaptive interaction, improves the ability to process sensation, thereby enhancing learning and behavior. (Bundy & Murray, 2002, p. 5)

These postulates reflect the predictive relationship between brain function and purposeful behavior. With the remarkable advances in neuroscience knowledge in the past several decades, revisiting the neuroscience literature is essential for validation and further refinement of the current postulates. The next section presents a summary of the systematic review of the neuroscience literature published between 1996 and 2008 (Lane & Schaaf, 2010). The review addressed the question, What is the neuroscience evidence that occupational therapy using a sensory integrative framework with children and adolescents will be effective?

Evidence-Based Review of the Neuroscience Literature

Level I Studies

Level I studies (Kempermann & Gage, 1999; Rosenzweig & Bennett, 1972; Rosenzweig et al., 1969; Stoeckel, Pollok, Schnitzler, Witte, & Seitz, 2004) include experiments using a randomized controlled methodology. Most studies were primarily with animal models and examined the effects of enriched environments on brain structure. Findings indicate that environmental enrichment alters brain structure in positive ways in animals. Specifically, dendritic branching and number of synapses increased, reflecting increased neuronal interactions and complexity in sensory and motor processing. These findings provide indirect support of at least one theoretical premise of occupational therapy using a sensory integration approach: Environments rich in appropriate sensory and motor opportunities facilitate neural changes. Of interest, the literature showed that active exploration was a necessary component of the brain changes described. This finding lends support for another central premise of occupational therapy using a sensory integration approach: that active engagement (of the child) is needed to facilitate integration of sensory information.

Finally, these investigations indicated that objects in the environment should be varied and that the exposure required is at least 1 hour per day over a few weeks. This finding provides some basic science data that may inform investigations related to the optimal length and frequency of intervention (also known as *dosage*). However, because behavioral measures were not included in many of the studies, no direct inference between brain changes and behavior changes can be made. Further, studies using enriched conditions were conducted using animal models; it is a long way from animal to human, even in the basics of sensory and motor processing. This review did examine human studies that capitalized on the provision of specific sensory input and examined changes in motor output. Of note, Lacourse, Turner, Randolph-Orr, Schandler, and Cohen (2004) studied human participants and found that changes in the nervous system resulted from engagement in sensory–motor practice, thus suggesting that the human brain has the potential to change in response to sensory and motor input. See Table C1 in Appendix C for more detailed information on the studies.

Level II Studies

Level II studies included two-group nonrandomized investigations using designs such as cohort and case controlled. There were 9 studies using human participants, 2 with nonhuman primate participants, and 16 using other animals (primarily rodent models, with some primate models). The studies used a variety of methods to examine the results of sensory input; some used enriched experiences, and others examined sensory alterations caused by congenital or induced lesions such as deafness and blindness. Overall, the Level II studies provided evidence that supports neuroplasticity in the central nervous system in response to sensory input. The animal data provided strong support that altered or enhanced sensory input changes the way the nervous system processes information (Bennett et al., 1964; Gordon & Stryker, 1996; Moses, Martin, Houck, Ilmoniemi, & Tesche, 2005; Recanzone, Schreiner, & Merzenich, 1993). The mechanisms for these changes included increased dendritic branching (Volkmar & Greenough, 1972), histological changes (in cell structure and function; Volkmar & Greenough, 1972), anatomical changes (in sensory and motor maps or reorganization of brain areas; Gordon & Stryker, 1996; Merzenich, Recanzone, Jenkins, & Grajski, 1990; Recanzone et al., 1993; Wu, van Gelderen, Hanakawa, Yaseen, & Cohen, 2005), changes in cellular activation patterns (Bennett et al., 1964; Recanzone et al., 1993), and most recently, Gómez-Pinilla, Ying, Roy, Molteni, and Edgerton (2002) demonstrated that neuroplasticity also occurs through upregulation of genes (increasing gene expression) via specific brain proteins and enzymes, including brain-derived neurotrophic factor.

As was the case for Level I studies, results from Level II animal studies most consistently support neuroplasticity in response to enriched conditions such as opportunities for sensory, motor activity, and social interaction (Bennett, Rosenzweig, Diamond, Morimoto, & Hebert, 1974; J. Brown et al., 2003; Kempermann, Kuhn, & Gage, 1998). Neuroplasticity was observed in the visual and auditory systems (Moses et al., 2005; Recanzone et al., 1993). Neuroplastic changes also are documented in the somatosensory cortex, but less consistently (Merzenich et al., 1990; Wu et al., 2005). The documented changes may not occur throughout the entire nervous system but rather may be specific to precise areas of the central nervous system—the hippocampus being one of these areas (Kempermann et al., 1998).

These same concepts are supported in the human studies, but the data are not as strong because of limitations in studying human brain tissue and processing (Bach-y-Rita, 2004; Mercado, Bao, Orduña, Gluck, & Merzenich, 2001). The human studies do, however, demonstrate that (1) the auditory system demonstrates plasticity both in its processing (activation patterns) and cortical representation in response to auditory input (Bangert & Altenmüller, 2003; Doucet et al., 2005; Moses et al., 2005); (2) the brain processes stimuli differently because of either training (e.g., piano playing) or enriched conditions (Röder, Rösler, & Neville, 2000); and (3) processing of sensory stimuli is dynamic and flexible, but also task-specific; that is, the sensory systems used during a task are flexible, but the processing systems activated are dependent on the task presented (Russo, Nicol, Zecker, Hayes, & Kraus, 2005). Additional human studies demonstrated plasticity in human sensory systems. For example, participants who had blindness demonstrated auditory system reorganization such that they became more efficient at processing auditory cues (Doucet et al., 2005). Sober and Sabes (2005) demonstrated that the use of sensory cues was dynamic, flexible, and dependent on availability of a sensory system. For example, participants could readily shift their degree of reliance on vision or proprioception, depending on what stimulus was available during a reaching task.

Level II studies involving humans reinforced outcomes related to the neuroplastic effects of enriched conditions identified in Level I and II studies involving animals and provided some interesting information about human sensory processing. These studies suggested that deficits in one sensory modality results in alterations in how the brain processes information in other modalities (Doucet et al., 2005) and that a typical nervous system can adapt to various types of sensory information available within the environment to complete a task (Sober & Sabes, 2005). Also, this last point offers some support for the assumption of sensory integration theory that a successful environmental interaction promotes processing and integration of sensory information. In Sober and Sabes's (2005) study, success depended on the subject's ability to blend visual and proprioceptive strategies. Both studies used adults as participants, and it is important to note that mature nervous systems may process information differently from developing nervous systems.

Level III, IV, and V Studies

Studies at Levels III, IV, and V are characterized as single group, nonrandomized (III); single-subject design, case series (IV); or case reports/expert opinion (V). Those reviewed here spanned 1967 to 2005 and included many human studies, as well as studies on monkeys, kittens, and rats. Early studies of the visual cortex in animal models demonstrated that the sensory systems had an innate and predetermined organization but that this organization was dependent on sensory input and experience for full expression of function (Wiesel & Hubel, 1965, 1974). Lesions resulted in reactive morphological and physiological changes in sensory systems, suggesting that the brain reorganizes when deprived of specific sensory input. Classic studies such as Hubel and Wiesel (1964) also showed that there were critical periods for development and restoration of function after lesion and that function did not necessarily return after a period of deprivation or lesion. Thus, time and critical period seem to be limiting factors to the degree of plasticity in organization and function.

Reactive neuroplasticity, documented behaviorally by Sober and Sabes (2005) and described earlier, was identified in the organization of the human somatosensory cortex (Schaefer, Heinze, & Rotte, 2005; Wu et al., 2005). This region of the brain was shown to adapt dynamically to requirements of a specific task, in that sensory input during a task resulted in changes in tactile discrimination ability. For instance, Schaefer and colleagues (2005) found more distant and distinct somatosensory cortical finger representation when digits 1 and 5 were stimulated during a fine motor/cognitive task than when participants were "at rest." The plasticity was highly task-dependent and dynamic, in that changes were shown during task performance. These investigators concluded that changes to the somatosensory cortex are dynamic and task-specific. Further, the fact that changes were greater during tasks that required cognitive processing suggested that dynamic plasticity can be facilitated by activation of the frontal and prefrontal cortex.

The integration of visual and auditory sensory input was investigated by Moses and colleagues (2005) by pairing visual and auditory stimuli and noting activation in expected brain regions. Subsequently, presentation of a visual stimulus alone resulted in specific responses in the auditory cortex, suggesting that the presentation of sensory information from one modality can produce brain activity in the primary cortex of another sensory modality when the sensations are initially paired. Because our world is not one of single-channel sensory inputs, pairing of sensation is the rule, not the exception. This rule is a foundation of occupational therapy using a sensory integration approach in which sensations are intended to be meaningfully paired such that input in one sensory modality can be used to influence processing in another modality. Because the Moses study was specific to the auditory and visual systems, application to other sensory systems must be done cautiously. Further, using single-case design, You and colleagues (2005) noted that training, either actual or via virtual reality, resulted in reorganization of cortical regions that were associated with changes in performance, again suggesting a role for feedback, either actual sensory feedback or virtual feedback.

Together, the findings suggest that neuroplasticity is dynamic and that the sensory systems interact such that pairing the presentation of several modalities influences neural processing in subsequent presentation of a single modality. Sensory strategies used are typically task- and experience-specific, and sensory processing strategies can be linked to the stage of motor performance. Globally, these findings support the tenets of sensory integration theory as proposed by Ayres (1972b).

Summary and Conclusions From Neuroscience Evidence

First, it is important to reiterate that many of the investigations reviewed here were conducted on animals, and those on humans typically used adults. Both of these facts limit the application of the findings to occupational therapy using a sensory integration approach with children. Nonetheless, many interesting parallels can be drawn between these basic science studies and Ayres's (1972b) sensory integration theory. First, several of the environmental enrichment studies (e.g., Bennett et al., 1974, 1996; Diamond, Rosenzweig, Bennett, Lindner, & Lyon, 1972; Rosenzweig et al., 1969) provide early evidence that neuroplasticity is possible and that the environment affects neural structure and function. This finding has tremendous implications for occupational therapy in general and occupational therapy using a sensory integration approach specifically.

Building on these classic studies, investigations of specific sensory interventions documented changes in central nervous system function, organization, and structure after sensory manipulations. Thus, there is little question that the nervous system is plastic and that sensory input is an important mediator of this plasticity. Motor activity and interest in task also appear to be important contributors, and active engagement is seen to enhance the effects. Further, the studies reviewed indicated that neuroplastic changes were developmental, dynamic (reactive), and task-specific. In this regard, these data provide indirect support for the use of occupational therapy using a sensory integration approach, which is built on the premise that active engagement in meaningful sensory–motor activities at the just-right challenge and in a playful and meaningful context, has a positive impact (by means of neuroplasticity) on processing in the nervous system (Ayres, 1972b). Beyond this support, the studies reviewed inform us that multisensory integration may be task-specific or dependent on task complexity. This finding warrants consideration in the provision of occupational therapy using a sensory integration approach.

Applied to occupational therapy using a sensory integration approach, the message is that tasks intended to tap into more than a single sensory processing system must do so naturally if integration is to occur. For instance, if we are hoping to integrate proprioceptive and visual inputs, then swinging on a trapeze over a bolster and targeting a pile of pillows as the drop point has the potential to be integrative; this activity combines proprioception (muscle contraction involved in hanging on and flexing the trunk to clear the bolster), vestibular (swinging/linear movement), and visual (identification of the target) inputs in a natural and highly motivating manner. Conversely, passive input (e.g., passive spinning, passively applied touch) would appear not to create the same affordance for integration.

Sensory Function and Dysfunction

Ayres's work provides occupational therapy practitioners with a model for understanding the contribution of sensation to development, assessment tools for understanding human behavior, a theory for interpreting assessment findings, and intervention techniques to address identified challenges in performance. The next section of this document provides background information about the influence of sensory functions in normal development, followed by sections describing Ayres's conceptualization of sensory integrative function, sensory integrative dysfunction, and approaches to intervention.

Development of Sensory Functions

The development and integration of sensory functions occurs rapidly in infancy and early childhood, with evidence of some sensory systems functioning in utero. Sensory integration begins in the prenatal period, with avoidant responses to touch occurring as early as 5 1/2 weeks and proprioceptive functions emerging by 9 weeks (Salihagic-Kadic, Kurjak, Medic, Andonotopo, & Azumendi, 2005). Studies also reveal that auditory processing begins at about 25 weeks of gestation (Graven & Browne, 2008a) and that visual responses to light are consistent by 34 weeks of gestation (Graven & Browne, 2008b). The vestibular system is the first to mature and is fully functional at birth (Maurer & Maurer, 1988). In the neonatal period, the tactile, olfactory, and vestibular system functions are used to help develop attachment between the infant and caregiver and are used for state regulation and feeding. Vestibular proprioception functions are evident as the infant begins to lift the head against gravity and mold his or her own body to the caregiver's (Parham & Mailloux, 2010; Spitzer & Roley, 2001). Continued growth and development of the nervous system lead to tactile–visual integration as the infant brings hands to midline, vestibular–proprioceptive integration evidenced in the emerging ability to maintain an upright position against gravity, and the emergence of praxis as the infant coordinates eye-to-hand movements. In the second half of the first year of life, integration of visual, vestibular, and proprioceptive inputs assists the infant in learning to crawl, creep, and pull to stand (Ayres, 1979). The tactile system contributes to the development of hand skills, and the auditory and visual systems interact as the infant combines gestures with emerging language.

Integration and use of sensory information as a foundation for environmental interaction continues throughout early childhood and is reflected in the increasing complexity of person–environment interactions. In the second year, the child developing typically demonstrates better integrated visual, vestibular, and proprioceptive inputs through improved balance and postural control (Ayres, 1979). Tactile, vestibular, and proprioceptive functions contribute to development of a more comprehensive body awareness, laying the foundation for body concept and image. The auditory system helps the child develop and use more complex language. Increased control over the body and coordination of limbs is apparent in more complex motor planning and success in physical skill. During the 3rd through 17th years of life, sensory integrative functions become more refined and are demonstrated through the child's ability to use tools with skill, gauge and grade own strength, coordinate actions to learn skills such as riding a bike, and discriminate visual or auditory stimuli for identification and localization (Ayres, 1979; Spitzer & Roley, 2001).

The adaptive response. Although typically discussed in the literature as physical or action-oriented, adaptive responses can take various forms. For example, adaptive responses seen in children developing typically include such things as caring for one's own body, using materials to create or build, maintaining emotional stability when disappointed, maneuvering skillfully around obstacles in the environment, engaging in group activities, using tools to accomplish a task, and developing complex play scenarios.

The adaptiveness of a response is determined by the context and the demand on the individual. A response that is adaptive in one context may not be in another. For example, maintaining attention to a book during reading time at school is an adaptive response for a child who might otherwise be distracted by the sound of other children moving about the classroom. However, continuing to read a book when the fire alarm sounds would not be adaptive. Adaptive responses can have varying degrees of complexity, quality, and effectiveness and bring meaning to a child's actions (Ayres, 1972b). Simple adaptive responses include reflexes and the ability to stand upright against the pull of gravity (Ayres, 1972b). More complex adaptive responses are produced when a child learns to coordinate his or her legs to push the pedals of a bicycle while balancing on two wheels or orient his or her fingers in the openings of scissor handles and move the thumb and fingers in opposition to open and close the scissors while simultaneously pushing the hand across a piece of paper. Through the process of interacting with a dynamic and ever-changing environment, the child has almost constant opportunities to respond to stimuli in increasingly complex ways.

Feedback and feedforward. As adaptive responses increase in complexity and quality, the child learns through feedback arising from the sensations produced by the body and from the effect of action on the environment. Physically, the child experiences the feelings of how the body moves, the amount of effort expended, and the coordination of parts of the body. Cognitively, the child develops a plan of action, gains awareness of whether the plan brought success, and forms ideas for modifying future efforts. Affectively, the child experiences feelings of success and achievement, gaining a sense of mastery and appreciating the power to act upon the world. The combination of these emotional and physical experiences with the sensory feedback provides a foundation upon which the child can make sense of the world, build skills, and learn.

Feedforward is another important aspect of performance recognized by Ayres for its contribution to motor skill but still is not fully understood. The hypothesis is that when a child prepares to perform a movement, a copy of the motor plan intended for use is compared to previous plans and their results and evaluated against the current sensory information in order to detect any planning errors that may interfere with success (Ayres, 1972b; Kandel, Schwartz, & Jessell, 2000; May-Benson, 2010). If errors are found, the plan can be adjusted before or during execution. Feedforward is especially important for anticipatory actions related to moving objects such as preparing to catch a ball or move out of the way of an oncoming car.

Sensory registration, modulation, and discrimination. The term *registration* refers to the detection of sensation (Kandel et al., 2000) and is the initial point of perception. The registration of sensory information tells the individual that something has occurred or something has changed. It is, therefore, a response to change or novelty in the sensory environment. *Modulation* has been defined as "the capacity to regulate and organize the degree, intensity, and nature of responses to sensory input in a graded and adaptive manner" (L. J. Miller, Reisman, McIntosh, & Simon, 2001). In other words, modulation is the active process by which an individual adjusts or otherwise adapts to incoming information (Lane, 2002). An imbalance in modulation is often apparent through disorganized behavior that does not match contextual demands (Ayres, 1979). Effective modulation is necessary for environmental interaction, social engagement, emotional regulation, self-regulation of behavior, and attention direction. At the behavioral level, modulation is reflected in interactions that "match the demands and expectations of the environment" (Lane, 2002, p. 103). The ability of the individual to demonstrate such organization is often referred to as "regulation of behavior." *Self-regulation* is often referred to in the literature as an organized behavioral state whereby the individual is able to successfully adapt to the demands of his or her environment (Boekoerts & Pintrich, 2005). More specifically, self-regulation is "the ability to monitor and modulate cognition, emotion, and behavior to accomplish one's goal and/or to adapt to the cognitive and social demands of specific situations" (Berger, Kofman, Livneh, & Henik, 2007, p. 257). Clearly, regulation of behavior is influenced by, even dependent upon, an individual's ability to adequately modulate responses to external and internal sensory stimuli. In fact, Porges (1995) underscored that regulation of behavior is dependent upon one's ability to adequately register and modulate sensory input. Thus, a regulated state is a consequence of adequate registration and modulation of sensory input.

Sensory *discrimination* is the ability to take in information from the physical environment and perceive qualities of stimuli, such as spatial or temporal features. Discrimination creates a foundation upon which sensory stimuli are interpreted and become meaningful. Sensory discrimination affords knowledge of similarities and differences among stimuli as well as awareness of concepts such as what and where something is (L. J. Miller, Anzalone, et al., 2007).

Registration, modulation, and discrimination are critical components of sensation processing. Dysfunction in any of these can be reflected through dysfunctional behavior, including poor self-regulation of behavior.

Sensory Integration Function

In describing the influence of sensation on behavior and learning, Ayres (1972b, 1979) discussed seven distinct forms (sight, sound, taste, smell, touch, movement, and resistance) and three sources of sensation (interoception, vestibular–proprioception, and exteroception). *Interoception* refers to sensations that arise from within the body and are used primarily for survival (Kandel et al., 2000). For example, organs and viscera produce sensations that inform the individual of needs related to hunger, pain, and body temperature. These sensations drive the individual to execute behaviors aimed at alleviating the hunger, removing the source of pain, and regulating body temperature.

Vestibular–proprioceptive information arises from receptors in the head and musculoskeletal system and provides information about the position and orientation of the body and speed and direction of movement (Kandel et al., 2000). The vestibular system receptors are located in the inner ear. This system detects position and movement of the head in relation to gravity. The proprioceptive system carries sensations from the muscles, joints, and tendons about joint position and movement. Together, vestibular–proprioceptive information provides an individual with information about the position of the body in space, the orientation of the body's parts in relation to each other, and the movement of the body through space.

Exteroception is the term used to refer to sensations arising from stimuli that are external to the body (Kandel et al., 2000). The sensations of touch, taste, and smell give an individual awareness of qualities of things with which the person comes into contact (e.g., smell is detected through tiny particles that come into contact with olfactory receptors). Vision and hearing do not require contact with an object and provide information about things that are in close proximity to or far from the body. The integration of interoception, vestibular–proprioception, and exteroception culminate to provide a person with an awareness of self as an individual, self as an agent of interaction with the environment, and self as a participant in a dynamic context in which others exist and interact. Adequate functioning of these three contributors to perception enable an individual to perceive, understand, and interact with others and the environment in an organized and purposeful manner (Smith Roley & Jacobs, 2008).

As the individual participates in daily life, sensation is experienced and the nervous system responds. The sensory input gives the individual information about the body, the environment, and person–environment interactions. When sensory input is accurately and effectively processed and integrated, the individual develops accurate and useful concepts of self, others, gravity, environment, and the interactions among these factors; together, these lay a foundation for successful occupational engagement and participation in context.

Sensory Integration Dysfunction

Ayres's view of sensory integrative dysfunction emerged out of her studies and her clinical practice with children with perceptual–motor dysfunction and learning disabilities. She described her clients' difficulty in recognizing that a sensation had occurred, inability to respond to a physical challenge, inefficient organization of the body for use, and emotional responses to sensation, among others, stating that the children seemed unaware of or unable to accurately interpret and use the sensations around them to interact with the environment (Ayres, 1972b).

Conceptualizations of dysfunction are based on the understanding that behavior and physical skills are affected by the qualities and types of sensory inputs, the individual's capacity to process and interpret stimuli, and the complexity of physical and social contexts in which the individual functions (Spitzer, 1999). Dysfunction in sensory processing and integration, including inadequate modulation and/or discrimination of the temporal and spatial qualities of sensory input, can interfere with adaptive behaviors and lead to limited engagement and performance in everyday occupations (Ayres, 1972b; Bar-Shalita, Vatine, & Parush, 2008; Bundy & Murray, 2002; Gal, Cermak, & Ben-Sasson, 2007).

Patterns of sensory integration dysfunction.
Ayres's conceptualization of sensory integrative dysfunction was shaped by her studies of the sensory–perceptual challenges experienced by the children in her clinic with learning and behavioral disorders (Ayres, 1965). Although Ayres's investigation of unusual sensory responsiveness did not include standardized assessment or psychobiological markers, she described behaviors reflecting sensory sensitivities as indicative of dysfunction in the ability to modulate responses to input (Ayres, 1972b). Among the behaviors she described were tactile defensiveness (Ayres, 1964) and gravitational insecurity (Ayres, 1979). Between 1965 and 1989, she conducted numerous studies using subtests of the assessments she developed, the Southern California Sensory Integration Tests (SCSIT; Ayres, 1972c) and the Sensory Integration and Praxis Tests (SIPT; Ayres, 1989). She completed several factor analyses and a cluster analysis to identify patterns in the test scores of these children and to determine whether the patterns recurred with sufficient frequency to be considered characteristic of sensory integrative dysfunction.

Ayres conducted 7 factor analytic studies using various groupings of SCSIT subtests and other measures with small samples of children with and without perceptual–motor or learning disabilities. Six relatively consistent patterns of dysfunction emerged from the results of these studies, 5 of which were considered related to sensory integrative dysfunction. These were designated "(1) disorder in postural, ocular, and bilateral integration; (2) apraxia; (3) disorder in form and space perception; (4) auditory-language problems; and (5) tactile defensiveness" (Ayres, 1972b, p. 94). Ayres revised and refined her theory, incorporating new hypotheses and knowledge based on the results of her research. Thus, the theory of sensory integration experienced a continual and dynamic evolution throughout Ayres's career. Just prior to her death in 1988, Ayres conducted an additional investigation of patterns of sensory integration dysfunction using both factor analysis and cluster analysis methods to examine the SIPT subtest scores of 125 children with typical development and 293 children identified with learning or sensory integrative disorders. The results of the cluster analysis were consistent with patterns identified through prior factor analyses. The cluster patterns that included typical and atypical children were (Ayres, 1989)

- Low average sensory integration and praxis,
- High average sensory integration and praxis,
- Low average bilateral integration and sequencing,
- Visuo- and somatodyspraxia,
- Dyspraxia on verbal command, and
- General sensory integrative dysfunction.

Of these six clusters, Ayres felt that dyspraxia on verbal command was not related to sensory integrative dysfunction due to the high language comprehension component of the tests that load on this factor.

Identification of these patterns helped clarify and add meaning to the interrelationships between the sensory systems and functional behavior. Findings from each individual study aided understanding of the way various sensations affected function. For example, these studies revealed that poor bilateral integration was related to processing of vestibular–proprioceptive input and that dyspraxia was associated with poor discrimination of tactile stimuli (Bundy & Murray, 2002).

Proposed models of sensory integration dysfunction. Over time, many theorists and researchers have continued to examine patterns of sensory integrative dysfunction; some have proposed other conceptual models, which are discussed briefly below. Because none of these models have been examined sufficiently or confirmed through empirical testing, each needs to be interpreted cautiously.

Dyspraxia and sensory modulation disorders— Fisher and Murray. In an expansion of Ayres's work, Fisher and Murray (1991) combined information from clinical observations with the data from Ayres's factor and cluster analyses to identify two primary categorizations of sensory integrative dysfunction, which they referred to as *poor modulation* and *poor praxis.* These categorizations have become widely recognized and are frequently referred to in the literature, and they are described briefly below.

Ayres (1979) used the term *dyspraxia* to refer to a disorder of integrating tactile, vestibular, and proprioceptive sensory information, resulting in interference with the ability to plan and execute skilled or nonhabitual motor plans (1972a). Dyspraxia can be observed in an individual's inaccurate or ineffective movements, despite the person's best efforts. For example, a child might inaccurately time the coordination of his or her hands when trying to catch a ball; misplace his or her foot when trying to kick a rolling soccer ball; be unaware of how to move his or her body to climb on playground equipment; and show a lack of ideas about how to play with toys, use tools, or participate in active games. Bundy and Murray (2002) suggested four substantial contributors to dyspraxia: postural deficits, deficits in tactile discrimination, deficits in bilateral integration and sequencing, and somatodyspraxia.

Bundy and Murray (2002) combined the findings from Ayres's factor and cluster analyses and her investigations of tactile defensiveness with the work of other theorists and researchers (e.g., Dunn, 1997; L. J. Miller et al., 1998; Wilbarger & Wilbarger, 1991) to describe four patterns of dysfunction in modulating sensory information. They described dysfunction in sensory modulation as relating to ineffective regulation of the facilitory and inhibitory neural activity involved in processing sensory stimuli (Bundy et al., 2002; L. J. Miller et al., 2001). They proposed that ineffective sensory modulation resulted in such high or low states of physiological arousal that the individual was unable to self-regulate behavior, emotion, and attention. Behavioral manifestations of poor sensory modulation include lack of response or poor adaptation to changing stimuli, difficulty directing and maintaining attention, emotional over- or underreactivity, and poor behavioral control (Smith Roley, 2006a). Dysfunction in sensory modulation can result in behaviors often described as aversive, avoidant, defensive, underresponsive, overresponsive, seeking, or withdrawal (Bundy et al., 2002).

Generalized dysfunction—Mulligan. In an effort to further examine the patterns of dysfunction in sensory integration as measured and identified through the SIPT (Ayres, 1989) and validate Ayres's five-factor model, Mulligan (1998) conducted an analysis of SIPT scores from 10,475 children, including a subset of scores of 995 children with learning disabilities. She used confirmatory factor analysis to compare her findings to the five-factor model that Ayres had proposed and found several weaknesses. Further examination using exploratory factor analysis revealed a second-order four-factor model with a more satisfactory fit. Mulligan labeled the higher order factor *generalized practic dysfunction* and the four first order factors *dyspraxia, bilateral integration and sequencing deficit, visuoperceptual deficit,* and *somatosensory deficit.* A subsequent confirmatory factor analysis supported the four-factor model, which also held up when tested using the data from the subgroup of children with learning disabilities. Mulligan's findings emerged from the data themselves and have yet to be tested on an independent sample. However, they help clarify the manner in which interrelationships between sensation processing and functional behavior are manifest and emphasize the need for ongoing research in this area. It is also important to note that the SIPT does not include scores that reflect sensory modulation, precluding the possibility of identifying disorders of modulation with that tool. Implications of Mulligan's work are presented in the next evidence-based review of literature, related to subtypes in sensory integration dysfunction.

Sensory thresholds and patterns of responding—Dunn. In another line of inquiry, Dunn (1997, 2001) proposed a model of sensory modulation based on the concepts of neurological thresholds and individual self-regulatory abilities. The model reflects an interaction between neuroscience and behavioral concepts such as temperament and personality and is aimed at characterizing the manner in which people receive and use sensory information to construct their daily lives. Dunn stated that people "characterize their experiences from a sensory point of view.... Sensation is the common language by which we share the experience of being human" (Dunn, 2001, p. 608).

Dunn's Model of Sensory Processing (Dunn, 1997, 2001) identifies *neurological thresholds* as the point at which "the proper amount of input has accumulated" and a response is triggered (Dunn, 2001, p. 609). Thresholds differ among individuals and result in persons noticing and responding to different intensities and amounts of stimulation. These differences are reflected in the choices people make for daily activities as well as their responses, such as mood, temperament, and self-organization (Dunn, 2001). Dunn also identified *responding strategies,* four observable behavioral profiles that she believed reflect an individual's patterns of sensory processing. Both the neurological thresholds and the responding strategies are described as existing along continua and are arranged in her model in a manner that reflects their interaction (Dunn, 1997, 2001). This arrangement is intended to illustrate how an individual's behavioral responses to sensory events reflect that person's neurological thresholds and responding strategies.

The four anchor points of Dunn's model are named for extremes in response patterns; however, individual responses can occur anywhere along the continua of the model. The anchor points are high threshold/passive responding, high threshold/active responding, low threshold/passive responding, and low threshold/active responding. Behavioral responses are interpreted as being in accordance with or serving to counteract the thresholds.

Data supporting Dunn's model are emerging from studies using questionnaires developed by Dunn and colleagues (Dunn, 1999, 2002, 2006). These data suggest that sensory-seeking behaviors are a prominent feature in the daily lives of individuals across the life span, including infants (Dunn, 2002; Dunn & Daniels, 2001), children and youths (Dunn, 1999; Dunn & Brown, 1997), and adults without disabilities (C. Brown, Tollefson, Dunn, Cromwell, & Filion, 2001). Examination of the data using factor analytic methods suggests that sensory-processing patterns among individuals cluster according to an individual's reactivity to sensory stimuli (i.e., thresholds), not by sensory system. Further support for considering sensory processing according to reactivity rather than by discrete sensory system functions comes from examination of psychophysiological studies showing correlation between behavioral responses to sensory stimuli and measurement of sympathetic nervous system activity via habituation (C. Brown et al., 2001; McIntosh, Miller, Shyu, & Dunn, 1999; McIntosh, Miller, Shyu, & Hagerman, 1999; L. J. Miller et al., 1998). Examination of behaviors believed to reflect sensory processing reactivity patterns among persons with clinical diagnoses suggests that these individuals process and respond to sensory stimuli differently than individuals without diagnoses (C. Brown et al., 2001; Ermer & Dunn, 1998; Kientz & Dunn, 1997; McIntosh, Miller, Shyu, & Dunn, 1999; Watling, Deitz, & White, 2001).

Sensory modulation disorder—L. J. Miller. Building on Ayres's work, L. J. Miller and colleagues conducted a variety of studies using physiological and behavioral measures to examine concepts related to the specific processes of sensory modulation (McIntosh, Miller, Shyu, & Hagerman, 1999; L. J. Miller et al., 1998). Investigators proposed using the term *sensory modulation disorder (SMD)* to describe the patterns of behavior characteristic of persons with disordered sensory modulation (Lane, Miller, & Hanft, 2000). SMD is described as being characterized by overresponsivity, underresponsivity, and fluctuating responses to sensory stimuli (Lane et al., 2000; L. J. Miller & Summers, 2001). *Overresponsivity* is described as an increased intensity, duration, or magnitude of a response to sensation. *Underresponsivity* is described as diminished intensity, duration, or magnitude of response to a sensation. Although each of these patterns can exist exclusively, fluctuations between hyper- and hyporesponsiveness also can be exhibited. L. J. Miller and colleagues asserted that when hyper-, hypo-, or fluctuating responsivity is present, an individual's ability to achieve and maintain a state that supports and allows optimal occupational functioning is impaired (McIntosh, Miller, Shyu, & Hagerman, 1999; L. J. Miller et al., 1998).

This line of research has included numerous investigations of physiological responses to sensation in conjunction with measures of behavioral reports and observations in children with and without clinical diagnoses (S. Reynolds, Lane, & Gennings, 2010; Schaaf, Miller, Seawell, & O'Keefe, 2003). Based on the findings of these studies, L. J. Miller and colleagues (2007) proposed a nosology for organizing and classifying the patterns of behavior indicative of disordered sensory integration and processing. The overarching construct of the nosology is *sensory processing disorder (SPD)*, which is defined as "impairments in detecting, modulating, interpreting, or responding to sensory stimuli" (L. J. Miller, Coll, & Schoen, 2007). The nosology proposes SPD as a primary disorder that can be divided into three distinct subtypes: *sensory modulation disorder (SMD)*, *sensory discrimination disorder (SDD)*, and *sensory-based motor disorder (SBMD)*.

In this nosology, SMD is further broken down into three subtypes: *sensory overreponsivity (SOR)*, *sensory underresponsivity (SUR)*, and *sensory seeking/craving (SS)*. SOR is characterized by faster and more intense responses to sensation that last longer than responses exhibited by people with normal sensory responsivity. SUR is characterized by a disregard for or lack of response to sensory stimuli, which can lead to diminished engagement with the physical and social environments. SS is evidenced by active engagement in activities that provide intense and frequent sensations and can include impulsive, aggressive, or explosive behaviors.

SDD is a dysfunction in the ability to interpret qualities of sensory stimuli as needed for identification and localization, as well as recognition of similarities and differences among stimuli (L. J. Miller, Schoen, James, & Schaaf, 2007). SDD can occur in any of the sensory modalities and may be present in one or more modalities for a given individual.

SBMD reflects dysfunction in the use of sensory input for motor output and is expressed in disorganized, ineffective, or inefficient postural and volitional movements. L. J. Miller's nosology conceptualizes SBMD as having two subtypes: postural disorders and dyspraxia. *Postural disorder* is defined as "difficulty stabilizing the body during movement or rest to meet the demands of the environment or of a given task" (L. J. Miller, Anzalone, et al., 2007, p. 138). *Dyspraxia* is defined as "an impaired ability to conceive of, plan, sequence, or execute novel actions" (L. J. Miller, Anzalone, et al., 2007, p. 138).

Evidence-Based Review of Subtypes of Children and Adolescents With Challenges in Processing and Integrating Sensory Information

A total of 57 articles were reviewed; however, only 4 articles provided direct evidence for subtypes (Davies & Tucker, 2010). These studies used a multivariate statistical approach that revealed a pattern of sensory sensitivities and sensory-based motor functions and dysfunctions. The remaining 53 studies examined a single sensory attribute and used univariate methods but were limited in usefulness in determining subtypes because they were not able to uncover a pattern of characteristics that distinguished different groups, a key concept for identifying and confirming subtypes. Thus, the discussion of the evidence reported in these latter articles will be briefly addressed in the "Implications for Clinical Practice and Research" section. First, we will summarize the evidence found in the 4 articles that directly tested the existence of subtypes.

Studies Directly Examining Subtypes

Mulligan (1998 [Level III]) used an existing database of SIPT (Ayres, 1989) scores obtained from Western Psychological Services to conduct a factor analysis of 10,475 cases, including a discrete group of 995 children with learning disabilities within that sample. The best fitting model for these data included a higher order model consisting of a general factor and four first-order factors that were all highly related and appeared to fall under one general concept. The general factor was described as a general practic dysfunction, later interpreted by Mulligan as sensory integration dysfunction (personal communication, July 30, 2007). The four first-order factors were visual–perceptual deficit, bilateral integration and sequencing deficit, dyspraxia, and somatosensory deficit.

A second study conducted by Mulligan (2000 [Level III]) used a cluster analysis on 1,961 heterogeneous cases, also from the Western Psychological Services SIPT scores database. A five-cluster result was considered most meaningful: Cluster 1, generalized sensory dysfunction and dyspraxia–severe (11.2% of the sample); Cluster 2, dyspraxia (29.6%); Cluster 3, generalized sensory dysfunction and dyspraxia–moderate (8.4%); Cluster 4, low-average bilateral integration and sequencing (36.6%); and Cluster 5, average sensory integration and praxis (14.2%). These five groupings appeared to be on a continuum of dysfunction severity; however, it is noteworthy that dyspraxia and bilateral integration and sequencing were identified as discrete subtypes. This finding helps to confirm earlier studies also finding these subtypes.

The third study included multiple assessments that evaluated sensory reactivity, adaptive behavior, and information-processing abilities such as memory and attention in children with autism spectrum disorders (Liss et al., 2006 [Level III]). In contrast to the previous two studies that used data from only one assessment tool (i.e., SIPT), this study included multiple assessment tools (i.e., Vineland Adaptive Behavior Scales [Sparrow, Balla, & Cicchetti, 1984], Kinsbourne Overfocusing Scale [Kinsbourne, 1991], and a 103-item sensory questionnaire designed for this study with 60 items from the Sensory Profile [Dunn, 1999]). An additional contrast is that this study focused on one group of children, those with autism. A cluster analysis conducted on data from 254 participants with autism revealed four clusters. Cluster 1 consisted of children (11.8% of the sample) who were oversensitive to sensory stimulation, had high scores on overfocused selective attention, and were most impaired on social skills. Cluster 2 included children (25%) who were considered to be relatively high functioning on the autism spectrum and exhibited few sensory problems. Cluster 3 consisted of children (30.6%) who were low functioning in communication and social skills, were sensory undersensitive, and exhibited sensory-seeking behaviors. Children in Cluster 4 (32.6%) were similar to children in Cluster 1, but their symptoms were less severe in comparison. These results suggest that children with autism may fall into different subtypes as identified by sensory reactivity.

Dunn and Brown (1997) conducted a factor analysis of the Sensory Profile scores collected on 1,115 children developing typically to analyze the relationship between items on this assessment. The results yielded nine factors: sensory seeking, emotionally reactive, low endurance/tone, oral sensory sensitivity, inattention/distractibility, poor registration, sensory sensitivity, sedentary, and fine motor/perceptual. These factors now are used by test administrators to interpret individual scores on this tool. A study conducted by Dunn and Bennett (2002 [Level II]) on the scores of children with ADHD revealed that most of the Sensory Profile items that significantly distinguished the children with ADHD from children with typical development fell into four of the nine factors: sensory seeking, emotionally reactive, inattention/distractibility, and fine motor/perceptual. Multivariate analyses are needed to confirm these findings.

Studies Indirectly Examining Subtypes

Although the 53 studies that examined a single sensory attribute within a specific diagnosis did not provide direct information about subtypes, these articles were reviewed because they provided some useful information regarding diagnosis-specific patterns related to sensory processing. The majority of these articles investigated children in four diagnostic groups: autistic spectrum disorder (ASD), ADHD, DCD, and learning disorders (LD). Many children may have more than one disorder, so these diagnostic categories are not necessarily discrete. This section is divided into the categories based on the primary diagnosis reported in the individual studies. When interpreting these results reported for the discrete diagnosis, it is important to consider that children may have comorbidities or characteristics of several disorders. These studies represent a variety of levels of evidence, which are recorded in Table C2 in Appendix C.

Sensory processing differences in ASD. Children with ASD demonstrated strengths in tasks requiring visual and auditory discrimination (Jarrold, Gilchrist, & Bender, 2005; O'Riordan & Passetti, 2006). Visual discrimination, such as visually searching for objects, was a strength, but only when other attention demands were not required (Jarrold et al., 2005). Therapists could capitalize on these visual and auditory processing strengths by incorporating other sensory systems or cognitive demands into intervention tasks to increase integration of sensory input (Davies & Tucker, 2010). Alternatively, for critical task performance, practitioners and teachers can allow children with ASD to capitalize on their visual and auditory strengths by presenting tasks that require the child to incorporate these skills. Related to sensory-based motor performance, children with ASD were shown to rely more on visual input than on vestibular, somatosensory, or proprioceptive input while maintaining balance (Minshew, Sung, Jones, & Furman, 2004; Molloy, Dietrich, & Bhattacharya, 2003). Several studies found that children with ASD have more disturbances in motor planning than with balance, equilibrium, or motor execution (Jansiewicz et al., 2006; Rinehart et al., 2006; Vernazza-Martin et al., 2005). Thus, when planning intervention for motor functioning in everyday activities for children with ASD, occupational therapy practitioners should be aware of these strengths, along with the deficits in praxis and balance when vision is occluded. For example, instead of focusing on execution of a motor skill such as balance, practitioners could engage the child in activities that require motor planning (e.g., maneuvering through an obstacle course, playing "Simon Says," jumping rope; Davies & Tucker, 2010).

Sensory processing differences in ADHD. Children with ADHD were shown to have sensory processing deficits across modalities (Dunn & Bennett, 2002; Parush, Sohmer, Steinberg, & Kaitz, 1997; Yochman, Ornoy, & Parush, 2006; Yochman, Parush, & Ornoy, 2004). One study found sensory-based motor deficits in preschool children with ADHD (Iwanaga, Ozawa, Kawasaki, & Tsuchida, 2006). However, other investigations demonstrated that children with ADHD did not have difficulties with fundamental sensory-based motor performance; rather, deficits were shown only in complex, higher level sensory processing abilities involving sustained visual attention to moving objects and discrimination of the duration of visual and auditory stimuli (Toplak & Tannock, 2005; Vickers, Rodrigues, & Brown, 2002). These higher level motor deficits would be evident in activities such as catching, throwing, or kicking a ball, all of which require timing and synchronization of limbs (Davies & Tucker, 2010). Thus, an occupational therapy practitioner should include these higher level motor tasks in assessment and intervention for children with ADHD.

Sensory processing differences in DCD. Children with DCD have been found to have difficulties in motor planning and praxis as well as specific difficulties processing visual information, such as in tasks that require visual perception and visual–motor coordination. Similar to children with ASD, children with DCD relied more heavily on their vision when performing tasks involving motor coordination and balance compared to children with typical development (Van Waelvelde et al., 2006). Occupational therapy practitioners can address this during intervention by providing visual cues during a task, especially difficult tasks, and grading the activity by decreasing the visual cues over time as the child becomes more proficient and independent. The studies that investigated sensory-based activities in children with DCD did not evaluate sensory modulation or sensory discrimination performance, which remains unexplored.

Sensory processing differences in LD. Finally, children with LD, similar to children with DCD, were found to have difficulties in visual processing, especially spatial visualization and visual–motor skills (Humphries, Krekewich, & Snider, 1996; O'Brien, Cermak, & Murray, 1988). Deficiencies in sensory-based motor function and motor coordination also were found in children with LD (O'Brien et al., 1988; Snow, Blondis, Accardo, & Cunningham, 1993; Stoodley, Fawcett, Nicolson, & Stein, 2005). Challenges in sensory-based motor function and motor coordination seen in children with both DCD and LD may be attributed to the lack of ability to predict consequences of their movement actions (Smits-Engelsman, Wilson, Westenberg, & Duysens, 2003). This inability could be caused by lack of sensory feedback, not slowness or limited information processing. Thus, occupational therapy practitioners should emphasize motor planning activities with children with LD and DCD and encourage them to predict certain outcomes of their movement or allow the children to experience and analyze the consequences of their movements prior to execution. Graphesthesia and stereognosis are areas of challenge for children and adolescents with LD for complex tactile tasks (Snow et al., 1993). Thus, tasks that involve more complex tactile discrimination skills should be addressed in assessment and, if indicated, considered in treatment when working with children with LD. As with children with DCD, sensory modulation performance was not evaluated in children with LD, and this area of sensory processing remains uncharted.

The results of this review suggest that some subtypes are being identified and supported by research. In addition, children in different diagnostic categories may present with diagnostic-specific patterns of sensory deficits. Collectively, these findings provide evidence to suggest that treatment strategies may need to vary depending on diagnostic categories and sensory-based subtypes, in addition to the specific sensory characteristics of the child.

Implications for Clinical Practice and Research

Mulligan's (1998, 2000) research found distinct subtypes of sensory integrative dysfunction consistent with Ayres (1972c, 1989), specifically, dyspraxia and bilateral integration and sequencing subtypes. Research on subtypes within particular diagnoses is beginning to uncover several discrete subtypes specific to a diagnosis. Liss and colleagues (2006) found four subtypes of sensory reactivity in children with autism. Two subtypes consisted of children who were hypersensitive to sensory input. Another group of children exhibited underresponsiveness to sensory input and were sensory seekers. The final subtype included approximately 25% of the children with autism in this sample who did not display sensory deficits. Dunn and Bennett (2002) found that children with ADHD had challenges in four discrete categories: sensory seeking, emotionally reactive, inattention/distractibility, and fine motor/perceptual. This evidence-based review suggested that the clinical diagnosis is associated with the subtypes found.

One limitation to these data is that the studies reviewed used different assessments to examine heterogeneous samples, making it difficult to identify subtypes. For example, the studies conducted by Mulligan (1998, 2000) and Ayres (1972c, 1989) used the SIPT subtest, which has a number of items assessing praxis and tactile discrimination, but no items directly assessing modulation. Thus, the subtypes that emerged are ones that include sensory discrimination/perception and praxis. On the other hand,

Dunn and Bennett (2002) and Liss and colleagues (2006) used parent questionnaires that had many items assessing sensory modulation, but very few items evaluating praxis. Because of this, Dunn and Bennett's research identified subtypes mainly related to sensory modulation with very few that identified praxis or sensory discrimination/perception. Researchers should be attentive to the assessments used in future research aiming to identify or confirm subtypes. As revealed in the 4 studies that directly examined subtypes, the different assessment items in each study yielded different clusters or groupings. This finding emphasizes the need for a comprehensive assessment of sensory function and sensory-based motor performance that includes sensory perception, discrimination, modulation, and praxis in a single study. In addition, studies that include multiple assessment items and tools also will increase our capability to capture patterns of sensory processing abilities that lead to function or dysfunction in everyday activities, provided these assessments are comprehensive in their scope.

Finally, more studies using multivariate methods are needed to confirm or dispute the existence of subtypes of sensory integrative dysfunction or sensory processing disorder. Since this review, an additional study completed by Mailloux and colleagues (in press) addressed some of these concerns and provided additional verification of the patterns of sensory integration dysfunction identified by Ayres. In this recent study, an exploratory factor analysis was conducted on data collected retrospectively from 273 children 4–9 years of age. Unlike previous studies, this study included data from several assessments: SIPT; Sensory Processing Measure: Home (SPM; Parham & Ecker, 2007); or an earlier version of the SPM, the Evaluation of Sensory Processing (ESP; Johnson-Ecker & Parham, 2000), and a behavior measure of attention/inattention and distractibility that was taken from descriptive data from the intake forms. Only tactile items that were included on both the SPM and ESP forms were included in the factor analysis. Thus, this study included measures of praxis (SIPT), modulation (tactile defensiveness from the SPM and ESP), and attention (intake form). The results of the factor analysis with 20 items from the four instruments yielded a six-factor solution. However, two of the factors had only one item, so a four-factor solution was the best fit. The four factors were visuo- and somatodyspraxia, vestibular/proprioceptive bilateral integration and sequencing, tactile and visual discrimination, and tactile defensiveness and attention.

Safety and Risk Issues

Fundamental information regarding sensory system development and functions and concepts of sensory integration theory are included in the entry-level education of many occupational therapy practitioners (S. Reynolds, Watling, Zapletal, & May-Benson, 2010). However, comprehensive assessment and intervention that focuses on sensory integration are considered advanced-level practice (Smith Roley & Jacobs, 2008). An advanced practitioner is knowledgeable in the safe application of occupational therapy using a sensory integration approach and the risks associated with a variety of intervention strategies used in treating children and adolescents with challenges in processing and integrating sensory information.

In a clinical setting, the physical environment when using occupational therapy with sensory integration intervention often has large, suspended equipment, and safety must be maintained within the therapy environment. Suspended equipment must be hung securely to a supporting beam or freestanding structure designed to suspend equipment. Mats, cushions, and pillows are used to pad surfaces around the therapy room and under any suspended equipment. All equipment must be checked routinely and monitored in order to maintain safety. The equipment is manufactured to provide tactile, proprioceptive, and vestibular input under the guidance of a trained therapist.

During intervention, the occupational therapy practitioner must stay close to the child and be ready to quickly move and stabilize the child and/or the equipment. Particular attention should be given when the child is in an inverted position to protect his or her head and neck position and when making fast rotary movements to ensure that the child is safe throughout the activity. The occupational therapy practitioner needs to closely monitor the child's response during participation in sensory-based activities. Activation of the vestibular system, although organizing for many children, may produce strong autonomic nervous system responses, including nausea or blanching, and can affect arousal, producing distractible, unfocused behavior (Parham & Mailloux, 2010). Weighted vests and weighted blankets may be used to provide the child with sustained deep tactile input; the child's response to this input must be monitored, and the therapist must be careful not to use excessive weight relative to the child's size. Currently, there is no standardized protocol that has demonstrated efficacy with weighted vest or blanket, use and the occupational therapist must have a clear occupation-focused rationale for using this equipment and monitor the child's individual response to this intervention. In a school-based context, occupational therapy using a sensory integration approach usually is provided in the natural context of the child's classroom or other school environments, and safety considerations should be customized to the nature of each environment. Advanced training should include safe use of equipment and monitoring of the child's response to sensory stimulation across contexts and environments.

Schaaf and colleagues (2010; Schaff & Smith Roley, 2006) make specific equipment recommendations for therapists who utilize the sensory integration frame of reference, including bouncing equipment, rubber ropes for pulling, therapy balls, various swings (disc, platform, net, tire, bolster), scooter board and ramp, weighted objects of various sizes, inner tubes, spandex fabric, crash pillows, ball pit, vibrating toys and massagers, various tactile materials, visual targets, climbing equipment, and props and materials to support engagement in play and practice in daily living skills (Schaaf et al., 2009, pp. 158–159). Specific interventions that use this type of equipment and are implemented by occupational therapy practitioners are described in the "Interventions" section beginning on page 31.

Mentorship and Training in Using a Sensory Integration Approach

The concepts underlying the theory of sensory integration are rooted in advanced knowledge of biology, physiology, neurology, psychology, and human behavior. As such, the ability to accurately recognize the signs and symptoms of dysfunctional sensory processing and integration require advanced skills. Recommendations of advanced training and mentorship were made as early as Ayres's original work, and such opportunities were developed and offered as early as 1977. Given the numerous advances in the neurosciences and the study of human behavior, recommendations for training and mentoring continue to be relevant for occupational therapists wishing to develop a thorough understanding of theories and intervention practices related to sensory processing and integration. A variety of training and mentoring opportunities are available throughout the United States and internationally. Among those activities recommended by experts in the field are

- Postgraduate training in sensory integration theory, assessment procedures and interpretation, and intervention techniques
- Certification in sensory integration theory and practice, including administration and interpretation of the SIPT (Ayres, 1989)
- Mentoring in using sensory integration intervention methods, including consultation and professional guidance in clinical reasoning and application of intervention methods
- Supervised use of sensory integration methods in a clinically based format for a minimum of 2 years
- Ongoing study and review of literature relevant to sensory processing, sensory integration, and the neurosciences supporting these constructs
- Ongoing dialogue and consultation with professional colleagues who are trained in sensory integration methods (Parham & Mailloux, 2010; Smith Roley, 2006b).

When pursuing mentorship, it is important to examine the mentor's specific educational experience and ongoing education, participation in contemporary practice, and participation in research activities. Identification of the mentor's specific philosophical orientation to sensory processing and integration is also important, given the breadth with which these concepts are currently interpreted and applied. Additionally, it is important to determine the extent to which the training being offered is occupation-based and consistent with the certification and licensure approvals of occupational therapy practitioners.

Summary of the Evidence-Based Literature Reviews and Recommendations for Occupational Therapy Interventions

The systematic reviews of the five focused questions include a total of 194 articles. Of these articles, 40 were at the highest level of evidence as Level I studies. Of the others, 96 were Level II studies, 37 were Level III studies, 17 were Level IV studies, and 3 were Level V studies. One qualitative study was incorporated into the review. Fifty-three articles were included in the subset of the two focused questions related to occupational therapy interventions. Twenty-seven were Level I studies, 6 were Level II studies, 7 were Level III studies, and 13 were Level IV studies. All studies included in the review, as well as those not specifically described in the evidence-based literature review section of this Practice Guideline, are summarized and critically appraised in the evidence tables in Appendix C, and full references are provided in the "References" section. Readers are encouraged to read the full articles for more details.

Recommendations for occupational therapy practice for children and adolescents with challenges in processing and interpreting sensory information can be found in Table 7. The recommendations are based on the strength of the evidence for a given topic from the intervention questions in combination with the expert opinion of the review authors and content experts reviewing this guideline. The strength of the evidence is determined by the number of articles included in a given topic, the study design, and limitations of those articles. Recommendation criteria are based on standard language developed by the U.S. Preventive Services Task Force of the Agency for Health Care Research and Quality. More information regarding these criteria can be found at http://www.uspreventiveservices taskforce.org/uspstf/standard.htm.

Although it is clear that additional investigation is needed to continue developing and examining interventions designed to ameliorate the effects of challenges in processing and integrating sensation, the available evidence-based literature is useful to inform current clinical decisions. The recommendations presented in Table 7 indicate that occupational therapy using a sensory integration approach, sensory-based interventions, and other occupational therapy interventions can be used effectively to improve the occupational performance of children and adolescents who have challenges in processing and integrating sensory information. For example, the literature reviewed provides evidence that occupational therapy using a sensory integration approach and sensory-based occupational therapy strategies can support client achievement of functional goals and lead to gains in play skills, motor and praxis abilities, sensory processing and perception, behavior, emotion regulation, social participation, attention, and engagement. Practitioners should use caution when considering using sensory strategies to target complex or general goals such as academic performance, organization, or language, because the evidence is not sufficient to recommend sensory interventions for these purposes. Some examples of how these guidelines can be used to guide the evaluation and intervention of children and adolescents with challenges in processing and integrating sensory information is provided in Table 8.

In summary, concepts related to using sensation to support health and participation through engage-

Table 7. Recommendations for Occupational Therapy Interventions for Children and Adolescents With Challenges in Processing and Integrating Sensory Information

	Recommended*	No Recommendation	Not Recommended
Areas of Occupation	• Occupational therapy using a sensory integration approach for performance on individual functional goals for children with problems in sensory processing (C) • A combination of sensory integration, sensory diets, and therapeutic riding to address performance on functional, parent-centered goals in children with problems with sensory processing (C) • Sensory integration for participation in active play for children with sensory processing disorder (C) • Sensory integration to address play skills and engagement for children with autism (C) • A cognitive and task-based approach to address participation in occupations for children with motor deficits characteristic of developmental coordination disorder (DCD) (B) • Movement therapy for on-task passive behaviors in children with autism (C)	• Sensory integration for academic and psychoeducational performance (e.g., math, reading, written language) (I) • Exercise for play behavior in children with autism (I)	

Performance Skills

Motor and Praxis Skills	• Sensory integration for gross motor and motor planning skills for children with learning disabilities (B) • A cognitive and task-based approach for motor skills for children with motor deficits characteristic of DCD (B) • Mental imagery to address performance on motor skills for children with attention and learning problems (C) • Motor imagery programs for performance on motor skills for children with problems in motor coordination (C) • Sensorimotor techniques to address motor performance and reduce falls in children with DCD (C)	• Perceptual–motor training for motor performance for children with learning problems (I)	
Sensory–Perceptual Skills	• Occupational therapy using a sensory integration approach to address sensory processing skills for children with problems in sensory processing (C) • Sensory integration approach for visual perception in children with DCD (C) • A combined sensory diet plus therapeutic listening program to address areas of sensory processing for children with sensory processing disorders and visual–motor delays (C) • Sensory integration combined with perceptual–motor curriculum for visual, auditory, and tactile perception for children with suspected neurological problems (C)	• Sensorimotor activities for sensory organization for children with DCD (I)	
Emotional Regulation Skills	• Sensory integration to address maladaptive behaviors in children with problems in sensory processing (B) • Sensory integration to address self-esteem in children with learning disabilities and sensory integrative dysfunction (B) • Occupational therapy using a sensory integration approach for decreasing externalizing and internalizing behaviors in children with problems in sensory processing (C) • A combination sensory diet plus therapeutic listening program for improvements in behavior for children with sensory processing disorders and visual–motor delays (C)	• Sound therapy to address behavior for children with autism (I)	

(Continued)

Table 7. Recommendations for Occupational Therapy Interventions for Children and Adolescents With Challenges in Processing and Integrating Sensory Information (cont.)

	Recommended*	No Recommendation	Not Recommended
Communication and Social Skills	• Occupational therapy using a sensory integration approach to address socialization in children with problems in sensory processing (C) • Sensory integration for engagement and reduced aggression in children with sensory modulation disorder (C) • A sensory integration approach for improved social interaction and reduced disruptive behaviors in children with autism (C) • Massage for social communication in children with autism (C)	• Sound therapy for improved language skills for children with autism (I)	
Client Factors			
Mental Functions	• Sensory integration for attention in children with autism (C) • Weighted vests to address attention in children with pervasive developmental disorder and sensory processing disorder (C)		
Sensory Function and Pain	• Occupational therapy using a sensory integration approach to reduce the amplitude of electrodermal responses in children with problems in sensory modulation, indicating a decreased stress response to repetitive and potentially noxious sensory stimuli (B) • Touch pressure/deep pressure and massage to address touch aversion and improved responsiveness to sound in children with autism (B) • Sensory integration to increase nystagmus in children with learning disabilities (C) • Sensory integration to address tactile discrimination for children with suspected neurological problems (C) • Physical exercise to reduce self-stimulatory behaviors for children with autism (C) • Movement therapy to decrease negative responses to touch for children with autism (C)	Sensory integration to increase nystagmus in children with reading delays and problems in sensory integration (I)	
Consultation	• Occupational therapy provided on a consultation basis was effective for service delivery for children with sensory integration dysfunction, DCD, and learning problems (A)		

*The terminology used for the recommendations is language used in the article from which the evidence is derived.

Note. Criteria for level of evidence (A, B, C, I, D) are based on standard language (see Agency for Healthcare Research and Quality, 2009). Suggested recommendations are based on the available evidence and content experts' clinical expertise regarding the value of using the intervention in practice.

A—There is strong evidence that occupational therapy practitioners should routinely provide the intervention to eligible clients. Good evidence was found that the intervention improves important outcomes and concludes that benefits substantially outweigh harm.

B—There is moderate evidence that occupational therapy practitioners should routinely provide the intervention to eligible clients. At least fair evidence was found that the intervention improves important outcomes and concludes that benefits outweigh harm.

C—There is weak evidence that the intervention can improve outcomes, and the balance of the benefits and harms may result either in a recommendation that occupational therapy practitioners routinely provide the intervention to eligible clients or in no recommendation because the balance of the benefits and harm is too close to justify a general recommendation.

I—Insufficient evidence to determine whether or not occupational therapy practitioners should routinely provide the intervention. Evidence that the intervention is effective is lacking, of poor quality, or conflicting and the balance of benefits and harm cannot be determined.

D—Recommend that occupational therapy practitioners do not provide the intervention to eligible clients. At least fair evidence was found that the intervention is ineffective or that harm outweighs benefits.

Table 8. Application of Practice Guideline to Cases: Examples of Evaluation and Intervention

Description of Child	Evaluation	Intervention
	• Is comprehensive, assesses performance across occupations, contexts, and interactions • Includes interview, observation, and standardized testing • Includes analysis of behavior with an emphasis on how sensory processing and the environment influence behavior	• Is intensive and comprehensive • Emphasizes processing and integrating sensation as preparation for engagement and participation • Emphasizes client and family priorities • Aims to support the client in context
• **Laurean is a 2-year-old girl** with difficulty in self-regulation with heightened responsiveness to sensations. • She is described as "emotionally fragile, always on the verge of breaking down." • She startles easily at unexpected noises, refuses to go near balloons or animals, and will not approach other children engaged in play. • She plays well independently and with her mother, but leaves her play abruptly if another child approaches. • Once she becomes upset, Laurean remains on edge for the rest of the day, which typically results in the family cancelling outings or errands in order to prevent breakdowns. • She requires at least 30 minutes of rocking and cuddling in order to fall asleep at night and sleeps only 2–3 hours at a time.	• Evaluation of sensory processing using the Infant/Toddler Sensory Profile (Dunn, 2002) or the Sensory Processing Measure–Preschool (SPM–P): Home (Ecker & Parham, 2010) • Caregiver interview using the Canadian Occupational Performance Measure (Law et al., 2005) to explore daily routines, engagement expectations, and priorities for the family • Clinical observations of sensory processing and integration during structured and unstructured activities • Other assessment tools as indicated to evaluate motor, play, self-care skills • Evaluation results reveal difficulties in processing auditory, visual, and tactile input. The parents' priorities are for Laurean to fall asleep more quickly, stay asleep for longer periods of time, and recover more effectively after being upset.	• Occupational therapy services are provided once weekly in a clinical setting with the parent present and once weekly in the family's home. • Services focus on improving self-regulation for calming and sleep. • Strategies include sensory integration techniques, with an emphasis on developing strategies for use within the home. • The occupational therapist helps the mother recognize when Laurean is becoming overaroused and provides training in implementing sensory strategies to help modulate her arousal. • The occupational therapist also helps Laurean's mother identify and implement strategies for modifying the home environment to support self-regulation and sleep.
• **Ty is a 5-year-old boy** enrolled in half-day kindergarten at the local public school. • His teacher has noted that he has difficulty staying seated for circle time and table work, is unable to locate materials needed for his work, has difficulty getting started on his work, and often looks around the room while others are working. • During recess, he runs aimlessly around the playground. • He is unable to pump himself on the swing, catch or kick a ball, or skip. • During free play, he wanders around the room engaging briefly with toys in simple ways and does not demonstrate complexity in his play. • The teacher discusses these concerns with Ty's mother, who reports similar behaviors in the home. The mother agrees to an occupational therapy evaluation at school, stating that the family does not have health insurance for private services.	• Evaluation of sensory processing using the Sensory Processing Measure (SPM): Home (Parham & Ecker, 2007), Main Classroom and School Environment Forms (Miller Kuhaneck, Henry, & Glennon, 2007), or Sensory Profile (Dunn, 1999) and Sensory Profile School Companion (Dunn, 2006) • Standardized measure of motor development such as Bruininks–Oseretsky Test of Motor Proficiency, 2nd ed. (Bruininks & Bruininks, 2005), Miller Function and Participation Scales (L. J. Miller, 2006), or School Function Assessment (Coster, Deeney, Haltiwanger, & Haley, 1998) • Structured observations across school environments to observe ideation, play, engagement, regulation, praxis, fine motor, gross motor, and visual skills • Assessment of visual–perceptual and visual–motor skills (possible tools include Beery–Buktenica Test of Visual–Motor Integration [Beery, Buktenica, & Beery, 2004], Test of Visual–Motor Skills–3 [Martin, 2010], and Test of Visual–Perceptual Skills, 3rd ed. [Martin, 2006]) • Evaluation results reveal deficits in auditory, visual, and tactile processing; visual–perceptual skills; visual–motor integration; and praxis	• Individual occupational therapy services are provided for 20 minutes per week in the school setting. In addition, ongoing consultation with the classroom teacher and family allows for generalization of strategies across home and school settings. • Strategies include Ayres's sensory integration intervention with an emphasis on processing tactile, vestibular, and proprioceptive inputs in the context of dynamic activities that are meaningful to Ty. • Play skills are addressed in individual sessions in which the therapist uses materials similar to those available in the classroom to help Ty develop play schemas he can use during free play. • The occupational therapist incorporates playground play into Ty's therapy sessions to increase his familiarity with the available equipment, help him learn strategies for using the equipment, and help build his ideation and self-confidence for playground play. The occupational therapist invites others on the playground to join in to promote social participation during play. • Ty is provided with a ball chair to use during seated table work and an air-filled cushion to sit on during circle time.

(Continued)

Table 8. Application of Practice Guideline to Cases: Examples of Evaluation and Intervention (cont.)

Description of Child	Evaluation	Intervention
Samantha is an 8-year-old girl who enjoys school, reading, and playing with her dolls. • She is able to perform all necessary tasks to care for her body and belongings at home with reminders and occasional assistance from her mother and is able to perform required activities at school without assistance. • Motorically, she slumps when seated, leans when standing, and fatigues easily. • She has difficulty keeping up in physical education (PE) class and avoids the sports-oriented sessions; she does not engage in physical play at recess or in after-school activities. • Samantha cannot coordinate the right and left sides of her body to perform jumping jacks or time her upper extremity movements to hit a ball with a racket or bat. • Because Samantha's difficulties do not interfere with her success at school, her parents pursue an evaluation at an outpatient pediatric therapy clinic.	• Sensory Integration and Praxis Tests (Ayres, 1989) • Caregiver report of sensory processing (SPM: Home [Parham & Ecker, 2007]) • Classroom teacher, PE teacher, and playground assistant report of sensory processing (SPM: Main Classroom and School Environment Forms [Miller Kuhaneck et al., 2007] or Sensory Profile [Dunn, 1999]) • Clinical observations based on sensory integration theory (Blanche, 2002) • Standardized measure of motor skills (Bruininks–Oseretsky Test of Motor Proficiency, 2nd ed. [Bruininks & Bruininks, 2005]) • Client and caregiver interview using the Canadian Occupational Performance Measure (Law et al., 2005) to determine main areas of concern and priorities for treatment • Children's Assessment of Participation and Enjoyment and Preferences for Activities of Children (King et al., 2005) • Perceived Efficacy and Goal Setting System (Missiuna, Pollock, & Law, 2004) • Evaluation results reveal deficits in praxis and gross motor skill development as well as poor body scheme awareness	• Occupational therapy services are provided twice weekly for 45 minutes in an outpatient therapy clinic using Ayres's sensory integration intervention. • Samantha attends the first session each week independently, and her mother joins in during the second. • Services focus on improving Samantha's body scheme through a variety of tactile, proprioceptive, and vestibular activities. • Suspended equipment and vestibular input are used to challenge Samantha's bilateral motor coordination, ideation, and praxis skills and to help her integrate multisensory experiences including tactile, vestibular, proprioceptive, and visual input. • Practitioners obtain information about performance in school, especially PE and recess, to be able to suggest strategies for school. Even though Samantha does not receive occupational therapy services in school, obtaining this information from school personnel as well as sharing information with school personnel leads to a collaborative approach.
Jared is a 7-year-old boy who is physically active in sports and intense in his activities. • He fidgets with his clothing, constantly tugs at his baseball jersey, refuses to wear short-sleeve shirts or short pants even in summer, and does not go barefoot. • Jared has a limited diet, preferring to eat hard crunchy food and avoiding all soft and creamy textures. • During his parent–teacher conference, the teacher described him as distractible and edgy. He is frequently off-task at school and is regularly sent to the principal's office for minor infractions such as yelling at other kids or being too rough. The teacher has moved him to the front of the class to be able to monitor him and keep him on task. • Jared has one friend with whom he plays well. Other friendships have been affected by his intensity in play and poor social interaction skills. • Jared's parents pursue an occupational therapy evaluation at a private clinic after hearing about sensory integration on a television program.	• Sensory Integration and Praxis Tests (Ayres, 1989) • Caregiver report of sensory processing (SPM: Home [Parham & Ecker, 2007]; Sensory Profile [Dunn, 1999]) • Main classroom teacher and other appropriate staff reports of sensory processing (SPM: Main Classroom and School Environment Forms [Miller Kuhaneck, Henry, & Glennon, 2007]) • Observations based on Sensory Integration Theory (Blanche, 2002) • Client and caregiver interview using the Canadian Occupational Performance Measure (Law et al., 2005) to determine main areas of concern and priorities for treatment • Behavior Rating Inventory of Executive Function–Preschool Version (BRIEF–P; Gioia, Espy, & Isquith, 2003) indicates difficulty with executive functions • The results of the evaluation reveal that Jared has difficulty processing tactile information and that this may be the reason for his distractibility and limited diet. In addition, poor integration of tactile and proprioceptive inputs may contribute to the intensity of his physical play and his difficulty with grading force curing interactions.	• Occupational therapy services using Ayres's sensory integration approach are provided for 60 minutes once each week. Jared's parents are included in each session. • Strategies include a range of activities that offer opportunities for Jared to receive proprioceptive, tactile, and vestibular input through intense physical play; collaboration with the therapist to create obstacle courses and imaginative play scenarios; and use of various tools and materials that require grading of force. • A sensory diet is developed for use within the home context. Jared and his parents are instructed in use of the sensory diet and they implement it while continuing with weekly appointments. The therapist monitors use of the sensory diet, and Jared's responses to it. Modifications are made as necessary. • Consultation with school personnel including the main classroom teacher and other appropriate school staff would be appropriate for discussing the implications of sensory processing challenges (tactile and proprioceptive) on school performance and to collaborate to assist in Jared's success at school.

Case	Evaluation	Intervention
Christian is a 12-year-old boy who has an interest in computers and history. Christian has always had difficulty with motor planning and avoided all participation in organized sports. He will often ask to go to the nurse's office during his gym period. Christian has transitioned to middle school and is having difficulty with organizing his materials and navigating the school environment to the point where he is now struggling in school. Christian has a history of being bothered by certain sounds and textures and has adapted to textures by not wearing wool, turtlenecks, and so on, but is still bothered by seams in socks and new clothes that don't feel "worn in." Christian has few friends and reports the noise of the group, when his peers gather, is distracting and overwhelming. The classroom teacher, who is familiar with sensory integration treatment through a friend who works in private practice, has made a referral for an occupational therapy evaluation, and Christian's parents have agreed to an evaluation by the school therapist because they are getting increasingly frustrated with his middle school performance.	• Adolescent/Adult Sensory Profile (C. Brown & Dunn, 2002) • Standardized measure of motor skills (Bruininks–Oseretsky Test of Motor Proficiency, 2nd ed. [Bruininks & Bruininks, 2005]) • Structured observations across school environments to observe impact of motor, regulation, and sensory processing on school performance • Client interview using the Canadian Occupational Performance Measure (Law et al., 2005) to determine main areas of concern and priorities for treatment • Evaluation results indicate difficulty processing tactile and auditory information, specifically exhibiting overresponsiveness to these sensations, and gross motor skill deficits, especially in the area of bilateral motor coordination and balance	• Individual occupational therapy services are provided for 20 minutes per week in the school setting. In addition, there is ongoing consultation with the classroom teacher and other appropriate school staff to allow for generalization of strategies to the classroom setting and other school environments such as PE. This also includes developing organizational skills for Christian's materials and assisting in navigating school environments such as hallways between classes, where it can be very noisy. • The focus of the individual occupational therapy services is using a sensory diet, specifically proprioceptive input that Christian reports "helps him relax" in the classroom, which includes chair push-ups, movement breaks, and deep breathing. • The sensory diet is extended into the home, with activities that are rich in proprioceptive, tactile, and vestibular input in naturalized contexts (e.g., gym, pool, treadmill, yoga) and designed to normalize the hyperresponse to touch and sound. • Specific exercises to improve Christian's bilateral motor coordination and balance are added to a home program, including reciprocal stride jumps and activities that incorporate two sides of the body and balance. • The occupational therapist brainstorms with Christian on coping strategies to use when he is in a group of his peers if the sound is bothering him, including pressing the palms of his hands together, deep breathing, and keeping one of his earphones in as he listens to the conversation.
Caroline is a 17-year-old girl who enjoys poetry, writing song lyrics, and cartoon artwork. She has received occupational therapy services both through the school system and privately over the years to address difficulties with sensory overresponsiveness to touch and auditory sensations. She is hypersensitive to sound and uses her headphones in noisy situations to cope. Caroline becomes anxious when she is in a new environment. Caroline prefers warm weather and does not like to wear most articles of winter clothing. She reports that she feels better if she exercises but can't organize a routine. Caroline receives special education resource assistance to help her manage her workload and organize her materials. She currently is not receiving direct services but as she prepares to transition to college, both school officials and parents have requested a more comprehensive occupational therapy evaluation to provide suggestions to be included in her transition plan.	• Client interview using the Canadian Occupational Performance Measure (Law et al., 2005) to determine main areas of concern and priorities for treatment • Adolescent/Adult Sensory Profile (C. Brown & Dunn, 2002) • Structured interview to assess contextual factors, including the environment, in order for Caroline to identify the potential impact her sensory issues may have, the coping strategies she can use, and her priorities for transition • Evaluation results show that Caroline continues to have a pattern of overresponsiveness to sound and touch. She has identified that she wants to be able to follow a predictable routine and try to get involved with more physical activities because those seem to help her reduce her anxiety. She enjoys the solitary aspects of writing and is looking forward to majoring in English, but is feeling overwhelmed with all of the upcoming changes, which have increased her anxiety.	• One occupational therapy session is scheduled with the occupational therapist for Caroline to self-identify and rate activities that provide proprioceptive input to help reduce anxiety and counter the hyperresponsiveness to touch and auditory sensation. • From this session, a sensory diet is recommended that Caroline can implement on a daily basis with activities she has identified as being most helpful, including using a weighted ball, brisk walking, and using headphones to listen to music when she is in crowded places. • It is also recommended that Caroline try gym and exercise routines that are in heated rooms (yoga, Pilates) because she has self-identified that she feels best when her body "feels warm." Enrolling in these types of classes on her college campus will help provide her with a structured routine. • A trial structured exercise routine is formulated and will be monitored by the occupational therapist for a 4-week period to assess whether Caroline can follow a routine and adjust accordingly.

ment in occupation emerged more than 4 decades ago. In the ensuing years, significant advances in the understanding of neuroscience and the manner in which sensation and functional behavior interact have informed theory development and application of concepts for evaluation and intervention. However, the specific mechanisms through which sensation and function interact are not well understood. At the present time, occupational therapy practice addressing challenges in processing and integrating sensory information continues to rely on behavioral measures and observations. Occupational therapy practitioners interested in using the theories and strategies addressed in this guideline are urged to obtain advanced training in these methods to ensure mastery of both theoretical and technical aspects of these concepts. It is only through the adequate preparation of personnel, reliable implementation of intervention methods, valid and detailed documentation of services, and persistent scientific investigation that these theories and methods will become further refined and a substantial evidence base established.

■ ■ ■

Appendix A. Preparation and Qualifications of Occupational Therapists and Occupational Therapy Assistants

Who Are Occupational Therapists?

To practice as an occupational therapist, the individual trained in the United States
- Has graduated from an occupational therapy program accredited by the Accreditation Council for Occupational Therapy Education (ACOTE®) or predecessor organizations;
- Has successfully completed a period of supervised fieldwork experience required by the recognized educational institution where the applicant met the academic requirements of an educational program for occupational therapists that is accredited by ACOTE or predecessor organizations;
- Has passed a nationally recognized entry-level examination for occupational therapists; and Fulfills state requirements for licensure, certification, or registration.

Educational Programs for the Occupational Therapist

These include the following:
- Biological, physical, social, and behavioral sciences
- Basic tenets of occupational therapy
- Occupational therapy theoretical perspectives
- Screening and evaluation
- Formulation and implementation of an intervention plan
- Context of service delivery
- Management of occupational therapy services (master's level)
- Leadership and management (doctoral level)
- Use of research
- Professional ethics, values, and responsibilities.

The fieldwork component of the program is designed to develop competent, entry-level, generalist occupational therapists by providing experience with a variety of clients across the life span and in a variety of settings. Fieldwork is integral to the program's curriculum design and includes an in-depth experience in delivering occupational therapy services to clients, focusing on the application of purposeful and meaningful occupation and/or research, administration, and management of occupational therapy services. The fieldwork experience is designed to promote clinical reasoning and reflective practice, to transmit the values and beliefs that enable ethical practice, and to develop professionalism and competence in career responsibilities. Doctoral-level students must also complete a doctoral experiential component designed to develop advanced skills beyond a generalist level.

Who Are Occupational Therapy Assistants?

To practice as an occupational therapy assistant, the individual trained in the United States
- Has graduated from an occupational therapy assistant program accredited by ACOTE or predecessor organizations;
- Has successfully completed a period of supervised fieldwork experience required by the recognized educational institution where the

applicant met the academic requirements of an educational program for occupational therapy assistants that is accredited by ACOTE or predecessor organizations;
- Has passed a nationally recognized entry-level examination for occupational therapy assistants; and
- Fulfills state requirements for licensure, certification, or registration.

Educational Programs for the Occupational Therapy Assistant

These include the following:
- Biological, physical, social, and behavioral sciences
- Basic tenets of occupational therapy
- Screening and assessment
- Intervention and implementation
- Context of service delivery
- Assistance in management of occupational therapy services
- Professional literature
- Professional ethics, values, and responsibilities.

The fieldwork component of the program is designed to develop competent, entry-level, generalist occupational therapy assistants by providing experience with a variety of clients across the life span and in a variety of settings. Fieldwork is integral to the program's curriculum design and includes an in-depth experience in delivering occupational therapy services to clients, focusing on the application of purposeful and meaningful occupation. The fieldwork experience is designed to promote clinical reasoning appropriate to the occupational therapy assistant role, to transmit the values and beliefs that enable ethical practice, and to develop professionalism and competence in career responsibilities.

Regulation of Occupational Therapy Practice

All occupational therapists and occupational therapy assistants must practice under federal and state law. Currently, 50 states, the District of Columbia, Puerto Rico, and Guam have enacted laws regulating the practice of occupational therapy.

Note. The majority of this information is taken from the *Accreditation Standards for a Doctoral-Degree-Level Educational Program for the Occupational Therapist* (AOTA, 2007a), *Accreditation Standards for a Master's-Degree-Level Educational Program for the Occupational Therapist* (AOTA, 2007b), and *Accreditation Standards for an Educational Program for the Occupational Therapy Assistant* (AOTA, 2007c).

Appendix B. Evidence-Based Practice

One of the greatest challenges facing health care systems, service providers, public education, and policymakers is ensuring that scarce resources are used efficiently. The growing interest in outcomes research and evidence-based medicine over the past 30 years, and the more recent interest in evidence-based education, can in part be explained by these system-level challenges in the United States and internationally. In response to demands of the cost-oriented health care system in which occupational therapy practice is often embedded, occupational therapists and occupational therapy assistants are routinely asked to justify the value of the services they provide based on scientific evidence. The scientific literature provides an important source of legitimacy and authority for demonstrating the value of health care and education services. Thus, occupational therapy practitioners, other health care practitioners, and educators are increasingly called on to use the literature to demonstrate the value of the interventions and instruction they provide to clients and students.

According to Law and Baum (1998), *evidence-based occupational therapy practice* "uses research evidence together with clinical knowledge and reasoning to make decisions about interventions that are effective for a specific client" (p. 131). An evidence-based perspective is based on the assumption that scientific evidence of the effectiveness of occupational therapy intervention can be judged to be more or less strong and valid according to a hierarchy of research designs and an assessment of the quality of the research. The American Occupational Therapy Association (AOTA) uses standards of evidence modeled from those developed in evidence-based medicine. This model standardizes and ranks the value of scientific evidence for biomedical practice using the grading system in Table B1. In this system, the highest levels of evidence include those studies that are systematic reviews of the literature, meta-analyses, and randomized controlled trials. In randomized controlled trials, the outcomes of an intervention are compared to the outcomes of a control group, and participation in either group is determined randomly. This design provides strength to the conclusion that the effect (dependent variable) was caused by the treatment (independent variable).

The evidence-based literature review presented within this document includes primarily Levels I–III of evidence. Level I evidence consists of meta-analyses, systematic reviews, and randomized controlled trials. Level II evidence consists of studies in which assignment to a treatment or a control group is not randomized (e.g., cohort study). Level III evidence consists of studies that do not employ a control group. In this review, if Levels I, II, and III evidence for occupational therapy practice are adequate, then only those levels are used to answer a particular question. If, however, higher level evidence is lacking and the best evidence provided for occupational therapy specifically only is ranked as Levels IV and V, then studies at those levels are included. Level IV studies are experimental single

Table B1. Levels of Evidence for Occupational Therapy Outcomes Research

Levels of Evidence	Definitions
Level I	Systematic reviews, meta-analyses, randomized controlled trials
Level II	Two groups, nonrandomized studies (e.g., cohort, case–control)
Level III	One group, nonrandomized (e.g., before and after, pretest and posttest)
Level IV	Descriptive studies that include analysis of outcomes (e.g., single subject design, case series)
Level V	Case reports and expert opinion that include narrative literature reviews and consensus statements

Adapted from "Evidence-Based Medicine: What It Is and What It Isn't," by D. L. Sackett, W. M. Rosenberg, J. A. Muir Gray, R. B. Haynes, & W. S. Richardson, 1996, *British Medical Journal, 312*, pp. 71–72. Copyright © 1996 by the British Medical Association. Adapted with permission.

case studies, with at least marginal manipulation of the independent variable. Level V evidence includes descriptive case reports in which therapists simply described what they did and what the outcome was for one or a few persons.

Since 1998, AOTA has instituted a series of evidence-based practice (EBP) projects to assist members in meeting the challenge of finding and reviewing the literature to identify evidence and in turn use the findings from the evidence to inform practice (Lieberman & Scheer, 2002). Following the evidence-based philosophy of Sackett, Rosenberg, Gray, Haynes, and Richardson (1996), AOTA's projects are conducted based on the principle that the EBP of occupational therapy relies on the integration of information from three sources: (1) clinical experience and reasoning, (2) preferences of clients and their families, and (3) findings from the best available research.

A primary focus of AOTA's EBP projects is an ongoing program of systematic review of multidisciplinary scientific literature using focused questions and standardized procedures to identify practice-relevant evidence and to discuss its implications for practice. Systematic reviews of literature relevant to children and adolescents with challenges in sensory processing and sensory integration strengthen our understanding of the foundations of this important area of practice and is the focus of this practice guideline.

Background

In May 2004, a motion was presented to the AOTA Representative Assembly (RA) to establish a task group for the purpose of developing a professionally published information packet to highlight the benefits of using a sensory integration (SI) approach for occupational therapy practitioners working in schools and other settings. This packet was to support the use of SI in practice and to provide support to occupational therapy practitioners and families of children with difficulty processing and integrating sensory information when faced with payment and reimbursement challenges. The motion was revised by the RA, calling for an evidence-based literature review of the efficacy of SI interventions. The RA passed the amended motion during its meeting at the May 2004 AOTA Annual Conference & Expo, and the review was integrated into AOTA's Evidence-Based Literature Review Project.

In August 2004, Carolyn Baum, PhD, OTR/L, FAOTA, AOTA president, expanded the RA motion to include evidence related to the basic sciences (e.g., neuroscience), social sciences, occupational science, and studies of clinical effectiveness. The intent was to ensure that the review provided the breadth and depth needed to guide present and future occupational therapy practitioners, researchers, and educators working in their respective areas. The working title of the project became "AOTA Evidence-Based Literature Review of Occupational Therapy for Children and Adolescents With Sensory Processing Disorder/Sensory Integrative Dysfunction." Six questions were developed for intervention, assessment, environment/context, occupational performance, and neuroscience. An advisory group was formed of practitioners, educators, researchers, and scientists; the advisory group included members of AOTA's Special Interest Sections and national and international content experts both within and outside of occupational therapy (e.g., neurology, neuropsychology, pediatrics). The members of the advisory group were sent drafts of questions that focused on each specific area and were asked to review and comment. They also were asked to rank the questions with respect to their importance to the profession. In addition, advisory group members were encouraged to solicit feedback from other content experts.

Project staff compiled the comments and tabulated the rank ordering. As a result of the comments, the environment/context question was combined with the intervention question because the literature was believed to be overlapping and one question would be sufficient. A decision also was made to eliminate the assessment question and target the reviews on intervention, neuroscience, and performance. During and after this review process, content and research experts were contacted regarding their interest in participating in this project as review authors for individual focused questions. During discussions with the experts, it was recognized that two distinct questions might be appropriate to examine the effectiveness of occupational therapy interventions for children and adolescents with difficulties processing and integrating sensory information. One question would examine interventions using an SI approach, and the second would examine non-SI interventions. This approach was taken not only to manage better what might have become a large volume of literature but also to ensure that all perspectives on the question were covered adequately and appropriately. As an outcome of discussions with the advisory group and experts in the field, the following questions resulted. These questions guided the selection of research studies for the review, synthesis, and interpretation of the findings:

1. *Neuroscience:* What is the neurophysiologic evidence that using a sensory-based approach in occupational therapy with children and adolescents will be effective?
2. *Neuroscience/Subtyping:* What is the evidence for the existence of different types of SI/sensory processing problems in children and adolescents?
3. *Occupational Therapy SI Intervention:* What is the effectiveness of SI interventions (including the effect of context) in creating, promoting, establishing, restoring, maintaining, modifying, and preventing future limitations in activities of daily living (ADLs), instrumental activities of daily living (IADLs), education/transition, play/leisure, and social participation in children and adolescents whose sensory processing patterns interfere with everyday life participation?
4. *Occupational Therapy Non-SI Intervention:* What occupational therapy interventions (including the effect of context) are effective in creating, promoting, establishing, restoring, maintaining, modifying, and preventing future limitations in ADLs, IADLs, education/transition, play/leisure, and social participation in children and adolescents whose sensory processing patterns interfere with everyday life participation?
5. *Occupational Performance:* What kinds of difficulties do children and adolescents with problems in SI/sensory processing demonstrate in ADLs, IADLs, education, work/transition, play/leisure, and social participation?

Methodology

Databases and sites searched included Medline, PsycINFO, CINAHL, ERIC, BIOSIS Previews, Science Citation Index, Social Science Citation Index, RehabData, and OTseeker. In addition, consolidated information sources, such as the *Cochrane Database of Systematic Reviews* and the *Campbell Collaboration,* were included in the search. These databases are peer-reviewed summaries of journal articles and provide a system for clinicians and scientists to conduct evidence-based reviews of selected clinical questions and topics. Moreover, reference lists from articles included in the systematic reviews were examined for potential articles, and selected journals were hand-searched to ensure that all appropriate articles could be included.

Search terms for the review were developed by the consultant to the AOTA Evidence-Based Literature Review Project and AOTA staff in consultation with the authors of each question and reviewed by the advisory group. The search terms were developed not only to capture pertinent articles but also to make sure that the terms relevant to the specific thesaurus were included. A medical research librarian with experience in completing systematic review searches conducted all searches and confirmed and improved the search strategies. In addition, a filter based on one developed by McMaster University (www.urmc.rochester.edu/hslt/miner/...library/.../cinahl_eb_filters.pdf) was used to narrow the search to research studies. In addition to these general steps, procedures specific to each question are described below.

Inclusion and exclusion criteria are critical to the systematic review process because they provide the structure for the quality, type, and years of publication of the literature incorporated into a review. The review of all five questions was limited to peer-reviewed scientific literature published in English. The review also included consolidated information sources such as the *Cochrane Collaboration.* Except as described here, the literature included in the review was published between 1986 and 2006. The review excluded data from presentations, conference proceedings, non–peer-reviewed research literature, research reports, dissertations, and theses.

The search strategy for Question 1 (neuroscience) included *neuronal plasticity or neuroplasticity or neural plasticity (limited to humans) PLUS sensory systems (vision, tactile, auditory, olfactory, gustatory, proprioception, vestibular, temperature) PLUS diagnoses (attention deficit hyperactivity disorder OR ADHD, autism, brain injury, stroke, learning disabilities, nonverbal learning disabilities, developmental coordination disorder)*. Studies were limited to those that included the following measures: *f*MRI, MRI, EDR, EDA, skin conductance, and EEG. In addition, the publication lists of authors of classic animal studies also were reviewed. Animal studies of these authors were included if the study focused on neuroplasticity, and the article was included in the review regardless of publication date. Authors included in the review were P. Bach-y-Rita, E. L. Bennett, C. Cotman, M. C. Diamond, D. E. Feldman, T. Field, W. E. Fordyce, F. Gage, W. T. Greenough, T. K. Hensch, D. H. Hubel, G. Kempermann, B. Kolb, N. J. Lenn, M. M. Merzenich, T. L. Petit, M. R. Rosenzweig, L. Rosselli-Austin, J. L. Rubenstein, M. P. Stryker, H. M. Van Praag, R. N. Walsh, and T. N. Wiesel. The citations of 2,499 human studies and 1,658 animal studies were reviewed, for a total of 4,157 citations. Sixty-six articles were initially reviewed, and 49 were incorporated into the systematic review presented in this issue.

The neuroscience/subtyping (Question 2) and performance questions (Question 5) both used the same search terms to identify and capture applicable articles. Search terms included in these reviews were *discrimination (sensory, tactile, visual/spatial, proprioceptive, and auditory), dyspraxia, emotional regulation, hypersensitivity, hypotonia, overresponsiveness, oversensitivity, postural disorder, sensation seeking, sensorimotor or sensory motor, sensory based motor disorder, sensory defensiveness, underresponsiveness*. The results for several of the search terms (*discrimination, hypersensitivity, hypotonia, sensation seeking, sensorimotor,* and *sensory motor*) were limited to those articles pertaining to diagnostic categories included in the intervention questions. A complete list of diagnostic categories and clinical conditions is included in Table B2. Five hundred and forty citations were reviewed for subtyping (Question 2) and performance (Question 5). For subtyping (Question 2), 95 articles were retrieved, and 57 were included in the final selection and review process.

The occupational performance review (Question 5) was completed, in part, as an academic partnership among the review author, graduate students, and AOTA staff and consultant. The review author worked on the review with a group of entry-level master's students for a project to fulfill requirements for a capstone research course. The 540 citations cited previously provided the initial group of articles for the review; searches through 2008 yielded additional citations. Other later modifications to the search strategy were the inclusion of articles specifically on developmental coordination disorder, because it is frequently used as a synonym for dyspraxia, and the limitation of articles on performance issues in autism spectrum disorder to those studies incorporating a measure of sensory performance.

Selected articles met the following inclusion criteria:
- Participant demonstration (through observation or assessment) of limitation in occupational performance
- Presence of a comparison group that included participants with relevant diagnostic categories or a sensory processing deficit affecting performance
- Descriptive articles that included data on performance deficits in areas of occupation.

Studies that lacked either an occupational performance component or an assessment of occupational performance were excluded. Thirty-five articles were included in the systematic review on performance.

The search terms for Questions 3 and 4 (occupational therapy interventions using SI and non-SI approaches) are listed in Table B2. Studies of intervention effectiveness were included if the described intervention was within the domain of occupational therapy, although it did not have to be a common occupational therapy intervention or administered by an occupational therapist or occupational therapy

Table B2. Search Terms for Occupational Therapy Sensory Integration (SI) and Non-SI Intervention Systematic Reviews

Category	Search Terms
Diagnoses and clinical conditions included	Children with handwriting problems; clumsy child syndrome; developmental coordination disorder; disorder of attention, motor, and perception; developmental dyspraxia; fine motor deficits; gross motor deficits; learning disabilities; perceptual motor deficits; sensory integrative dysfunction; sensory modulation disorder; sensory modulation dysfunction; sensory motor deficit; sensory processing disorder
Diagnoses and clinical conditions (only if a sensory motor/perceptual motor component is included in the study)	Attention deficit disorder, attention deficit hyperactivity disorder, autism spectrum disorder (including autism, Asperger syndrome, and pervasive developmental disorder), deprivation—sensory deprivation (excluding deafness and blindness), dyslexia, fetal alcohol syndrome, fragile X syndrome, learning disabilities, prematurity, specific language disorder
Diagnoses and clinical conditions excluded	Acquired brain injury, cerebral palsy, childhood stroke, deafness/blindness, mental retardation, regulatory disorder, seizure disorders, spina bifida, stroke, traumatic brain injury
Interventions	Activities of daily living (also self-care and instrumental activities of daily living), activity, activity groups, adaptive behavior, antisocial behavior, assistive technology, attention, augmentative communication, behavior modification, behavioral interventions (e.g., Applied Behavioral Analysis—Lovaas, discrete trial training), comprehensive behavioral programs (e.g., **T**reatment and **E**ducation of **A**utistic and Related **C**ommunication Handicapped **CH**ildren, Learning Experiences—An Alternative Program for Preschoolers and Parents), consultation, cooperative behaviors, decision-making skills training, environmental modification, executive function, exercise, family coping/coping skills, floor time, friendship, functional approaches, handwriting, intervention, job training, massage, natural environment intervention, neurodevelopmental treatment, neuromotor occupational therapy, oral sensorimotor programs, parent/teacher mediated, perceptual–motor learning, peer group, peer interaction, peer mediated, play, prevocational, priming, problem-solving skills training, relationship-based intervention, routines-based interventions, sensory diet, SI, sensory integrative, social competence, social participation, social skills training, social stories, tactile stimulation, therapeutic listening/auditory integration training, time management, token economy, touch pressure, transitioning, vestibular stimulation, weighted vests/weighted materials, Wilbarger protocol, work

assistant. The following inclusion criteria were specific to this review: Participants in the intervention study were age 21 and younger; the search was limited to 1996 to 2006, but earlier systematic reviews and classic articles that may or may not have been incorporated into a systematic review also were included; and selected articles published in 2007 were recommended by experts in the field and included in the review. A total of 1,079 citations were reviewed. Thirty-two articles were included in the systematic review of SI approaches, and 20 articles (reporting on 21 studies) were included in the review of non-SI intervention approaches.

The teams working on each focused question reviewed the articles according to their quality (scientific rigor and lack of bias) and levels of evidence. In addition to Level I, II, III, IV, and V evidence, 2 qualitative studies were included in the occupational performance review. The team abstracted each article included in the review using an evidence table that provides a summary of the methods and findings of the article and an appraisal of the strengths and weaknesses of the study based on design and methodology. The evidence tables of all articles included in the review can be found in Appendix C. Review authors also completed a Critically Appraised Topic (CAT), a summary and appraisal of the key findings, clinical bottom line, and implications for occupational therapy of the articles included in the review for each question. AOTA staff and the EBP project consultant reviewed the evidence tables and CATs to ensure quality control. All review authors were either doctoral-level trained occupational therapists with expertise in the content area examined by the focused question or graduate students or master's-level trained occupational therapists under the guidance and direction of the review author.

The findings from studies included in the systematic reviews also were used to develop evidence-based recommendations. These recommendations for occupational therapy practice for children and adolescents with challenges in processing and integrating sensory information can be found in Table 7. The recommen-

Table B3. Number and Levels of Evidence for Articles Included in Each Review Question

Review Question	Number of Articles Included in Review						
	Level I	Level II	Level III	Level IV	Level V	Qualitative	Total in Each Review
Neuroscience	9	27	11	1	1	0	49
Neuroscience/Subtyping	4	44	8	1	0	0	57
Occupational Therapy SI Intervention	18	4	4	6	0	0	32
Occupational Therapy Non-SI Intervention	9	2	3	7	0	0	21
Occupational Performance	0	19	11	2	2	1	35
Total for Each Level	40	96	37	17	3	1	
						Total in All Reviews	194

dations are based on the strength of the evidence for a given topic from the systematic reviews in combination with the expert opinions of the review authors and content experts reviewing this guideline. The strength of the evidence is determined by the number of articles included in a given topic, the study design, and limitations of those articles. The review authors and other context experts provided clinical expertise regarding the value of using a given intervention in practice. Recommendation criteria are based on standard language developed by the U.S. Preventive Services Task Force of the Agency for Health Care Research and Quality. More information regarding these criteria can be found at http://www.uspreventiveservicestaskforce.org/uspstf/standard.htm.

A total of 194 articles were included in the review of the five focused questions. The review was broad, incorporating not only evidence regarding intervention effectiveness but also evidence on neuroscience, subtyping, and performance issues for children and adolescents with difficulties processing and integrating sensory information. Although the review included published literature from occupational therapy and related fields, all studies provided evidence within the scope of occupational therapy practice. One hundred and thirty-six (70%) of the articles were at Level I or Level II, indicating that the review incorporated evidence at the highest levels. Table B3 presents the number of studies included in the complete review, those included in each focused question, and the composition of the articles included in the review by level of evidence.

The articles included in the systematic reviews have several overarching limitations. Several of the studies in all five systematic reviews had small sample sizes, which reduced the power of the statistical analysis. In addition, there was a lack of blinding, and group (both intervention and control) characteristics frequently were not described in enough detail to allow for replication. In some studies, it was difficult to distinguish the intervention and control groups because of the similarity of the groups. Many studies included in the reviews did not control for medication use, and variations in medication use by participants may have affected the results. Outcomes were based on parent report in several studies, and the variety of outcome measures used in the studies may make it difficult to group the results of studies. Where heterogeneous populations have been noted, the authors indicated that the results must be interpreted with caution. In addition, studies that included a select or limited diagnosis could reduce the generalizability to other populations. Studies at lower levels of evidence lacked randomization and a control group, making it difficult to generalize results to other samples.

■ ■ ■

Appendix C. Evidence Tables

Table C1. Neuroscience Evidence for the Effectiveness of Using a Sensory-Based Approach in Occupational Therapy With Children and Adolescents

Author/Year	Study Objectives	Level/Design/ Participants	Intervention and Outcome Measures	Results	Study Limitations
Bach-y-Rita (2004)	The objective was to review work on sensory substitution.	Level not indicated; many studies were summarized.	Use of tactile vision substitution systems on motor performance of participants without sight. Vibrotactile substitution to provide meaningful information regarding postural control. Exploration between somatosensory input and environmental exploration.	Tactile input, once the coding of it is understood, was successfully used by people without sight to enable them to engage in activities such as perceiving a ball rolling toward them; reaching for a drink; and playing rock, paper, scissors. Postural stability could be produced with the use of a head accelerometer and vibrotactile input coding on the tongue. Study demonstrated that active exploration is required for tactile discrimination of texture and spatial temporal touch.	Sensory substitution paradigms are very lab-oriented and generally not practical for clinical use.
Bangert & Altenmüller (2003)	The objective of the study was to examine EEG of auditory and motoric features of piano performance separately; examine two 5-wk training paradigms for beginners, one a conventional "map" group, the other a "no-map" group in which notes were randomly assigned to keys after each trial; and examine the same paradigms for professional piano players.	Level II Nonrandomized controlled trial *Design* Three group repeated measures (baseline, after 1st practice session, before 6th practice session, after 10th practice session). Nonrandomized cohort. Professional group was measured only once. *Participants* Inexperienced (*n* = 17) and professional musicians (*n* = 9), grouped into map (*n* = 9), no-map (*n* = 8), and professional (*n* = 9)	*Intervention* Listen to 3-s piano melodies, wait 4 s, and attempt to replay the melodies as accurately as possible. *Two inexperienced groups*: Map group practiced music that was mapped consistently to the keys, so there could be carryover from one session to another. For no-map group, notes were randomly assigned to piano keys each session; participant had to relearn the location of notes each session, and there was no carryover between sessions. Professionals engaged in the same training paradigm of listening and reproducing melodies. Sessions lasted 20 min, 2×/wk; training spanned 5 wk *Outcome Measures* Event-related DC–EEG during auditory probe (passive listening) and motor probe (silent finger movement)	*Auditory and Motor Probes* • *Map group*: Changes in the pattern of activation were noted across the test sessions, but statistical significance was not delineated. • *No-map group*: No pattern differences were noted across time. Professionals and inexperienced groups differed in overall EEG pattern, but this appears to be a function of two groups of beginners. Between beginner groups at 5 wk, differences were noted in activation of left central and right fronto-temporal region.	Small sample; group assignment not described; group characteristics not described in detail, but author refers reader to previous manuscript.

(Continued)

Table C1. Neuroscience Evidence for the Effectiveness of Using a Sensory-Based Approach in Occupational Therapy With Children and Adolescents *(cont.)*

Author/Year	Study Objectives	Level/Design/Participants	Intervention and Outcome Measures	Results	Study Limitations
Bavelier et al. (2001)	The objective was to examine the effects of early deafness and early acquisition of American Sign Language on the organization of neural systems important in perception of visual motion (lateralization of motion processing) and visual attention (peripheral visual attention, visual orienting).	Level II 3 groups: deaf signers (*n* = 11); typical control participants (*n* = 11); ages 18–27; comparison group (*n* = 8), adults with hearing ages 22–42, born to deaf parents (hearing signers). All were right handed.	*Intervention* 7 scans, each 4 min 16 s during which displays viewed had 12 alternating blocks of static dots and motion flow fields. Participants were asked to fixate on central point. In luminance conditions, participants monitored either static or moving blocks for increased luminance. In velocity condition, participants monitored motion blocks for abrupt changes in velocity. *Outcome Measures* fMRI: regions of interest identified on the basis of anatomical and functional criteria: visual areas 1, 2, and 3a; visual area 5, motion-sensitive region, posterior parietal cortex, and frontal eye fields. *Behavioral performance:* Participants were asked how many blocks contained ≥3 changes in luminosity or velocity.	There were no robust behavioral differences, but there was a trend for deaf signers to better detect peripheral changes and for hearing people to better detect central changes. fMRI: • MT–MST recruited more strongly in hearing people when the task required monitoring motion and when attention was directed centrally. • Greater recruitment of MT–MST in left hemisphere in deaf and hearing signers, but in right hemisphere in hearing control participants; thus, early signing modifies motion processing into a robust left-hemisphere advantage. Early deafness, not signing, leads to heightened sensitivity in posterior parietal cortex, a major center of selective attention. Deaf signers also showed greater recruitment of posterior superior temporal sulcus area, an area associated with processing of biological motion and socially relevant body signals. Findings may point to enhanced attention, especially with regard to motion features.	Lab conditions may limit generalizability. This study will not generalize to other disruptions of sensory processing.
Bennett, Diamond, Krech, & Rosenzweig (1964)	This article is a summary of several studies examining responses of the brain to experience and the relationship of intelligent behavior in animals to brain chemistry.	Level II Control and 1 or 2 experimental groups of rats	*Control (SC):* standard lab housing (3/cage, no special treatment) *ECT:* housed in groups of 10–12, provided toys, exposed daily (30 min) to open field environment in which patterns of barriers was changed; challenged "after some weeks" by mazes *IC:* 1 animal/cage, dimly lit, quiet room, could not see or touch another animal Exposure time: 80 days *Outcome Measures* • Acetylcholine • AChE • Weight of cortex	*ECT vs. IC and SC:* There was greater growth of cortex, especially in visual area and to a lesser extent in somesthetic region, not reflecting increased body weight. There was increased AChE activity, with the greatest gain in visual region. Alterations were not due simply to handling. In repeat studies on "old" rats, the weight of cortex and AChE mimicked these results. Repeated in several lines of rats, with some rats showing more and others less change, but all showing change.	Animal study limits generalizability. Classic, but older, studies mean that chemical analysis methods are dated and perhaps less accurate than optimal. No blinding for histology or behavioral testing could bias results.

Bennett, Rosenzweig, Diamond, Morimoto, & Hebert (1974)	This study investigated persistent cerebral effects of enriched vs. impoverished environmental conditions and effects of switching from EC to IC.	Level II 3 groups: EC throughout, EC–IC, IC throughout	Two studies: 1. *EC:* housed 12/cage; 6 toys added to environment, some new ones added each day while others were removed. Exposure to maze each day. *IC:* housed in separate cages in quiet, illuminated room; no handling. Exposed to EC for 30 or 80 days; then switched to IC. 2. 3 different EC conditions and 1 IC condition.	Cerebral effects of EC begin to dissipate when animals are removed from enriched environment, although significant differences persist. Degree of persistence varies with length of initial exposure and length of second exposure, as well as brain region studied. Findings suggest that long-term changes both behaviorally and enzymatically indicate possible effect on memory storage.	Classic studies cited, but the relative age of studies cited may be problematic. Animal study limits generalizability. These were "normal" nervous systems, limiting application to the central nervous system in the face of disease or dysfunction. No blinding for histology or behavioral testing could bias results.
Braun et al. (2001)	The objective was to characterize the effects of motor action on the organization of the somatosensory cortex in normal adults.	Level III 1 group nonrandomized participants: 9 men and 3 women, ages 24–43, all right handed	*Intervention* Presentation of tactile stimuli to first (D1, thumb) and fifth (D5, little finger) digits of hand, right × 2 blocks, left × 2 blocks within a session, random block application within block to D1 or D5, each finger receiving 500 stimuli. 2 sessions separated by 1 wk of time. Behavioral measure during application of input was writing without vision or rest. *Outcome Measures* Whole head MEG for somatosensory-evoked magnetic field measurement. Motor activity measured from finger flexors and extensors. Electro-oculograms used to control for eye movement artifacts. Changes in functional organization of somatosensory cortex were assessed by calculating the distance changes between representations of D1 and D5.	Electromyographic activity was greater during writing than rest conditions—an expected finding. EMG in the stimulated hand was increased only during the writing condition in which stimuli were applied to the digits. MEG showed significant reduction of global field activity of somatosensory-evoked field during writing. Motor activity exerts a gating influence on the processing of somatosensory input. The distance between D1 and D5 representation grew larger during writing and immediately became smaller during rest. This finding and other data suggest that input to the digits is processed separately during fine motor tasks, minimizing cross-talk. Thus, functional organization of somatosensory cortex adapts dynamically to requirements of a specific task. Task in this case was highly trained task of handwriting. Findings similar for left and right hands.	Although a functional task (handwriting) was used, the situation in which it was tested was not contextually grounded. This situation may limit generalizability. Because this study was done on typical adults, there may be limited generalizability to children or adults with disability. Task-specific activation of cortical connectivity patterns may be reflective of how cortical networks support optimal performance.
J. Brown et al. (2003)	The objective of the study was to determine the effects of enriched environment and physical activity on neurogenesis in olfactory bulb and dentate gyrus in mice.	Level II Nonrandomized controlled group *Subjects* N = 42 mice divided into 3 groups	*Intervention* Enriched and standard environment exposure; in enriched exposure, there was no dietary supplementation to control for olfactory stimulation. Exposure for 43 days. *Outcome Measures* Cell number, type in olfactory bulb and dentate gyrus	Enrichment and physical activity did not produce changes in cell proliferation in olfactory bulb or ventricular wall.	Animal study limits generalizability. No blinding for histology or behavioral testing could bias results.

(Continued)

Appendix C. Evidence Tables

Table C1. Neuroscience Evidence for the Effectiveness of Using a Sensory-Based Approach in Occupational Therapy With Children and Adolescents (cont.)

Author/Year	Study Objectives	Level/Design/Participants	Intervention and Outcome Measures	Results	Study Limitations
Carey et al. (2004)	The objective of the study was to determine whether joint-movement tracking training at the ankle produces functional gains and brain reorganization (as has been found for finger tracking).	Level IV *Design* Single-subject with multiple baseline (4 pretest) and follow-up (4 posttest and 2 follow-up) *Participant* $N = 1$ 50-yr-old man, 20 mo after right-sided (left pons) stroke; slower than normal ambulation, use of cane, catching of right ankle throughout day, more so when tired	*Intervention* Joint movement tracking training at the ankle *Outcome Measures* Self-rating of ease of performance (put on right shoe, ankle on level ground when rested, walk on level ground when tired, walk on stairs when rested, walk on stairs when tired) Walk time: fastest comfortable 50-ft walking speed Ankle ROM Ankle tracking accuracy fMRI	*Self-rating:* Improvement in all areas immediately after training, with some loss of improvement at follow-up *Walk time, ROM, tracking accuracy, and peak dorsiflexion:* No significant change *fMRI:* Immediately after intervention, increased active voxel count and signal intensity in many regions, with precentral gyrus (motor cortex) most profound; return to baseline at follow-up even though self-ratings remained high	Single-subject design and inherent variability in fMRI measurement may limit generalizability. Participant also had near-normal walk time and ROM preintervention; thus, changes in these measures might not be expected.
Diamond, Rosenzweig, Bennett, Lindner, & Lyon (1972)	The objective was to determine the effects of environmental enrichment and impoverishment on the rat cerebral cortex. This study expands previous work by 1. Determining whether age at start of EC affects results, 2. Adding a third condition (SC) to determine whether the previous findings are caused by EC, and 3. Comparing cortical depth measures with cortical weight values.	Level I 2-group randomization (littermates were randomized to EC and IC). Age and duration were the independent variables.	*Intervention* EC, IC, or SC: • 31 pairs (EC vs. IC = 1 pair) were started in condition at 25–55 days old (mean = 30 days). • 18 pairs were started at 105–185 days (mean = 60 days). • 50 pairs were started at 60–90 days (mean = 30 days).	Cortical depth and weight were greater in EC rats. *25–55 Day Cohort* EC rats showed pronounced differences in occipital cortex and somesthetic cortex. *60–90 Day Cohort* This group showed the most positive results, with differences in occipital cortex significant at the .001 level. *105–185 Day Cohort* Cortical depth changes were not as marked as with the other groups. Effects of EC are similar for two 80-day groups (EC and IC) in which the age at onset differed. The caudal region of the cerebral cortex, including the occipital cortex, showed the greatest effects. The second series of studies in which they included SC data showed different effects depending on the age of animals and segments of cortex studied. Active exploration is the critical component responsible for the changes in cortical depth (not visual stimulation).	Animal study limits generalizability. Studies demonstrate improvements in cortical weight and depth, but the changes are not related to behavioral or learning improvements.

Author (Year)	Study Objectives	Level/Design	Intervention and Outcome Measures	Results	Study Limitations
Doucet et al. (2005)	The objective was to examine the possibility that participants with blindness are more efficient at processing spectral acoustic information to solve a task.	Level II *Design* 3 groups, cohort design *Participants* Normally sighted humans ($n = 5$) • Blind participants "without bias" (could accurately localize sound both monaurally and binaurally; $n = 5$) • Blind participants "with bias" (localized sound presented monaurally on the side of the open ear only; $n = 5$) Groups were defined post priori on the basis of auditory testing.	*Intervention* Stimuli were 30-ms noise bursts ranging from 2–16 kHz broadband, 2–3 kHz (low-pass), and 5–16 kHz (high-band) presented at 40dB SPL. Sound was presented binaurally; monaurally to the right ear (with left ear obstructed with a soft foam plug and covered by hearing protector or muff); and binaurally with the contours of the ear pinna filled with acoustical paste (petroleum jelly) to equalize the convolutions of the pinna. *Outcome Measure* Pointing with the dominant hand toward the perceived source of sound	Blind participants fell into 2 groups on the basis of bias. Group membership was not linked to etiology of blindness or presence of residual vision. Findings were robust; previously shown with psychophysiologic and PET techniques. Spectral alterations negatively affected blind participants' ability to localize sound, suggesting they make better use of spectral information in the sound localization process. Authors suggested that plasticity underlies the supranormal performance of participants with blindness.	Small sample size and a post priori group assignment limit generalizability. The link to neuroplasticity is assumed, but there was no measure of this.
Gómez-Pinilla, Ying, Roy, Molteni, & Edgerton (2002)	The objective was to examine the possibility that exercise induces an integrated response of brain-derived neurotrophic factor and its receptor that may result in synaptic modification or adaptation.	Level II Nonrandom assignment to voluntary exercise or sedentary groups Exposed to 3 or 7 days running Rat model	*Outcome Measures* Total and mRNA for brain-derived neurotrophic factor and its receptor, protein in soleus muscle and lumbar cord	Voluntary exercise increased expression of molecules associated with brain-derived neurotrophic factor action on synaptic function and neurite growth in lumbar cord and soleus muscle. Paralysis (botox) resulted in reduced brain-derived neurotrophic factor in cord and muscle, although there was some mediation of this effect in the cord by exercise.	Animal study limits generalizability. No blinding for histology or behavioral testing could bias results.

(Continued)

Table C1. Neuroscience Evidence for the Effectiveness of Using a Sensory-Based Approach in Occupational Therapy With Children and Adolescents (cont.)

Author/Year	Study Objectives	Level/Design/Participants	Intervention and Outcome Measures	Results	Study Limitations
Gordon & Stryker (1996)	The objective of the study was to extend the findings of plasticity in cats, mammals, and rats to mice because the mouse model offers the experimental advantage of having many transgenic and knockout techniques to allow control over genetic makeup.	Level II Nonrandomized controlled trial *Design* 2 groups *Subjects* N = 60 mice of various ages	*Interventions* Study 1: MD; suture right eye Study 2: AMD, slightly different suturing process Study 3: BD for 4 days Normal controls were used for comparison. Visual deprivation for varying lengths of time and at varying ages between 12 and 40 days Visual cortices were exposed, and recordings were made from cortical cells *Outcome Measures* • Cell electrophysiological recordings; histological examination of visual cortical cells in nondeprived animals and comparisons made between ipsilateral and contralateral deprived eye • Recordings made in binocular zone and surrounding monocular areas of V1	*Normal:* Strong bias toward contralateral eye even in binocular region *4-day MD:* Dramatic ocular dominance changes in hemispheres both ipsilateral and contralateral to deprived eye • During critical period, the maximal effects of 4-day MD seen starting Postnatal Day 28, falling off after Postnatal Day 32 • *Duration of MD around Postnatal Day 28:* 2 day had little effect, 4 day was as effective as longer deprivation • BN (4 day) resulted in essentially typical cell function • *AMD:* 4–6 days at about Postnatal Day 28 resulted in shift toward contralateral eye representation in binocular V1; MD followed by AMD resulted in most cells being monocular, with many driven by ipsilateral eye • Histological assessment indicated that changes noted occur both subcortically and intracortically • Extends plasticity findings to another species and furthers understanding of the generalizability of this concept. Within the normal visual system, there is drive toward contralateral dominance that can be altered by relatively brief periods of monocular deprivation; this shift is very profound during critical periods.	Use of mouse as model may not be directly applicable to humans.
Grüsser et al. (2004)	The objective of the study was to examine sensation referred to as *phantom arm* after stimulation of lower body.	Level IV *Design* Single-subject design with repetition *Participants* Participant 1: 61-yr-old man; right arm amputation after bone cancer, 14.5 years prior. Reported pricking and cutting phantom limb pain in hand and digits and nonpainful sensation for arm and digits (pressure,	*Outcome Measure* Neuroelectric source imaging and fMRI to assess reorganization in primary somatosensory cortex	*Participant 1:* Reorganization of mouth into deafferented hand region in primary sensory cortex, so did not match referred sensation pattern; likely the result of other mechanisms *Participant 2:* Primary sensory cortex	Single subject, so generalizability is limited.

		tingling, numbing, warmth); combined sensations present about 60% of time; referred sensations elicited with nonpainful application of sensation to lower ipsilateral limb *Participant 2:* 37-yr-old man; right arm amputation after bone cancer, 22.7 years prior; used prosthetic for cosmetic purposes. Cramping and knocking phantom pain in all 5 digits present 4–6 hr each day; nonpainful sensation (pressure, itch, tingling, feeling of cold). Reported telescoped phantom located in residual limb and crawling, nonpainful sensation and residual limb pain. Referred sensation from chest, shoulder, ipsilateral calf and 1st toe, aspects of foot both ipsi- and contralateral.		
Guest & Spence (2003)	This was a series of studies designed to move prior work with abrasive textures into the realm of "ecologically appropriate" textures of pilled fabrics. In addition, the authors examined hypothesis that attention is distributed between vision and touch during many texture-based tasks.	Level III Humans, 1 group	*Intervention* *Experiment 1:* 4 textures of pilling fabric; participants determined which of pair was "rougher" using touch, vision, or both. Each approach occurred in different session. Pairs were randomized within sessions. 40 trials occurred for each stimulus pair with correct choice on first stimulus for 20 trials and second for 20 trials ($n = 10$). *Experiment 2:* Same overall design, but 1 stimulus was presented unimodally and the other was presented bimodally (touch paired with vision–touch; vision paired with vision–touch) ($n = 15$).	*Experiment 1:* Neither individual system dominated. Bimodal enhancement was not consistently found. *Experiment 2:* No evidence of consistent bias was found toward bimodal intervals. *Experiment 3:* Study of attention found that visual and tactile inputs act as independent sources of information and both contribute to discrimination process. Thus, vision and touch interact but do not show integration. These multiple sources of input appear potentially redundant.	Small sample sizes with lack of control group, lab setting, and use of typical adults limit generalizability.

(Continued)

Table C1. Neuroscience Evidence for the Effectiveness of Using a Sensory-Based Approach in Occupational Therapy With Children and Adolescents *(cont.)*

Author/Year	Study Objectives	Level/Design/Participants	Intervention and Outcome Measures	Results	Study Limitations
			Experiment 3: All stimuli were presented bimodally. Identification was of rough–smooth for both stimuli. Specific stimuli were identified for each participant to be within 60%–80% accuracy range. Participants ($n = 10$) were not naïve to experimental protocol as they were for Experiments 1 and 2. *Outcome Measures* Correct/incorrect identification		
Halder et al. (2005)	The objective was to examine the effects of simple movement repetition on corresponding brain activity in humans.	Level III 1 group, nonrandomized *Participants* 10 students (6 men and 4 women) with a mean age of 24.5 yr All participants were right-hand dominant with no history of medical or psychiatric disease. *Design* Pretest, during, and post-test measure *Setting* Laboratory	All participants first practiced the task by squeezing a ball at 40% maximum force with their right hand while visual feedback was provided about the amount of force. Next, the task was divided into 13-min parts with 10-min breaks in between to minimize the effects of fatigue and loss of attention. Participants were instructed to squeeze the ball as hard as needed to match the force shown on the screen. Force was measured using a sphygmomanometer bulb connected to a blood pressure transducer that translated air compression into an analog signal that was digitized. A continuous-force trajectory channel was calculated. Event-related potentials were recorded via EEG using an electrocap with 64 channels. There were 4 main event-related potential measures: Microstate 1 was attributed to visual target processing; Microstate 2 is related to movement execution; Microstate 3 appears during the release phase, ends after movement execution, and reflects feedback processing or visuomotor integration. Microstate 4 was attributed to changes in general attention but was small, and authors did not consider it further.	Controlled repetition of the same movement leads to rapid cortical plasticity within 30 min. The finding that there are differential repetition effects (EEG changes) on each stage of the task (preparation, movement execution, and feedback integration) suggests that "partly distinct neural mechanisms of cortical plasticity operate on different stages of information processing" (during motor learning; p. 2276). Movement variability decreased significantly over trials, indicating that the motor system optimizes behavior by increasing consistency, despite constant effort. Effects of repetition were observed at multiple stages and did not correlate, suggesting that motor learning occurs in stages. For example, there appears to be a consolidation period in promoting repetition-induced plasticity (this means that the brain has distinct stages of neural processing during motor learning; 1 stage is consolidation that has a specific neural correlate). There was a change in activity (temporal decoupling) between visual and motor processing with practice, suggesting a decreased dependence on visual information as movement automation progresses. It is suggested that changes in the extent of lateral inhibition mediated by γ-amino butyric acid underlie plasticity in motor areas and may be the physiological correlate of the pattern observed here.	The sample size was small and a 1-group design. Participants were all young, so findings cannot be generalized to other age groups.

Hodzic, Veit, Karim, Erb, & Godde (2004)	This study investigated alterations in cortical topography and task specificity of learning in a protocol that used passive tactile coactivation without attention to stimuli.	Level III 1 group 11 right-handed adults Pretest–posttest design	*Intervention* Conducted premapping fMRI, coactivation procedure, postmapping fMRI mapping of somatosensory (SI and SII) representation of right index finger (compared with left or control) *Coactivation*: Tactile input was applied to the fingertip to coactivate all receptive fields within area. Applied with varying interstimulus intervals to prevent habituation over the 3-hr application. *Spatial discrimination*: Grating orientation task featured 8 domes with gratings cut in the surface rubbed on fingertip, randomly orienting grooves to parallel or orthogonal to axis of fingertip. Outcome was discrimination threshold based on width of bars and grooves. *Temporal discrimination*: Vibrotactile stimuli were played via speakers attached to the computer and applied to the fingertip. Participants were given 500 ms. Two alternative forced-choice paradigms were used to determine whether the frequency of test stimulus was higher or lower than reference stimulus.	After passive coactivation, the grating orientation task discrimination was improved. Improvement was strongly correlated with reorganization in contralateral SI. Reorganization also seen in SII, but not linked to improved grating orientation task. Findings suggest that SI has a predominant role in processing and discrimination. Temporal discrimination did not improve; in some participants, it worsened. Findings may be linked to the drive of the brain to create the most behaviorally useful representation of sensation, which in this case may have been spatial. Alternatively, increased spatial responsiveness may have been accompanied by prolonged duration of response, thus impairing temporal discrimination.	The study lacked a control group, although each subject had a control finger. Lab setting limits generalizability.
Hubel & Wiesel (1964)	The objective of the study was to influence cortical connections in the visual system in a way that would rule out deficits of retinal and lateral geniculate processing.	Level II Nonrandomized controlled trial *Design* 3 groups, nonrandom assignment; groups not matched in number or on age *Subjects* Kittens used in Studies A and B; compared with typical adult cats	*Intervention* A: 4 kittens, ages 8–10 days; surgical manipulation to cut medial rectus, inducing squint (to mimic strabismus); recording data for 3 kittens took place at 3 mo; for the 4th, at 1 yr B: 2 kittens given opaque contact to occlude 1 eye one day, the other eye the next day; recorded at 10 wk C: 2 adult cats used as controls *Outcome Measures* For each kitten in Study 1, 7 cortical penetrations conducted to examine cortical cell activity; cellular recordings from 384 cells; histological sections	• Amount of binocular interaction between eyes far less than normal (cells more typically driven by both eyes were driven by one eye, either ipsilateral or contralateral) • Amount of binocular interaction even less than seen in Study A • Concluded there is decreased effectiveness of the nondominant eye	Animal study limits generalizability. Plasticity demonstrated is likely to be limited to early months of life. In addition, this plasticity is induced by damage or imposed disability and may not reflect what would happen under typical conditions.

(Continued)

Table C1. Neuroscience Evidence for the Effectiveness of Using a Sensory-Based Approach in Occupational Therapy With Children and Adolescents (cont.)

Author/Year	Study Objectives	Level/Design/ Participants	Intervention and Outcome Measures	Results	Study Limitations
Kempermann & Gage (1999)	The objective was to examine how experience-dependent neurogenesis in adult mouse hippocampus is modulated by long-term stimulation (Enr) and long-term simulation and withdrawal (Enr–WD).	Level I At age of weaning (21 days), mice were randomized to control, Enr, and Enr–WD conditions; $n = 12$/group.	Enrichment involved 1 large cage with toys, tunnels, and running wheels; periodic extra treats (fruits and crackers) were provided. Standard housing was 3/cage with ad libitum food and water. Exposure was 68 days, withdrawal for 28 days. Outcome Measures Overall activity and habituation to new environment Body and brain weight Motor coordination, physical fitness, procedural learning on rotarod Spatial learning using water maze testing, immunohistochemistry, and immunofluorescence for cell count	Sedentary mice were heavier but their brains were not. The Enr mice were less active when in activity chamber, indicating better habituation. Rotarod performance was better in Enr mice and improved with practice. No difference was observed between groups on swim maze, although Enr mice had faster swim times. Previous work had shown Enr resulted in increased number of progenitor cells in hippocampus. This study showed that longer exposure may preserve acute changes. Withdrawal tends to reverse changes, although this was not significant in the current study. Enr did increase new neurons and cells not differentiated between neurons and astrocytes. Thus, Enr might increase the potential for neurogenesis. Introduced the concept of novelty rather than simply enrichment as being important in hippocampal changes.	Animal study limits generalizability. No blinding for histology or behavioral testing could bias results.
Kempermann, Kuhn, & Gage (1998)	The objective was to examine the effect of living in an enriched environment on neurogenesis in dentate gyrus of mice at ages 6 mo and 18 mo (midlife and senescence).	Level II Control ($n = 12$ for each condition) and enriched environments ($n = 13$ for each condition), ages 6 mo and 18 mo	Enriched environment: Social interaction (13 mice/cage), exploratory options (toys, rearrangeable tunnels, activity wheel), food treats (cheese, crackers, fruit) in addition to food and water ad libitum Standard environment: Food, water ad libitum, 3 animals/cage All animals exposed to environment for 40 days when 5 from each group were sacrificed for study. Others stayed in the environment for an additional 28 days for behavioral water maze testing; sacrificed at age ~8 and 20 mo. Water maze testing: 2×/day for 10 days Immunohistochemistry, phenotype analysis, and stereology of granule cells conducted.	68-day exposure led to more cells differentiating into neurons: a threefold increase in labeled neurons in 20-mo-old mice and a more than twofold increase in 8-mo-old mice compared with littermates living under standard laboratory conditions. Astrocytes not affected.	Animal study limits generalizability. The underlying mechanism remains to be delineated and could not be derived from this study. The relationship to neurogenesis of astrocytes needs further exploration because although they did not appear to be equally affected by the environmental experience, a chance remains that the neuronal outcome was related to an effect on glia. The possible influence of glutamate is of interest, but it was not elucidated in this study. The extent to which the actual activities influencing spatial learning might have contributed to the noted behavioral improvements in water maze activity is undefined by this study.

Author	Study Objectives	Level/Design/Participants	Intervention and Outcome Measures	Results	Study Limitations
Kourtzi, Betts, Sarkheil, & Welchman (2005)	The objective was to investigate neural plasticity mechanisms that mediate shape learning in cluttered scenes across stages of visual processing in the visual cortex and examine the effect of regularities present in natural scenes that determine the distinctiveness of targets in a noisy background.	Level III 1 group, pre–post training $N = 26$ college students	*Intervention* *Baseline Day 1:* 100 trials of high or low salience, depending on study. *Training Days 2–4:* 400 trials with error feedback each day. Posttraining testing Day 5. *Experiment 1:* Low-salience stimuli (difficult to distinguish from background) *Experiment 2:* High-salience stimuli fMRI of V1, V2, VP, V4 (early retinotopic visual areas), and lateral occipital complex *Outcome Measures* fMRI: Responses were evoked when participants detected novel shapes vs. nontrained shapes. Responses occurred when salience of target shapes was altered in distinctiveness. Behavioral (right/wrong) responses were tracked.	Significant behavioral and fMRI differences occurred before and after training for low-salience trained shapes, but not for untrained shapes. Significant difference in percentage correct was found using high-salience shape, but lower fMRI responses were found with trained shapes (contrast to Experiment 1). This finding was especially apparent in later processing regions. Conclusions indicate humans learn novel objects in complex backgrounds by taking advantage of natural image features that allow organization. This process is influenced by the challenge of the task, such that with easier-to-recognize visual images, there is sparse coding, and with those more difficult to recognize, image features are stored in greater detail.	Generalization of findings limited by use of homogeneous population (all college students), and lack of specific information about the participant pool (gender, age) might influence findings.
Kujala et al. (2003)	MMN is an index of permanent auditory cortical representation of native-language speech sounds. When a new type of communication system is acquired (such as Morse coding skills), new representations must be formed. This study aimed to examine the development of the cortical memory traces for the Morse-coded acoustic language units in relation to existing memory traces for native-language speech sounds (plasticity) using MEG.	Level III 1 group, nonrandomized Convenience sample: • 7 participants from Finnish navy • Ages 19–23 • Right handed • Native speakers of Finnish *Setting* Laboratory	After a training period in Morse code, spoken and coded syllables were binaurally delivered by means of plastic tubes and earpieces at 60 dB above the participants' hearing level with a constant interstimulus interval of 490 ms. The participants were instructed to ignore the auditory stimulation and to watch a silent self-selected movie. MEG measurements were taken before the first session and after the training course. Training in Morse code lasted approximately 2 hr/day, 5 day/wk.	Initially, the MMN to Morse-coded syllables was stronger in the hemisphere opposite the 1 dominant for the MMN native-language speech sounds (4 participants were left-hemisphere dominant and 3 were right-hemisphere dominant). After the 3-mo training period, the pattern reversed, and the MMN for Morse code became lateralized to the hemisphere that was predominant for the speech sound MMN. This study provides neurophysiological evidence that "new memory traces" and brain reorganization occur in response to auditory sensory stimuli.	Small, nonrandomized sample limits generalizability.

(Continued)

Table C1. Neuroscience Evidence for the Effectiveness of Using a Sensory-Based Approach in Occupational Therapy With Children and Adolescents (cont.)

Author/Year	Study Objectives	Level/Design/Participants	Intervention and Outcome Measures	Results	Study Limitations
Lacourse, Turner, Randolph-Orr, Schandler, & Cohen (2004)	The objective was to determine whether physical performance of a learned task (pushing a button in a sequence with different fingers) differs from mental practice in terms of areas of cortex and cerebellum activated and performance level.	Level I Participants randomly assigned to 3 groups: physical performance, mental practice, or no practice. 39 boys, 21 girls; mean age = 23.3 (standard deviation = 5 yr) IV = practice group, test (pre or post), and sequence (A or B) Brain activation and movement sequence performance	Sequential button-press task with right hand during 2 test sessions and daily practice. 2 different sequences practiced. Movement activation was measured by BOLD fMRI. Movement performance was measured by counting the number of completed sequences and errors during repetitive 30-s epochs of the button-press task.	Physical performance demonstrated the most improvements in behavior (121% improvement). Mental practice demonstrated 86% improvement. No practice improved 38% for Sequence A (similar but smaller improvements for Sequence B). Physical performance improvements were associated with an increase in contralateral primary motor and sensory areas. Mental practice activated similar areas but also activated other brain areas, suggesting that somewhat different mechanisms may be at play with physical performance vs. mental practice.	Possible design limitation in that both physical performance and mental practice were performed as rapidly as possible during practice, whereas the task was visually paced at 2 Hz during the test sessions. Control of rate may have created a secondary confounding effect by varying the spatiotemporal requirements of the task between practice and test conditions.
Mercado, Bao, Orduña, Gluck, & Merzenich (2001)	This study determined whether pairing basal forebrain stimulation with the presentation of complex sound resulted in spectrotemporal response sensitivity and selectivity changes in rat auditory cortex.	Level II Single groups in 2 separate studies were both compared with nontreated rats (n = 10). All animals received electrical stimulation of the nucleus basalis.	*Intervention* Experiment 1 (n = 2): Stimulation paired with upsweep sound train Experiment 2 (n = 4): Stimulation paired with upsweep and no stimulation paired with downsweep sound trains, random presentation of paired and unpaired Background white noise: Studies delivered electrical stimulation randomly every 8–40 s, 400–500×/day, for 10–20 days. *Outcome Measures* Multiple-unit or single-unit extracellular recordings from right auditory cortex (ipsilateral to site of stimulation)	Previous studies demonstrated that pairing basal forebrain (nucleus basalis) stimulation with short-duration, pure-tone sounds mediated experience-induced changes in auditory cortical responses. This study adds to an understanding of auditory cortex plasticity. The auditory cortex regions responsive to sounds were larger, magnitude of response was greater, and number of neurons responding selectively was greater with paired stimulation. These findings were identified in mature rats, indicating continued plasticity even in the mature brain.	Animal study limits generalizability. Response of "typical" nervous system and application to systems after damage or disease may be limited. Lab setting may further limit generalizability.
Moses, Martin, Houck, Ilmoniemi, & Tesche (2005)	This study used MEG to investigate the spatial and temporal properties of associative plasticity during "magnetocerebral" conditioning.	Level III 1 group, nonrandom assignment Convenience sample of 4 men and 4 women ages 24–31, no known pathology	*Intervention* Participants were exposed to various experimental conditions. *Outcome Measures* MEG activity was recorded during a habituation phase, delay conditioning training, extinction, and trace conditioning. CS was an achromatic square, CS+ included a diagonal or vertical striped pattern, and CS– had a checkerboard pattern.	After pairing auditory and visual stimuli, auditory activation was found with a visual stimulus even in the absence of auditory input. Activation was found in and near Heschl's gyrus. These findings support other findings using fMRI and PET scans and are similar to paired and unpaired findings using somatosensory and auditory inputs.	Convenience sample, small sample size, and use of typical adults limit generalizability.

			Unconditioned stimulus was 100 ms binaural white noise. Stimuli within each phase were randomized. MEG data were averaged and filtered. Regions of interest were identified for each MEG, corresponding to regions around Heschl's gyrus. Peak response amplitudes for CS+ and CS− were compared for trace and delay conditioning. Peak amplitude and latency of response were compared for paired CS+ and unpaired CS− in the left hemisphere. Position and orientation of regions of interest in paired CS+ and unpaired CS− were compared. Pupil diameter after delay and trance sessions was documented to verify that the stimulus parameters produced autonomic responses.	MEG may be useful in understanding the dynamics of conditioned response across multiple sensory modalities. Pairing visual and auditory input results in activation of regions of the auditory cortex with visual stimulus only after a learning process. Thus, this study showed carryover in associative plasticity.	Use of adults limits application to children. Very tightly controlled paradigm limits application to an intervention session, such as would be used for SI.
Nakahara, Zhang, & Merzenich (2004)	In light of studies that show that exposure of kittens or rat pups to modulated tonal stimuli during an early postnatal period resulted in expansion of the representation of the exposed sound frequency in auditory cortex (A1), the purpose of this study was to clarify how the cortical representation of the dynamic aspects of complex sound are specifically shaped by the spectrotemporal patterns of auditory input during development.	Level II 2 groups nonrandomized litters of 9–12-day-old rat pups Stimuli consisted of 2 sets of tone sequences with distinct temporal orders Recordings taken from A1 and frequency/intensity response areas were reconstructed in detail to create cortical maps. Detailed maps were obtained from groups of ≥5 experimental and control rats at each postnatal benchmark age	Rat pups were exposed to a tone sequence with 2 specific spectrotemporal patterns during a critical period epoch from Postnatal Day 9–12. Each tone lasted 30 ms with an intensity of 65 dB.	Exposure to specific complex acoustic stimulus in the early postnatal critical period resulted in large-scale remodeling of the A1 neuronal response selectivity. The tonotopic organization of A1 was changed so that responses to specific sound stimuli were elaborated and wakened to the representations of others. An unresponsive zone emerged between the cortical zones of representation of the hypothetically competitive low- and high-tone stimulus sequences. Neurons responded more reliably to the elements of these complex input sequences when they were delivered in the order that was applied in the exposure protocol. Changes endured into adulthood without significant change (even though sound stimuli were terminated at end of critical period).	Animal study limits generalizability. The study was not randomized.

(Continued)

Table C1. Neuroscience Evidence for the Effectiveness of Using a Sensory-Based Approach in Occupational Therapy With Children and Adolescents (cont.)

Author/Year	Study Objectives	Level/Design/Participants	Intervention and Outcome Measures	Results	Study Limitations
Orduña, Mercado, Gluck, & Merzenich (2005)	The objective of the study was to explore the relationship between neural activity and perceptual sensitivities to sound. Do neural responses predict behavioral performance in perceptual tasks? *Hypothesis:* The degree of similarity in the cortical representations of complex sounds can be related to differences between those sounds.	Level III One-group, nonrandomized *Subjects* 6 adult male rats approximately 3 mo old	*Intervention* Stimuli delivered to left ear at pseudorandom sequence of frequency–intensity combinations. After this, responses to frequency-modulated stimuli were recorded. *Outcome Measures* Neural responses were recorded. Studies were designed to evaluate perceptual sensitivities by testing rats' capacity to discriminate complex sounds with various degrees of acoustic similarity.	• Demonstrated that there are neural activation patterns in response to sensation and discrimination of sensation on the basis of differential patterns of neural activity. • Sounds with similar cortical representations are more difficult to discriminate behaviorally than those with more differentiated representations, thus showing that perceptual sensitivities to sensory stimuli are proportional to the degree of overlap in their neural representation.	Animal study limits generalizability. No control group. Lack of randomization.
Pantev et al. (2003)	The objective was to examine the effects of music-induced cortical plasticity, specifically (1) effects of short-term laboratory training involving learning to perceive virtual instead of spectral pitch, (2) cross-modal plasticity when lips of trumpet players are stimulated at the same time as a trumpet tone, and (3) automatic encoding and discrimination of pitch contours and internal info are specifically enhanced in musicians compared with nonmusicians.	Level III 1 or 2 groups; nonrandomized: • *Group 1:* 10 nonmusicians • *Group 2:* 10 musicians (trumpeters), 3 women and 7 men age 26 (± 2.9), and 9 nonmusicians (3 women and 6 men age 25 ± 3.9). • *Group 3:* Neural coding of melody—is it affected by training? 12 musicians (8 women) and 12 nonmusicians (9 women) matched in age (20–40)	Musicians and nonmusicians learned short melody tones. Tactile and auditory stimuli were presented separately and together (bimodal). Sequence of note melodies: Intervals were changed from trial to trial. Interval condition and standard stimuli condition consisted of the same 5-note melody. Magnetic MMN field was used to investigate the neural mechanisms for the automatic encoding of melodic features. Control stimulus was frequency deviation to single tone.	Plasticity can be induced through relatively short-term training. All participants demonstrated a sudden switch from spectral to virtual mode of pitch perception, indicating higher synchronization of the cortical networks. Plastic reorganization processes occurred. Multimodal interaction was more pronounced in the musicians ($p = .012$) and significantly larger on the left ($p = .037$). Cross-modal musical training leads to remarkable modifications in cross-modal processing because of the behaviorally relevant somatosensory and auditory modalities and the increased use of these modalities during training. In general, the magnetic MMN field was significantly larger in musicians than in nonmusicians (ANOVA $p < .01$) for both contour and interval conditions. Performance of musicians was better than that of nonmusicians. Findings support the hypothesis that musical experience leads to specific changes in the neural mechanisms for processing abstract melodic information and that long-term musical training enhances the processing of pitch between notes of melody.	Sample size was small. No measures of brain morphologic changes were associated with behavioral changes observed.

Ptito, Moesgaard, Gjedde, & Kupers (2005)	The objective was to examine the cerebral correlates of cross-modal plasticity using sensory substitution (where information acquired with 1 sensory modality is used to accomplish a task that is normally subserved by another sensory modality). Tactile stimuli were substituted on tongue for vision in congenitally blind and sighted blindfolded control participants.	Level II 2 groups: Congenitally blind ($n = 6$; all men) and sighted blindfolded ($n = 5$; mean age = 38; mean age = 29; 2 men and 3 women)	*Behavioral training occurred over 7 consecutive days.* Participants learned to use the tongue display unit to detect the orientation of a Snellen pattern applied to the tongue. Laboratory setting with examiner *Outcome Measure* Cerebral blood flow in visual cortex area before and after training via PET	After training, participants with blindness activated large areas of the occipital, parieto-occipital, and occipitotemporal cortices, whereas control participants showed no activation of visual cortex. Control participants showed a significant deactivation of visual cortex during orientation task, before and after training, possibly suggesting increased activity in somatosensory cortex to perform a tactile-based orientation task.	Small sample size and lack of randomization limit the study.
Ragert, Schmidt, Altenmuller, & Dinse (2004)	The objective of the study was to determine whether skill-induced behavioral improvement seen in professional piano players is paralleled by other perceptual changes not directly related to the specific demands of piano playing.	Level II 2-group cohort design *Participants* Professional piano players ($n = 14$) and nonmusicians ($n = 16$)	*Intervention* Tactile coactivation protocol in which coactivation was applied for 3 hr to activate large number of receptive fields on right index finger *Outcome Measure* 2-point tactile discrimination tested between two groups	• Pianists showed lower discrimination thresholds on the tip of index fingers for both hands than did nonpianists; no gender differences. Authors indicated this demonstrates high spatial tactile acuity in the professional pianists. • Pianists also showed greater variability within their group in discrimination than the nonpianists, which was shown to be related to the degree of sensory and motor training they received. • Pianists also could be trained to improve tactile discrimination using the coactivation protocol to a greater extent than improvement could be seen in nonpianists. Influencing this outcome was the amount of training and practice the pianists had engaged in. • *Proposed mechanism:* At cellular level, could be related to changes in synaptic transmission, n-methyl-d-aspartate receptor function changes, or greater representation of finger in cortical sensory and motor regions. • The synaptic efficiency at the fingertips is greater, driving cortical reorganization. Further supported by training effect; no evidence of increased receptor density leads to the conclusion that it is cortical reorganization.	Small, nonrandom sampling; no direct measure of plasticity was used, but interpretation was based on links to existing literature.

(Continued)

Table C1. Neuroscience Evidence for the Effectiveness of Using a Sensory-Based Approach in Occupational Therapy With Children and Adolescents (cont.)

Author/Year	Study Objectives	Level/Design/Participants	Intervention and Outcome Measures	Results	Study Limitations
Recanzone, Schreiner, & Merzenich (1993)	This study is similar to study reported by Nakahara, Zhang, & Merzenich (2004). Adult owl monkeys were used. The objective was to determine whether the tonotopic organization of the primary auditory cortex is altered as a result of training on an auditory frequency discrimination task.	Level II Group design 10 adult owl monkeys— 5 trained, 5 not trained	5 monkeys were trained to detect a difference in the frequency of sequentially presented pairs of tones. Stimuli were delivered at pseudorandomized intervals.	The auditory frequency discrimination abilities of the 5 trained monkeys improved progressively with training. Improvements occurred in relatively a short and steep phase (large improvements early on) followed by a longer period with smaller gains. Largest gains were in the initial 5 sessions. Functional organization of primary auditory cortex (A1) was altered as a consequence of training. Changes correlated with behavioral performance. Changes not observed in untrained monkeys.	Animal study limits generalizability. Study was not randomized.
Renier et al. (2005)	The objective was to investigate the neural substrates of depth perception when a device substituting vision with audition was used. Using PET, the authors examined whether 2-dimensional or 3-dimensional perception with sensory substitution device recruited similar brain areas as in vision.	Level III 1 group, nonrandomized 9 male volunteers (mean age = 29.4 ± 12 yr)	A training session was held to learn the system to locate and estimate the distance of an object. *Outcome Measure* PET scan	Activation in visual association areas during both the target search task and the depth perception task were found. The findings suggest that some brain areas of the visual cortex are relatively multimodal and may be recruited for depth perception by means of senses other than vision. The study supports brain plasticity in response to sensory-based training.	No control group and no long-term testing limit generalizability.
Röder, Rösler, & Neville (2000)	The objective was to determine whether blind people process language differently than sighted people.	Level II 2 groups n = 11 in each group; matched in age, gender, handedness, and education 6 men and 5 women congenitally blind (mean age = 35; range = 25–48). Mean age of sighted people = 35; range = 23–48.	Event-related potentials (N400) In language context, the N400 effect is a centroparietal-distributed negative wave that is sensitive to semantic and lexical processes.	N400 distribution was different in blind vs. sighted people, and the effect started earlier in blind people. N400 had a left-lateralized frontocentral scalp distribution in the sighted participants, but a symmetric and broad topography in the blind participants.	Study was not randomized. Because this was a human study, findings are highly applicable.

Rosenzweig & Bennett (1972)	The objective was to define environmental conditions that bring about cerebral differences (EC vs. IC), specifically whether social grouping and exposure to EC during light or dark were essential components.	Level I 6-group randomized study of rats IC = home cage; EC = enriched condition	*Intervention* 6 experimental conditions and 1 control group: 1. IC, saline injection 2. EC, saline injection, light exposure 3. EC, saline injection, dark exposure 4. IC, methamphetamine 5. EC, light exposure, methamphetamine injection 6. EC, dark exposure, methamphetamine injection Control: IC EC exposure for 2 hr/day Intervention phase = 30 days 2-way ANOVA: Litter × Treatment *Outcome Measures* Brain weight and chemical analysis of brain tissue, specifically AChE, a byproduct of esterase activity on AChE	Light is not needed to obtain results from EC, but rats in the light condition showed results in occipital cortex. The most significant increase in brain weight in EC was in rats injected with methylphenidate (this action facilitated movement and play during EC in both dark and light). Social condition (being in the EC with other rats) showed a moderate change, but the addition of methylphenidate showed a more dramatic change, presumably because the rats were more active. Methylphenidate only did not produce an effect. All 5 groups showed a significant difference from control group on AChE:ChE ratio (a sensitive measure of effects that cancels out variable of brain weight).	Animal study limits generalizability. Impossible to determine whether similar findings will be shown in social conditions with humans, who are social beings.
Rosenzweig et al. (1969)	The objective was to study the exact nature and extent of the differences in rat cortical structure and function when animals were exposed to enriched experiences and impoverished experiences.	Level I Random assignment with 3 conditions: ECT, EC, and IC *EC:* brightly lit rooms, housed in groups, provided toys, etc. *ECT:* same as EC with exposure daily (30 min) to open field environment in which pattern of barriers was changed Blind analysis of results	Dissection, weighing, and chemical analysis of brain	Rats exposed to EC developed significantly greater cortical tissue weight, total AChE activity, total ChE, and cortical depth. Results occurred as clearly in adult rats as in young rats. Visual experience is not a necessary component of the conditions that evoke change. Tissue weights and cortical size = significant differences between ECT and IC, with greatest difference in occipital cortex and the least for somesthetic cortex. AChE activity greatest change (decrease) was in the occipital area. ChE activity greatest change was in the occipital area. ChE:AChE ratio (measure of glial cell) was greatest in the occipital region, although present in all regions. Cortical depths were greatest in occipital area in EC rats.	Animal study limits generalizability. Measures were only of brain, and the authors did not provide concurrent measures of behavior, so it is not possible to relate brain changes to behavioral changes.

(Continued)

Table C1. Neuroscience Evidence for the Effectiveness of Using a Sensory-Based Approach in Occupational Therapy With Children and Adolescents (cont.)

Author/Year	Study Objectives	Level/Design/Participants	Intervention and Outcome Measures	Results	Study Limitations
Russo, Nicol, Zecker, Hayes, & Kraus (2005)	The objective was to determine whether auditory training targeted to remediate perceptually based learning problems would alter the neural brainstem encoding of the acoustic sound structure and speed in such children.	Level II 9 experimental participants diagnosed with a language-based learning problem (such as dyslexia) and 10 control participants Age = 8–12 IQ > 85	*Intervention* Training using perceptual auditory training software: Earobics *Setting*: Labcratory *Outcome Measure* Pretraining and 3 mo posttraining brain stem responses to the syllable "da" were recorded in quiet and with background noise. Evaluated transient and sustained components of the brain stem responses. Transient = <11 ms after stimulus onset; sustained response = 11–50 ms after stimuli onset. Differences between groups were assessed using repeated measures ANOVA with test session as the within-subject factor and training group as the between-group factor.	Transient response did not demonstrate plasticity. Sustained response increased significantly in the trained participants, reflecting improved stimulus encoding precision (control participants did not exhibit this change). Concurrent changes in perceptual, academic, and cognitive measures were found. Children in the trained group demonstrated significant gains on listening tests. Gains in listening comprehension were related to changes in the brain stem response. Auditory training appears to alter the brain stem response to speech sounds. Specifically, neural encoding became more resistant to the deleterious effects of background noise. Increases in quiet-to-noise interresponse correlations represent greater timing precision in the frequency following response in noise after training.	Lack of randomization is a concern. The authors did not test beyond 3 mo posttraining; there is no way to know whether the findings persisted long term.
Schaefer, Heinze, & Rotte (2005)	The objective was to test the hypothesis of top-down influence on frontal areas of the primary sensory cortex; that is, test the hypothesis that prefrontal–cortical sensory gating is responsible for tactile maps in SI of the fingers during an activity.	Level III 1 group, 3 task conditions (Tower of Hanoi, control, rest) during imaging N = 10 male volunteers ages 18–30, healthy	MEG imaging of cortical representation of stimulated fingers (Digits 1 and 5) during the 3 task conditions	Cortical areas of D1 and D5 were more distant during a task that required cognitive function (Tower of Hanoi) than the same motor task not requiring cognitive function. Authors concluded that frontal or prefrontal regions can facilitate neuronal responsiveness in the primary sensory cortex, depending on the task demand. Differences were seen between the digits, and future studies will be needed to examine other digits. Authors also suggested that this "short-term" neuroplasticity indicates that somatopic representations can be altered dynamically and in a task-specific manner.	Earlier reported findings of other investigators were not supported, and the current study did not explain these differences. Subject pool was small and not well described.
Schapiro & Vukovich (1970)	The objective was to assess the effects of environmental stimulation on the development of rat cortical pyramidal cell synaptic loci (dendritic spines) and the number of such cells.	Level I Randomized selection of rats for experimental and control groups	Stimulation 3–5×/day from day of birth to Day 16 Stimulation = handling, stroking, shaking on a mechanical shaker, placement in warm and cold water, and subjecting to noise and flashing light and short periods of electrical shock	Increased number of spines per micrometer in 8-day-old animals and increased number of neurons at 8–16 days	Animal study limits generalizability. In the absence of behavioral measures, it is not possible to correlate anatomical changes with behavioral changes. Stimulation was passive. Unable to determine whether changes noted continued after stimulation.

Sober & Sabes (2005)	This study investigated the weighting of visual and proprioceptive feedback on production of motor response.	Level II There was a single group for each study, using control and experimental trials. In both studies, participants had visual feedback from reaching arm that disappeared once arm began to move.	*Experiment 1 (n = 7)*: 2 conditions of reach, 1 to a visual target, the other to a proprioceptive target identified as position of the left index finger (which had been passively positioned). 8 reaches to each of 6 targets, each with visual shift, to total 144 reaches. *Experiment 2 (n = 10)*: Investigation of information content of visual feedback; visual feedback representing arm and joint configuration or just location of fingertip. All reaches to visual target. No outcome measures; rather, results: • *Experiment 1*: Brain weights, sensory feedback to minimize adverse effects of transforming arm position to reach target. • *Experiment 2*: When feedback represents only fingertip position, movement is driven by proprioception; when feedback is whole arm, vision and proprioception contribute equally. Suggestion that this means that key difference between 2 conditions is information about configuration of joints. During movement toward target, same sensory signals can be given different weightings at different stages of reach planning or at same stage of planning for different tasks. Thus, sensory integration for reach planning is dynamic and driven by task demands.	Integration of sensory information is determined not only entirely by features of sensory input, but also by the computations required for task execution.	Experimental conditions are difficult to link to typical environments.

(Continued)

Appendix C. Evidence Tables

Table C1. Neuroscience Evidence for the Effectiveness of Using a Sensory-Based Approach in Occupational Therapy With Children and Adolescents (cont.)

Author/Year	Study Objectives	Level/Design/ Participants	Intervention and Outcome Measures	Results	Study Limitations
Stoeckel, Pollok, Schnitzler, Witte, & Seitz (2004)	The objective was to study use-dependent plasticity of human somatosensory cortex. Study 1 was to determine any differences in accuracy of localization of tactile stimuli on toes between participants who (1) used feet to accomplish simple tasks, (2) used toes to accomplish everyday activities such as writing and eating, and (3) were control participants. Study 2 was to determine any differences in somatosensory activation patterns to tactile stimuli on toes between the 3 groups.	Level I 3 groups randomized 23 thalidomide-affected participants with malformed upper extremities Mean age = 39.8 yr (range = 39–42). Setting Clinic-type environment	Not an intervention study 3 groups: 1. Used feet for certain actions only ($n = 10$) (F1) 2. Used feet extensively for everyday activities such as writing and eating ($n = 3$) (F2) 3. Control group: thalidomide-damaged extremities but normal hands; feet not used for any unusual actions ($n = 10$). 2 studies: 1. Tested accuracy of localization of tactile stimuli on toes; examined cortical representation between groups. • Threshold for detection of tactile stimuli on each toe determined • Threshold monofilament was chosen to evaluate localization for all toes. 2. Determined differences in activation of somatosensory area during tactile stimuli.	*Study 1:* Participants using their feet for everyday activities had significantly fewer errors (6%) on the tactile localization test than the comparison group (1-tailed $p = .003$). *Study 2:* Activation in Study 1 of somatosensory cortex was significantly stronger in F2 participants (participants who used feet for everyday activities; $p = .002–.137$).	Small experimental group size (F2: $n = 3$) may limit generalizability.
Stryker & Sherk (1975)	The objective of the study was to reexamine earlier findings that limiting the early visual environment of cats to simple vertical or horizontal stripes results in orientation selectivity of cells in visual cortex.	Level II Nonrandomized controlled trial Design 3 groups (one control), no random assignment. Sample size not specified. Cell recordings conducted using regular intervals to identify cells for recording; quantitative measurement of each unit's orientation-tuning curve; recorders were kept blind to exposure of the cats being tested. Subjects $N = 7$ cats	*Intervention* Cats kept in total darkness except for period of restricted exposure to either horizontal or vertical stripes *Outcome Measures* Recordings obtained from 456 sites in visual cortex of experimental animals; 359 sites for controls	• No experimental animal showed a bias in distribution of preferred orientations that differed from what was seen in control animals.	Animal study limits generalizability; link between human and cat visual system not clear. Methodology only briefly reported in this study, making it difficult to determine flaws.

Study	Objective	Design	Intervention/Outcome Measures	Results	Limitations
Trachtenberg & Stryker (2001)	The objective of the study was to establish an anatomical substrate paralleling the rapid physiological changes that had been previously identified in visual cortical processing after manipulation of visual input in kittens.	Level II Nonrandomized controlled trial *Design* 5 cats exposed to strabismus for 2 days between Postnatal Days 31 and 35; 2 exposed to strabismus for 1–2 wks, induced Postnatal Days 28–30; 2 with normal vision *Subjects* $N = 9$ cats	*Intervention* Varying exposure to strabismus or normal vision *Outcome Measures* Ocular dominance ratios, retrograde and anterograde labeling to look at connectivity	• Substantial changes in horizontal connections within the upper layers of visual cortex at the height of the critical period, apparent after 2 days of strabismus. Not clear whether changes seen were result of rapid addition of new connections to same-eye zones or loss of connections to zones dominated by other eye. • These rapid changes are in contrast to relatively slower changes previously documented to occur in thalamocortical pathways.	Animal study limits generalizability. Relatively small sample size, although with cellular recordings, this may be less critical.
van Praag, Kempermann, & Gage (1999)	This study separated aspects of enrichment to look at socialization, larger housing, physical activity, and forced activity-related learning in promoting hippocampal neurogenesis.	Level II 5 groups, $n = 14$/group; mice.	*Groups* • Control subjects • Learners (daily training in water maze) • Swimmers (placed in water without specific task) • Runners (in cage with wheel) • Enriched (14 mice/cage, access to environmental toys) *Outcome Measures* Progenitor cell proliferation and survival of progeny	Cell proliferation increased in mice housed with unrestricted access to running wheel. Both runners and enriched mice showed increased survival of progeny neural cells. Researchers were able to rule out additional food or treats or social groupings in promotion of neurogenesis, although enriched mice showed better survival of new cells and potential long-term effects.	Animal study limits generalizability.
Volkmar & Greenough (1972)	The objective was to examine the differences in higher-order dendritic branching in visual cortical cells in young rats reared in 3 different environments.	Level II Enriched environment, standard environment, impoverished environment Animals ages 22–25 days	*Intervention* EE: 12/cage; wood, metal, and plastic toys changed daily; 30 min "free play" daily in another environment IE: standard cages SE: pairs in standard cages Intervention for 29–31 days *Outcome Measure* Investigation of dendritic branching in 4 types of cortical cells	Profound differences in all 4 cell types. Substantially greater higher-order dendritic branching in enriched environment condition than in impoverished environment condition. Differences between SC and IC were less clear but still apparent. Data suggest that regulation of neuronal growth is through "use" related to the environment in which the animal is reared.	Animal study limits generalizability.
Walsh, Cummins, & Budtz–Olsen (1971)	The objective of the study was to determine whether changes in anteroposterior growth of rat cerebrum are significant and region specific.	Level II Nonrandomized controlled trial *Design* Half assigned to enriched and half to isolated conditions *Subjects* $N = 44$ rats	*Intervention* Enriched condition involved addition of toys to a group cage. Exposure for 30 days. *Outcome Measures* Growth in anterior region of brain	Enrichment led to growth of cerebrum attributable to growth in anterior region of brain.	Animal study limits generalizability. Little interpretation possible due to vagueness of anterior vs. posterior. No functional measures or associations.

(Continued)

Table C1. Neuroscience Evidence for the Effectiveness of Using a Sensory-Based Approach in Occupational Therapy With Children and Adolescents (cont.)

Author/Year	Study Objectives	Level/Design/Participants	Intervention and Outcome Measures	Results	Study Limitations
West & Greenough (1972)	The objective was to examine whether rats reared in groups in complex environments have longer postsynaptic regions in the occipital lobe.	Level I 2-group randomized design matched for body weight	*Intervention* EC = reared in groups with toys and play time; $n = 12$ IC = cage reared in isolation, $n = 12$ Age during experiment = 0–40 days Measure—after 35 days, rats were given 5 trials/day on a maze *Outcome Measures* Electron microscope used to analyze synaptic size in visual cortex. Synaptic bouton diameter and length of the postsynaptic thickening were measured. 23–51 synapses/animal were measured.	EC group performed significantly better on the maze. The length of the postsynaptic opaque region was significantly greater for the EC animals. There was a tendency for Type 1 synaptic boutons to be larger in EC animals, but it was not significant.	Animal study limits generalizability.
Wiesel & Hubel (1965)	The objective of the study was to determine the extent of recovery of visual functioning after eye sutures.	Level III *Design* One-group, nonrandomized (although eye suturing was mixed) *Subjects* 7 kittens whose eyes were sutured at birth for 3 mo (6 unilaterally and 1 bilaterally). Crossed design whereby 6 kittens had only 1 eye sutured and some had opposite eye sutured after 3 mo and others had both eyes open. 1 kitten had both eyes sutured and then unsutured.	*Intervention* Eyes sutured *Outcome Measures* Behavioral observations; morphological analysis of lateral geniculate; physiological recordings from visual cortex	*Behavioral findings* All kittens showed some slight behavioral recovery during the first 3 mo, but all animals remained severely handicapped and never learned to move freely using visual cues. *Morphological findings* No improvement in lateral geniculate body; atrophy remained. *Cortical physiology (recordings)* Cells' responses were abnormal and remained abnormal.	Animal study limits generalizability.
Wiesel & Hubel (1974)	The objective was to determine whether ordered sequences of orientation columns are present in very young, visually naïve monkeys.	Level II *Design* 2 groups, nonrandomized *Subjects* Macaque monkeys ($n = 6$)	*Intervention* $n = 4$ monkeys with eyes sutured shut at various times close to time of birth; 2 control participants *Outcome Measures* Recordings from Area 17 (occipital cortex)	Highly ordered sequences of orientation shifts were present and were not different from what is seen in adults, suggesting that the organization of the columns of the visual system is innately determined and NOT the result of early experience. In addition, there was deterioration of innate connections subserving binocular convergence, suggesting that deprivation results in deteriorating effects.	Animal study limits generalizability.

Author/Year	Study Objectives	Level/Design/Participants	Intervention and Outcome Measures	Results	Study Limitations
Wu, van Gelderen, Hanakawa, Yaseen, & Cohen (2005)	The objective was to examine effects of somatosensory stimulation (by means of direct stimulation of nerve) on brain activation/excitability in primary motor cortex, somatosensory cortex, and dorsal premotor cortex to determine whether this is a mechanism of neuroplasticity.	Level II 1 group, nonrandomized ($n = 19$) under 3 experimental conditions: (1) electrical stimulation of median nerve; (2) electrical stimulation of skin over deltoid; (3) no stimulation. Setting: laboratory	*Intervention* 2-hr electrical stimulation applied to median nerve at wrist, to skin overlying deltoid, and no stimulation *Outcome Measures* • fMRI • BOLD • Perfusion images of primary motor cortex, somatosensory cortex, and dorsal premotor cortex	Brain activation is measured by the number of voxels activated. *fMRI:* There was an increase in number of voxels activated in primary motor cortex, somatosensory cortex, and dorsal premotor cortex after median nerve stimulation activated by performance of thumb movements for up to 60 min. Results suggest that median nerve stimulation can lead to an expansion of the thumb representation in somatosensory cortex—a form of plasticity that may underlie the influence of somatosensory stimulation on motor cortex function.	No control group and passive input limit generalizability. No behavioral measures included, so the reader is unable to determine whether brain changes are related to behavioral change. A strength is that the number of voxels activated was comparable across sessions using fMRI, BOLD, or perfusion.
You et al. (2005)	The objective was to determine whether virtual reality therapy would promote practice-dependent plasticity in a child with cerebral palsy, leading to enhanced motor skills and overcoming nonuse.	Level V Case report Single-subject study with pre- and posttesting Intervention conducted by therapist unaware of research *Participant* 8-yr-old boy with hemiparetic cerebral palsy on right side	*Intervention* Virtual reality games that included bird-ball, conveyor, and soccer Intervention was 60 min/day, 5 day/wk, over 4 wk *Outcome Measures* • fMRI • Bruininks–Oseretsky Test of Motor Proficiency, Item 6: touching a swinging ball • Modified Pediatric Motor Activity Log • Upper limb subtest of Fugl-Meyer assessment	Bruininks–Oseretsky Test of Motor Proficiency score changed from 1 to 5. Pediatric Motor Activity Log showed increased amount of use and quality of movement. Fugl-Meyer assessment score improved from 39 to 52, showing enhanced active movement control, reflex activity, and coordination in the upper extremity. fMRI showed a change in activation pattern such that preintervention activation involved bilateral primary motor and sensory cortices, sensorimotor cortex, and ipsilateral supplemental motor areas with no activation of the premotor cortex. Postintervention showed loss of aberrant activation and primary activation of the sensorimotor cortex and contralateral primary sensory and motor cortices.	Single-subject design; use of isolated items from standardized assessment tools without substantiation of their ability to stand alone and intensity of intervention preclude its reimbursement potential. However, study suggests that using actual body movement and virtual reality feedback for knowledge of results (visual and proprioceptive feedback) in a manner that was perceived as playful and gamelike (controlled sensory environment) can result in a combination of functional changes and neuroplastic changes in critical cortical regions.

(Continued)

Table C1. Neuroscience Evidence for the Effectiveness of Using a Sensory-Based Approach in Occupational Therapy With Children and Adolescents (cont.)

Author/Year	Study Objectives	Level/Design/ Participants	Intervention and Outcome Measures	Results	Study Limitations
Zhang, Bao, & Merzenich (2001)	The objective was to examine structural and functional development of auditory cortex as modified by early environmental and learning experiences.	Level II Experimental and control conditions Adult rats and rat pups were used to map primary auditory cortex.	*Intervention* Experience exposure for pups and dams involved placement in sound-shielded and calibrated chamber for 10–16 hr/day, postnatal days 9–28, and exposure to a 25-ms monotone at 60–70 dB, at 6 pulses/s with 1-s intervals. Tone frequency included 4 kHz and 19 kHz. *Outcome Measure* Auditory mapping in adults and immature rats	In adults, monotone presentation did not induce organizational changes. Changes in the organization of rat pup cortex appeared as both tone frequency–dependent effects (which argues for the important role of sound environment in early development) and tone frequency–independent effects (general degradation of tonotopic organization and response selectivity suggests that tonotopic development requires temporally patterned input). Differences exist between these findings and those in other sensory systems. Investigators concluded, "acoustic environments are very important and potentially crucial in instructively defining the basic functional organization and processing capabilities of the auditory cortex" (p. 1128).	Laboratory situations and animal study limit generalizability.

Note. AChE = acetylcholinesterase; AMD = alternating monocular visual deprivation; ANOVA = analysis of variance; BD = binocular deprivation; BOLD *f*MRI = blood-oxygen-level-dependent functional magnetic resonance imaging; ChE = cholinesterase; CS = conditioning stimulus; DC-EEG = DC electroencephalogram; EC = enriched condition; ECT = enriched control with training; EE = enriched environment; EEG = electroencephalogram; EMG = electromyography; *f*MRI = functional magnetic resonance imaging; IC = impoverished condition; IE = impoverished environment; MD = monocular visual deprivation; MEG = magnetoencephalography; MMN = mismatch negativity; mRNA = messenger ribonucleic acid; MT–MST = medial temporal–medial temporal superior area, motion selective area; PET = positron emission tomography; ROM = range of motion; SC = social control; SE = standard environment; SI = sensory integration; SII = secondary sensory cortex; SPL = sound pressure level; V1 = primary visual cortex.

This table is a product of AOTA's Evidence-Based Practice Project and the *American Journal of Occupational Therapy*. Copyright © 2010 by the American Occupational Therapy Association. May be freely reproduced for personal use in clinical or educational settings as long as the source is cited. All other uses require written permission from the American Occupational Therapy Association. To apply, visit www.copyright.com.

From S. J. Lane and R. Schaaf (2010). Examining the neuroscience evidence for sensory-driven neuroplasticity: Implications for sensory-based occupational therapy for children and adolescents (Suppl. Table 1). *American Journal of Occupational Therapy, 64*, 375–390. Copyright © 2010, by the American Occupational Therapy Association.

Table C2. Summary of the Evidence Supporting Subtypes of Children With Difficulty Processing and Integrating Sensory Information

Author/Year	Study Objectives	Level/Design/Participants	Intervention and Outcome Measures	Results	Study Limitations
Ameratunga, Johnston, & Burns (2004)	The objective of the study was to investigate perceptual–motor abilities regarding vision, kinesthesia, and cross-modal judgment. These were examined in children both with and without DCD.	Level II *Design* Cross-sectional group comparison 2 groups The first group consisted of 9 children age 6. All these children had DCD. This was determined by having a score lower than 15% on the M-ABC. The second group had 9 typically developing children, matched for age and gender. Children were excluded from the study if they reported having any of the following: • Neurological disorder or PDD • Intellectual disability • Oncological, musculoskeletal, sensory, or skin disorders.	No intervention was used. 4 different visual–kinesthetic aiming conditions were used while a child was asked to point to an aiming target. The targets were either on the preferred, middle, or nonpreferred side. The conditions were as follows: • V:VK—Child visually inspects target, child aims at target with eyes open. • V:K—Child visually inspects target, child aims at target with vision occluded. • VK:K—Child visually inspects, reaches to, and feels target. Child aims at target with vision occluded. • K:K—Child's finger is guided to target (child's vision is occluded). Child aims at target with vision occluded. The aiming was measured using an electromagnetic position tracker using a sensor on the index finger of the child's preferred hand.	Children with DCD produced greater endpoint errors than the typically developing children when aiming at the target in all tasks and target positions. The children with DCD produced longer trajectory length ratios than the children without DCD. The children with DCD were slower at aiming at all target positions in all tasks. In each group, performance was significantly less accurate and efficient when not using both the visual and kinesthetic feedback.	Study is of good quality.
Antrop, Roeyers, Van Oost, & Buysse (2000)	The objective of this study was to investigate the evidence for the existence of different types of sensory processing/SI problems in children and adolescents.	Level I *Design* Randomized controlled trial with 2 groups Group 1 members had a clinical diagnosis of ADHD without comorbidity. They also had extreme scores on a *DSM–IV*–based questionnaire, the CBCL, the Teacher Report Form, and the IOWA Connors Teacher Rating Scale. Participants were ages 6–12, had normal intelligence, and were free of medication.	The intervention involved children either watching a video while waiting for 15 min or having no video to watch during the 15 min. An experimenter gave the instructions and then left the room for the duration of the time. This intervention occurred once while the child was being tested. *Outcome Measures* Target behaviors were observed during the 15 min, which were divided into 5 categories: gross motor activity (e.g., walking),	When looking at just the condition alone (video or no video), significant effects were found. Specifically, more activity was shown during the waiting period in certain behaviors in the no-video waiting condition. When looking at the group alone (children with ADHD vs. children without ADHD), significant effects were also found. These results indicated that children with ADHD showed increased activity in certain	None noted.

Appendix C. Evidence Tables

(Continued)

Table C2. Summary of the Evidence Supporting Subtypes of Children With Difficulty Processing and Integrating Sensory Information (cont.)

Author/Year	Study Objectives	Level/Design/Participants	Intervention and Outcome Measures	Results	Study Limitations
		Group 2 served as a control. Members were determined to have normal intelligence, were free of medication, were ages 6–12, and attended ordinary school.	minor motor activity (e.g., movement of arms), sounds (e.g., talk), self-occupation (e.g., nonintentional movement), and situation-specific behavior for this study (e.g., leaving the room).	behaviors compared with children without ADHD, regardless of the condition. The Group × Condition interaction was significant for 2 variables: trunk movements and touching objects. Specifically, when there was no video, children with ADHD showed increased trunk activity and touching of objects when compared with children with ADHD when watching a video and children without ADHD in either waiting condition (video or no video).	
Baranek (1999)	The objective of this study was to investigate the usefulness of sensory–motor measures in addition to social behaviors as early predictors of autism in infancy.	Level II *Design* Group comparison 3 different groups of children participated in the study. All the participants were viewed on videotape that had been recorded between the ages of 9 and 12 mo. There were 11 children in the first group (A), all of whom had the diagnosis of autism (10 boys, 1 girl). They were all diagnosed using *DSM–IV* criteria by a licensed psychologist. They also had to score >30 on the CARS. There were 10 children in the second group (DD), all of whom had DD (3 boys, 7 girls). All of these children had a documented DD or mental retardation either in medical or school records and included children with syndromes such as Down syndrome. There were 11 children in the third group (T), all of whom were typically developing (6 boys, 5 girls). All of these children were functioning in the average range on the VABS.	No intervention was used. The following measurements were used to place the children in appropriate groups: CARS and VABS. *Outcome Measures* Outcome measures were obtained from viewing home videotapes obtained from the parents of the children. Raters coded the tapes for the following categories of behavior: • Affective expressions • Looking • Gaze aversion • Responsiveness to name • Social touch • Anticipatory posture (later eliminated because of too few incidences) • Motor stereotypies • Object stereotypies • Tactile modulation • Auditory modulation • Visual modulation • Vestibular modulation (later eliminated because of too few incidences)	The level of mental retardation was not significantly different between the DD and A groups. Differences in the scores obtained on the VABS were not significant between the DD and A groups. The DD group demonstrated significantly more inappropriate play and significantly less looking at the camera than either of the other 2 groups. A discriminant analysis was conducted to determine whether the 9 variables could distinguish the 3 groups. Correct group classification was 93.7%. 2 functions were significant, and the first function distinguished the children with autism from the children in the other 2 groups. The most important items in this function were as follows: mouthing, social touch aversions, orientation to visual stimuli, and number of name prompts. The second function distinguished the children in the typical group from the children in the DD group. The variables most important in this	The raters' potential awareness of the distinguishing features of Down syndrome could have altered their ratings for some of the children in the DD group.

| | | | function were as follows: posturing, object play rating, looking at the camera, visual object stereotypy, and affect rating.

A second discriminant analysis was conducted to determine whether the 2 groups of children with disorders could be distinguished. The results were significant, and 6 of the variables most important in the separation of the groups were as follows: mouthing, orientation to visual stimuli, social touch aversions, posturing, number of name prompts, and affect rating. The classification rate was 95%. | |
|---|---|---|---|---|
| Baranek et al. (2002) | The objective of the study was to examine the relationship of sensory processing and occupational performance in school-age boys with Fragile X syndrome. | Level III

Design
Correlational

15 boys participated in the study. All had full mutation, Fragile X syndrome (confirmed by genetic testing). Their ages ranged from 53 to 126 mo. 13 of the children were white, and 2 were black.
The children had a mean Brief IQ composite score (Leiter International Performance Scale–Revised) in the mild range of mental retardation (*mean* = 60, *SD* = 14.29). | No intervention was used. All participants were tested at 1 time.

Measures of Sensory Processing
Parent report: Sensory Profile.
Observational Measures: TDDT–R and the Sensory Approach–Avoidance Rating.
The following measures were used to assess occupational performance:
• VABS
• The School Function Assessment
• A measure of play duration with the toys | The TDDT–R internal control score and the Sensory Approach–Avoidance Rating were correlated.
On the Sensory Profile, the average score fell >2 *SD*s below the mean.
The School Function Assessment criterion scores and the VABS standard scores both fell below the range of typical performance.
There was a significant negative relationship between TDDT–R internal control score and the VABS score.
The Sensory Approach–Avoidance Rating was significantly negatively correlated with all 3 of the School Function Assessment variables.
The Sensory Approach–Avoidance Rating was significantly negatively correlated with play duration. Thus, children with greater internally controlled aversion (avoidance) to toys with sensory features (TDDT–R and Sensory | Children's IQ scores, as well as socioeconomic status, covered a wide range, which could contribute to confounding variables.
A larger sample is needed to make the study more generalizable.
Better assessments of play across multiple contexts would add more to the results.
Because many of the findings rely on the validity of the Sensory Approach–Avoidance Rating, conclusions must be drawn with hesitation until that information is available. |

(*Continued*)

Table C2. Summary of the Evidence Supporting Subtypes of Children With Difficulty Processing and Integrating Sensory Information (cont.)

Author/Year	Study Objectives	Level/Design/Participants	Intervention and Outcome Measures	Results	Study Limitations
				Approach–Avoidance Rating) had lower levels of participation and performance in school, had less independence in self-care at home, and engaged for shorter duration in play. The Sensory Profile indicated that 11 of the 15 participants had definite sensory modulation deficits. The Sensory Profile scores did not relate to occupational performance.	
Baranek, David, Poe, Stone, & Watson (2006)	The objective of the study was to investigate properties of the SEQ and explain the nature of sensory patterns, prevalence, and uniqueness in children with autism and related disorders.	Level III *Design* In this comparison study, SEQ data were obtained from 258 children. 56 of the children had autism; the mean age of this group was 40.47 mo (86.8% boys and 13.2% girls). 24 had PDD; the mean age of this group was 39.14 mo (82.6% boys and 17.4% girls). 33 had DD or mental retardation; the mean age was 33.72 mo (75.8% boys and 24.2% girls). 35 children formed a group with other children with DD (76.5% boys and 23.5% girls). The mean age was 33.4 mo. The final group had 110 children, all typically developing. The mean age was 29.3 mo (46.8% boys and 53.2% girls). Exclusion criteria included no comorbid conditions such as fragile X syndrome or tuberous sclerosis. Participants also had to have intact vision and auditory functions.	No intervention was used. SEQ was given to measure behavioral responses to sensory experiences.	The SEQ scores were found to be inversely related to mental age; as mental age increased, sensory symptoms decreased. The SEQ mean scores varied significantly across groups. The children with autism had significantly higher scores on the SEQ than did the typically developing children or DD group. The only gender effects found involved the boys in the DD group; they scored significantly lower on the SEQ than did the girls. Compared with the typically developing group, the group with autism and the PDD group had higher SEQ symptoms on all 4 subscales, whereas the DD group had higher scores on 3 subscales. When comparing the group with autism to the group with DD, the group with autism showed greater hyporesponsiveness across contexts.	The cross-sectional approach used in this study provided limited understanding of the developmental nature of this problem. A longitudinal study would be a better way to address it.

Ceponiene et al. (2003)	The objective of this study was to investigate the sensory and early attentional processing of sounds differing in complexity in high-functioning children with autism using event-related potentials.	Level II *Design* Group comparison 2 groups The first group was made up of 9 children (8 boys, 1 girl). All of these children were diagnosed as having high-functioning autism using the *DSM–IV* (mean age = 8.9, range = 6.3–12.4). CARS was used on the children who were ages 5–9. The Reynell Developmental Rating Scale was used for the children ages 5–11. The second group was made up of 10 children (9 boys, 1 girl, mean age = 8.4, range = 6.6–12.4). This group served as the control participants, and they had no hearing or academic problems.	No intervention was used. The CARS and the Reynell Developmental Rating Scale were both used as diagnostic testing criteria. Brain responses (electroencephalogram) were recorded while the children were presented with auditory stimuli. There was 1 standard and 1 deviant stimulus for each of the following 3 stimulus classes: simple tones, complex tones, and vowels. 86% of the tones heard were standard, and the rest were of the deviant class. Participants were instructed to ignore the auditory stimuli and focus on watching silent videos.	In both groups of children, significant brain responses were elicited. The P1 was the only peak to be significantly reduced in the children with autism. A significant mismatch negativity was found in both groups of children. The complex tone mismatch negativity was significantly larger than the simple tones in both groups of children. Thus, in this study children with autism were able to discriminate frequency changes in tones of simple or complex orientation at the same level of accuracy as their peers. In the group of typically developing children, the P3 was significant in all stimulus conditions. In the children with autism, no P3 was elicited by changes in the vowel, whereas changes by both types of tones elicited P3s.	Study is of good quality.
Coleman, Piek, & Livesey (2001)	The objective of the study was to examine whether children identified as being at risk for DCD have worse kinesthetic ability than age-matched typically developing children.	Level II *Design* Longitudinal 2 groups The first group of 31 children (18 boys and 13 girls) was identified as being at risk of having DCD. This identification was determined by scoring <15th percentile on the M–ABC. The 31 children in the control group (matched for age, gender, and verbal IQ) all scored >50th percentile on the M–ABC. All the children were between the ages of 4 and 5. They were tested once and then again 1 yr later.	No intervention was studied. The M–ABC was used to identify which children were at risk for DCD. The WPPSI was given to determine cognitive ability. The KAT was also used; the children had to identify which of 16 different zoo animals they were touching (with no visual cues).	The KAT number correct, KAT positional error, block design, geometric design, and object assembly as a group significantly predicted M–ABC scores. Individually, all of the previously mentioned tests were significant predictors, except block design. 23 of the 30 children retested the second time were still at risk for DCD. There was a significant main effect for group and time with the KAT number correct, KAT positional error, block design, geometric design, and object assembly, but no significant interaction effect.	Study is of good quality.

(Continued)

Table C2. Summary of the Evidence Supporting Subtypes of Children With Difficulty Processing and Integrating Sensory Information *(cont.)*

Author/Year	Study Objectives	Level/Design/Participants	Intervention and Outcome Measures	Results	Study Limitations
				The children at risk for DCD had significantly more KAT positional errors and fewer numbers correct than did the control group. Object assembly, block design, and geometric design were significantly lower for the group with DCD than for the control participants. All children made fewer correct responses and more positional errors on the KAT at Time 1 than at Time 2.	
Davis, Bockbrader, Murphy, Hetrick, & O'Donnell (2006)	The objective of this study was to investigate visual processing in children who have autism compared with typically developing children. Specifically, the relationship between subjective reports of visual-processing difficulties to actual performance on several psychophysical measures was evaluated.	Level II *Design* Group comparison 2 groups The first group consisted of 9 children who were all clinically diagnosed by a psychologist using *DSM–IV* criteria as having autism and were considered high functioning. The age range was 10–18. The second group was made up of 9 age-matched typically developing children ages 7–15.	No intervention was used. The similarities and picture completion subscales of the WISC–III and the SIAPA–CV were administered. Psychophysical tests were administered: • Form and Motion Perception • Discrimination • Matching tasks • Contrast Sensitivity for Pattern and Flicker Detection	The children with autism scored higher than the control participants on all measures of the SIAPA–CV. Each child with autism reported ≥1 sensory anomaly; however, this sensory anomaly differed across children and modality. In the discrimination tasks, children with autism performed significantly worse than the typically developing children only for the 1,000-ms motion condition. The children with autism had significantly worse contrast sensitivity for pattern detection than did the typically developing children. There was a statistically significant relationship between psychophysical sensitivity and frequency of sensitivity-related visual anomalies measured by the SIAPA–CV. This relationship was negative, indicating that worse performance on the psychophysical tests was associated with greater frequency of visual sensitivity.	The sample size was small. Only high-functioning children with autism were used; therefore, generalization to the entire autism spectrum is not possible.

Dunn & Bennett (2002)	The objective of this study was to compare sensory responsiveness of children with ADHD and that of typically developing children.	Level II *Design* Group comparison 1 group consisted of 70 children, ages 3–15, who were diagnosed as having ADHD by professionals according to the *DSM–IV*. The second group consisted of 70 age- and gender-matched children who were typically developing and were randomly selected from a national standardization sample.	No intervention was used. *Outcome Measures* The Sensory Profile was used to measure sensory processing, modulation, and behavioral outcomes of sensory processing, as reported by the children's parents.	The children with ADHD performed significantly differently than the typically developing children on all 14 sections of the Sensory Profile, including auditory, touch, multisensory, emotional/social responses, and behavioral outcomes of sensory processing, and specifically on 118 of 125 items. In each case, the children with ADHD displayed the behavior more frequently, with 57 of these 118 items showing >1 raw score point difference between the means. This analysis revealed that most of the items that were significantly different between the 2 groups fell into 4 of the 9 previously defined factors (Dunn & Brown, 1997): sensory seeking, emotionally reactive, inattention/distractibility, and fine motor/perceptual.	A convenience sample was used. Some of the children (approximately half) also had a secondary diagnosis. Some of the children in the ADHD group were on medications and some were not. The children from the national standardization sample were not matched to the ADHD sample on characteristics like socioeconomic status and ethnicity.
Dunn, Myles, & Orr (2002)	The objective of this study was to investigate the evidence for the existence of different types of sensory processing/SI problems in children and adolescents.	Level III *Design* Group comparison 2 groups In Group 1, all the children, ages 8–14, attended public school and were diagnosed as having AD by a licensed professional. Group 2, the control group, consisted of a random sample of 42 children, ages 8–14, from the Sensory Profile standardization sample (these were data previously collected). They had no disabilities.	No intervention was used. *Outcome Measures* The Sensory Profile was used to measure responses to sensory events in daily life. It measures problems in the following areas: sensory processing, modulation, behavioral and emotional responses, and responsiveness to sensory events.	Children with AD performed more poorly than typically developing children in all the section scores of the Sensory Profile except for modulation of visual input affecting emotional responses and activity level. The children with AD also performed more poorly than typically developing children on all the factor scores: sensation seeking, emotionally reactive, low endurance/tone, oral sensory sensitivity, inattention/distractibility, poor registration, sensory sensitivity, sedentary, and fine motor/perceptual.	The Sensory Profile standardization sample uses a convenience sample. The impact of differences in sensory processing was not evaluated in the children's daily lives.

(Continued)

Table C2. Summary of the Evidence Supporting Subtypes of Children With Difficulty Processing and Integrating Sensory Information (cont.)

Author/Year	Study Objectives	Level/Design/Participants	Intervention and Outcome Measures	Results	Study Limitations
Ermer & Dunn (1998)	The objective of the study was to determine which items on the Sensory Profile best discriminate between children with autism or PDD, children with ADHD, and typically developing children.	Level II *Design* Group comparison The first group was made up of 38 children with autism or PDD, ages 3–13. The second group consisted of 61 children with ADHD, ages 2–15. The third group included 1,075 children ages 3–15 from a previous study. The children in this third group were not receiving any special education or taking any medication. Only 671 children from this third group were included in the data analysis because data were missing.	No intervention was used. *Outcome Measures* The Sensory Profile was used to measure sensory processing, modulation, and behavioral outcomes of sensory processing, as reported by the children's parents. The Sensory Profile measures the degree to which each child responds to everyday activities that involve the following sensory experiences: auditory, visual, taste/smell, movement, body position, touch, activity level, and emotional/social.	A discriminant analysis was conducted with the diagnostic groups as the dependent variable. The independent variables were the factor subscales (see Dunn & Brown, 1997). The discriminant analysis resulted in 2 significant functions. The first function discriminated children with disabilities from children without disabilities. The most significant factor was Factor 5: inattention/distractibility. The second function separated children with ADHD from the children with autism or PDD. 3 factors were significant in distinguishing Factors 1 (sensory seeking), 4 (oral sensory sensitivity), and 9 (fine motor/perceptual). Typically developing children had a high incidence of sensory-seeking behaviors and a low incidence of oral sensory sensitivity, inattention/distractibility, and fine motor/perceptual. Children with autism or PDD had a high incidence of behaviors in oral sensory sensitivity, inattention/distractibility, and fine motor/perceptual and a low incidence of sensory seeking. The children with ADHD had a high incidence of behaviors in sensory seeking and inattention/distractibility and a low incidence of oral sensory sensitivity and fine motor/perceptual. The overall correct classification was 89.9%, with 90.8% correct classification for typically developing children, 76.6% for children with ADHD, and 78.9% for children with autism.	This study used a convenience sample. The sample sizes varied quite a bit. Homogeneity of variance was violated, so these results must be interpreted with caution.

Forseth & Sigmundsson (2003)	The objective of the study was to investigate static balance on 1 leg in children with and without HECP. The broader goal was to better understand DCD.	Level II *Design* Group comparison All 9–10-yr-olds in a school were evaluated ($n = 88$). The summed scores on the 5 eye-hand coordination subtests of the M–ABC were used to classify the children. The 12 children with the highest scores (indicating HECP) were put in 1 group, and the 12 children with the lowest scores were put in the control group. The mean age was 10.6 in the group of children with HECP (3 boys, 9 girls). The mean age of the control group was 10.7 (5 boys, 7 girls).	No intervention was used. The M–ABC test was administered to identify children with motor coordination problems. 3 different static balance tasks were used: (1) stork stand, (2) balance on beam, and (3) 1-board balance. Within each task were 4 trials: 1. With vision, preferred foot 2. With vision, nonpreferred foot 3. Without vision, preferred foot 4. Without vision, nonpreferred foot	Significant differences were found between the groups for all 3 tasks, with and without vision. The role of vision appeared to be more important for the control group because significant differences were found between their tasks with and without vision. The HECP group performed significantly worse on both the preferred and nonpreferred leg in all conditions compared with the control group. On the stork stand with vision, when using the preferred leg, there were no group differences. However, group differences were found (the HECP group performed worse) when using the nonpreferred leg.	The children in the HECP group had not been identified as having a clinical motor coordination disorder. The study tried to make assumptions about which cortical hemisphere was involved in the coordination difficulties using only behavioral measures. No brain imaging techniques were used in this study.
Geuze (2003)	The objective of this study was to address the developmental and clinical differences in the control of static balance between typically developing children and children with DCD in 3 different experiments.	Level II *Design* Group comparison This study had 3 groups of participants. The first group consisted of 24 children classified as DCD with balance problems (DCD–BP). They had to have an M–ABC score <15th percentile. They also had to have a balance subscore of >2 and a static balance score of >1. The second group also had 24 children and was matched for age to serve as a control group. They had to score >15th percentile on the M–ABC to be included in this group. The age range for both of these groups was 6–12.	The M–ABC was used to select participants. The WISC–III was used to determine IQ. *Experiment 1*: A force-plate (Advanced Mechanical Technology, Inc.) was used to determine the displacement of COP during quiet stance. COP was recorded during 2 conditions, eyes open and eyes closed, both during 2-leg or 1-leg stance. *Experiment 2*: EMGs were recorded around the ankle, knee, and hip joint. The children then did the same procedure as in Experiment 1. Afterward, two 30-s trials were recorded on the nondominant leg with eyes open.	*Experiment 1*: All children were able to stand on 2 legs for 20 s with eyes open and eyes closed. 1-leg stance was more difficult for the younger group and the DCD–BP group. The DCD–BP group performed at the level of the younger age-matched control participants. The area of the COP was larger for the younger group, and a main effect of group was found to be significant. A main effect for age was found in both the areas of COP and maximum excursion of COP. The DCD–BP group showed a significantly larger area of COP, and the difference was greater in the 1-leg condition.	Data were collected over a long period of time (1998–2001), which could introduce events that were not controlled for in the study. Within-subject and between-subject variability was larger for Experiment 3.

(Continued)

Table C2. Summary of the Evidence Supporting Subtypes of Children With Difficulty Processing and Integrating Sensory Information *(cont.)*

Author/Year	Study Objectives	Level/Design/Participants	Intervention and Outcome Measures	Results	Study Limitations
		The third group was formed to serve as a cross-sectional developmental study and consisted of 25 children randomly selected from Grade 3 (ages 6–7) and 16 children from Grade 7 (ages 10–11). All of the children had an IQ of ≥80, and none had any known neurological problems. Only 13 children from the DCD–BP group and 13 children from the control groups participated in Experiment 3. The mean age was 9 yr 4 mo for the DCD–BP group and 9 yr 2 mo for the control group.	*Experiment 3*: Force-plate and EMG signals were recorded during 2-leg stance while the children crossed their arms and fixated on a dot. A mechanical perturbation of stance was applied randomly during the trial by a light ball hitting them from behind just below their waist. The children were told in advance to expect the ball.	The DCD–BP group had larger maximum COP values in lateral direction when standing on 1 leg with eyes closed. *Experiment 2*: Results indicated improved balance control with less muscle activation in the older group. The children in the DCD–BP group showed significantly more muscle activity than the children in the control group. *Experiment 3*: All children maintained stance without stepping away or any major movement. Only small differences were found between the groups. The children in the DCD–BP group showed longer duration of force-plate and muscle reactions only in the first unexpected perturbation.	
Geuze (2005)	The objective of this study was to examine the balance problems that children with DCD have in different situations.	Level II *Design* Group comparison Children were identified as having DCD by the classroom teacher and in some cases a physical education teacher. The group consisted of 13 children (10 boys, 3 girls) with an age range of 6–11. This group also had balance problems. The control group of 13 children was matched for age (9 boys, 4 girls). The criteria for being included in the group with DCD were as follows: • M–ABC score <15th percentile • M–ABC balance score >2 • M–ABC static balance score >1	Using EMG, the children were measured on their control of balance on 1 leg for 10 to 30 s.	Strong correlations were found in each group for lateral control. The older participants showed, on average, a stronger lateral control for the leg muscles than the younger children did. The children with DCD showed a weaker lateral control for leg muscles than the control group did, indicating less efficient control.	Study is of good quality.

Author/Year	Study Objectives	Level/Design/Participants	Intervention and Outcome Measures	Results	Study Limitations
Gomez & Condon (1999)	The objective of this study was to examine central auditory processing abilities of children with ADHD, ADHD + LD, and children with no disabilities.	Level II *Design* Group comparison 3 groups, each with 15 participants The first group was made up of children with a sole diagnosis of ADHD (11 boys, 4 girls). The second group consisted of children with a diagnosis of ADHD + LD (12 boys, 3 girls). The third group consisted of all typically developing children to serve as a control group (12 boys, 3 girls). All the children attended mainstream schools. All participants were screened for LD, and LD was determined by a discrepancy of >15 standard points between the child's IQ score and reading ability.	No intervention was used. 2 tests were used to measure central auditory processing: • Screening Test for Auditory Processing Disorders, consisting of 3 tests presented on audiotape: Filtered Words Test, the Auditory Figure Ground Test, and the Completing Words Test • Lindamood Auditory Conceptualization Test: sound discrimination and sequential order of pattern.	When examining reading scores, the ADHD + LD group had lower scores than the ADHD group, and both groups were lower than the children without disabilities. For ratings of inattention, the ADHD group scored higher than the ADHD + LD group, and both groups scored higher than the children without disabilities. For both the Completing Words Test and the Screening Test for Auditory Processing Disorders composite score, the ADHD + LD group scored significantly lower than the ADHD group and the children without disabilities. The degree of correct classification was much higher for the ADHD + LD and non-LD children than it was for the children with ADHD. When grouping the children as LD or non-LD, the correct classification rates were higher still. This finding implies that central auditory processing is associated with LD rather than ADHD.	Study is of good quality.
Humphries, Krekewich, & Snider (1996)	The objective of this study was to examine the sensorimotor basis of nonverbal learning disability syndrome.	Level II *Design* Group comparison An initial group of 90 boys was referred to a clinic for coordination or school-related difficulties. To be included in the first group, they had to have a significantly lower performance than verbal IQ score on the WISC–R and a WRAT arithmetic score significantly lower than the reading score, indicating a nonverbal learning disability. This group had 13 boys in it. The other group had 19 boys and	No intervention was used. *Outcome Measures* The Producing Model Sentences subtest from the Clinical Evaluation of Language Functions; the Number Recall subtest of the Kaufman Assessment Battery for Children, the Perceptual Quotient of the Test of Visual–Perceptual Skills; the Gross Motor Composite Score of the BOTMP; the Developmental Test of Visual–Motor Integration; and the Space Visualization, Motor Accuracy–Revised, and Design Copying subtests of the Southern	The group with the nonverbal learning disability performed significantly worse on Space Visualization and the Developmental Test of Visual Motor Integration.	Study is of good quality.

Appendix C. Evidence Tables

(Continued)

Table C2. Summary of the Evidence Supporting Subtypes of Children With Difficulty Processing and Integrating Sensory Information (cont.)

Author/Year	Study Objectives	Level/Design/Participants	Intervention and Outcome Measures	Results	Study Limitations
		showed no significant discrepancy of IQ or WRAT subtest scores. All participants of both groups had SI dysfunction and a learning disorder as defined as a score on 1 subtest of the WRAT ≥1 standard deviation below the IQ score on the WISC.	California Sensory Integration Tests were selected because they had the reliability to make group comparisons.		
Inder & Sullivan (2005)	The objectives of this study were to assist in understanding of DCD relative to different sensory conditions; to examine the performance relative to age-matched peers by means of multidimensional profiles and highlight difficulties they experience in ADLs, school, sports, and play; and to assist in the design of interventions. The Sensory Organization Test, which was used in this study, examines different sensory aspects of balance, such as visual, somatosensory, and vestibular.	Level IV *Design* Single-subject, multiple-baseline descriptive study 4 participants who had previously participated in a university-based movement clinic were recruited for the study (2 girls, 2 boys). Inclusion criteria were as follows: • Ages 8–12 • Motor coordination below expected for age • Motor impairment affecting school or ADLs • Motor difficulties not caused by medical condition or neurological, mental, or behavioral disorder	This was a descriptive study and not an intervention study. The instrument used for the multiple baseline was a dynamic posturography test in the form of the Sensory Organization Test. This test was used to measure postural stability under varying sensory conditions. Other measures were developed: • A parent/caregiver questionnaire was constructed seeking information on medical and family background. • A teacher questionnaire was constructed seeking curriculum performance and reading age. • Academic ability was assessed with Standard Progressive Matrices and the Peabody Picture Vocabulary Test–Revised. • The BOTMP was used to assess the child's current motor performance. • Selected questions from the All About Me Scale—performance and participation in gross motor activities (children, parents, and teachers).	The children displayed varying levels of motor performance. School performance also varied, but indicated poor performance in all the participants. Scores on equilibrium were 2 *SD*s below scores of the mean of peers for 2 participants and 1 *SD* below scores of the other 2 participants. There was increased sway in conditions with sensory conflict, and the greatest amount of sway and falls occurred in the most challenging conditions.	The Sensory Organization Test was conducted in an unnatural environment. The repetition of the Sensory Organization Test did potentially allow the children to learn the trial order. This problem could lead to enhanced performance.
Iwanaga, Ozawa, Kawasaki, & Tsuchida (2006)	The objective of the study was to describe sensorimotor, verbal, and cognitive abilities of children with ADHD, as measured by the Japanese version of the Miller Assessment for Preschoolers.	Level II *Design* Group comparison 46 boys were selected to participate in this study because they had a diagnosis from a	No intervention was used. The Japanese version of the Miller Assessment for Preschoolers is a restandardized version of the Miller Assessment for Preschoolers for use with	22 of the 46 boys with ADHD combined type were judged to be at risk (<5th percentile) for motor and cognitive abilities and should be further evaluated.	Only boys from Japan were included in this study, so generalization to other populations is not possible. Only boys with ADHD combined type were included, so generalizations

		professional of ADHD combined type using *DSM–IV* criteria. The mean age was 62.8 mo. All had symptoms for ≥6 mo, and all were unmedicated. A matched control group was made up of 46 typically developing boys. They were matched on age and IQ.	Japanese children. It includes the following indexes: • Foundation Index • Coordination Index • Verbal Index • Nonverbal Index • Complex Index • Total score	90% of the boys with ADHD scored in the caution or at-risk range (>25th percentile). The ADHD group was significantly lower than the control group on the total score and each of the indexes except the Nonverbal Index. The items that the boys with ADHD consistently had the most trouble with were standing balance and walks line (50% and 35%, respectively, fell <5th percentile).	to other types of ADHD (e.g., inattentive) are not possible. Children who refused to take the test were excluded, which could lead to bias toward children with less inattention or fewer hyperactive characteristics; thus, results must be interpreted with caution.
Jansiewicz et al. (2006)	The objective of the study was to investigate the full range of subtle neurological signs to examine the neurological systems involved in motor control in autism.	Level II *Design* Group comparison 2 groups (ages 6–17) The first group was made up of 40 children with a mean age of 11.35. All the children in this group had an ASD. All had a WISC–III full-scale IQ of ≥80 (with the exception of 1 child who had a large discrepancy between verbal and performance and was still included). Stimulants were discontinued 24 hr before testing. The control group was made up of 55 children with a mean age of 11.6. They had no neurological or psychiatric disorders. None of the children were taking medications.	No intervention was used. *Outcome Measures* The Physical and Neurological Exam for Subtle Signs was used to assess motor function.	The control group had a significantly higher IQ score than the group with autism. There was a significant difference between the groups on all of the following measures: balance, speed of repetitive and patterned timed movements, dysrhythmia, and overflow. In all cases, the autism group showed reduced performance. The only variable in which the children with autism who were taking stimulant medication differed from those not taking stimulant medication was the gait variable. There was a significant difference between the children in the autism group not on stimulant medication and the control group for the gait variable. A regression analysis showed that diagnosis had a significant effect on the gait variable. The ability of this model to predict autism was fairly high when using the following Physical and Neurological Exam for Subtle Signs variables: overflow, gait, balance, speed of patterned timed movements.	Some of the children in the group with an ASD were on medications (different kinds), whereas others were not. There was a statistical difference in IQ between the group with ASD and the control group (the control had a higher mean).

(Continued)

Table C2. Summary of the Evidence Supporting Subtypes of Children With Difficulty Processing and Integrating Sensory Information (cont.)

Author/Year	Study Objectives	Level/Design/Participants	Intervention and Outcome Measures	Results	Study Limitations

Jarrold, Gilchrist, & Bender (2005)	The objective of this study was to compare the importance of detection processes underlying visual search tasks in children with autism compared to typically developing children. Ability to visually search for objects is a specific type of sensory processing.	Level II
		
		Design
		Group comparison
		
		18 children with autism and 18 typically developing children were recruited.
		
		Autism: Mean age = 149 mo (range = 8 yr 4 mo–15 yr 0 mo).
		Typical: Mean age = 77.9 mo (range = 5 yr 2 mo–7 yr 8 mo).
			No intervention was administered. Baseline measures to match on mental age:
			• British Picture Vocabulary Scale: Baseline measure used to determine verbal and nonverbal skills.
			• Raven's Colored Progressive Matrices: Baseline measure used to match control participants to the children with autism.
			
			Experimental tasks:
			• Children's Embedded Figures Test
			• Search task:
			  – Feature (e.g., match color or size)
			  – Conjunction (e.g., involves attention in addition to feature "map")
			
			Manipulation:
			• Feature vs. conjunction trials
			• 3, 6, or 9 distracters
				The results confirmed that the 2 groups were matched on mental age (Raven's Colored Progressive Matrices and British Picture Vocabulary Scale).
				
				Children with autism were significantly faster at finding embedded figures than were the control participants.
				
				Children with autism who had better embedded figures scores were also faster in search tasks, but the relationship was not true for control participants. This finding relates only to the feature search.
				
				The opposite is true for the conjunction search; control participants who had better embedded figures scores had faster search times in the conjunction trials. This finding was not true for the children with autism.
					The children with autism were not high functioning; therefore, control participants were matched in mental but not chronological age, leading to a different age range for the groups. Because the participants were matched for mental age, some of the differences found could be because of maturation differences in search behavior.
					
					The predominant analyses used were correlations, and the sample size is smaller than what would typically be thought of as ideal for that kind of statistic.

Kagerer, Bo, Contreras-Vidal, & Clark (2004)	The objective of this study was to examine motor adaptation in children with DCD.	Level II *Design* Group comparison This study consisted of 2 groups. The first group had 7 children in it (1 girl, 6 boys) ages 6–8. These children had to have an M–ABC ≤25th percentile, normal cognitive ability, and a physician's diagnosis of DCD. The second group consisted of 7 typically developing children who were matched for age and gender. They had to score >40th percentile on the M–ABC and demonstrate normal cognitive intelligence.	No intervention was used. Children were diagnosed with DCD with the M–ABC, the Woodcock–Johnson Revised Cognitive Ability Early Development Scale, and the Physical and Neurological Examination for Soft Signs. Participants sat at a computer with their dominant hand holding a pen on a digitizing tablet. Vision of the hand was occluded. Custom software collected data on the position of the pen. Visual feedback on the pen movements was given in real time on the computer screen. Participants drew a line between a home position and a target position that occurred in 1 of 4 different positions around the home.	The children with DCD had slower movement times across the 4 baseline blocks. The DCD group appeared to be less affected by the visual feedback perturbation than the children in the control group. The control group members reduced their variability during exposure, whereas the group with DCD did not. Significant aftereffects were only present for ML in the control group and not at all in the group with DCD. Both groups showed a reduction of movement time, normalized jerk, and movement length, indicating improvement as a result of an adaptation process.	This study had a small sample size. The number of trials used may not have been enough to establish aftereffects in the groups with DCD.

			The task was performed under 3 conditions: 1. 20 trials under normal visual feedback 2. 60 trials in which the orientation of the feedback was rotated clockwise 45° 3. 20 trials under normal visual feedback *Outcome Measures* • Movement time • Initial directional error • Normalized jerk • Movement length • Root-mean-square error	
Kaplan, Wilson, Dewey, & Crawford (1998)	The objective of the study was to explore some of the issues surrounding DCD as a specific learning disability and more specifically to look at the overlap between the 3 disorders: reading disability, DCD, and ADHD.	Level II *Design* Group comparison 224 children with learning and attention problems participated in the study. 155 typically developing children also participated in the study. No child was referred to this study because of motor problems specifically. The main control group was made up of 112 control participants matched on age, gender, and socioeconomic status. The remaining 43 control participants were from a separate study and they had identical data. All children were between ages 8 and 18. Any child with an estimated IQ <75 was excluded from the study.	No intervention was used. All participants were tested 1 time. The WISC–III was administered to test IQ, and any participant with an IQ of <75 was excluded. *Outcome Measures* • BOTMP: Some of the children were tested on the M–ABC, but not all because it was not available until 1995. • DCD Questionnaire, filled out by the parent, was also given. To access the children's reading ability, the following tests were given: • Woodcock–Johnson Psychoeducational Battery–Revised • Woodcock Reading Mastery Test • WRAT–Revised • Auditory Analysis Test The following tests were given to assess whether the child had ADHD: • Diagnostic Interview Schedule for Children • CBCL • Abbreviated Symptom Questionnaire	Using test scores and standards from the BOTMP, 21.4% of the children were deemed as having DCD (scored <15th percentile on ≥2 of the 4 subtests). Of the 81 children who were diagnosed as having DCD, 61 came from the referred sample and 20 from the control group. The best agreement among tests was the BOTMP Battery Composite and Gross Motor Composite and the M–ABC. The DCD Questionnaire had poor agreement with the other tests. The BOTMP–short form had the most agreement with other tests (79%), followed by the 3 composite scores of the BOTMP. The DCD Questionnaire and the M–ABC had the lowest average agreement. Comorbidity was examined for a sample of 162 children for whom all the data were available. 53 children had a "pure" diagnosis of only reading disability ($n = 19$), ADHD ($n = 8$), or DCD ($n = 26$). 47 did not meet criteria for any of the diagnoses. 62 were comorbid cases (39 met criteria for 2 of the 3 diagnoses, and 23 met criteria in all 3 categories).	The large testing window could have introduced many confounding variables (1992–1997).

(Continued)

Appendix C. Evidence Tables 121

Table C2. Summary of the Evidence Supporting Subtypes of Children With Difficulty Processing and Integrating Sensory Information (cont.)

Author/Year	Study Objectives	Level/Design/Participants	Intervention and Outcome Measures	Results	Study Limitations
Kern et al. (2006)	The objective of the study was to better understand the extent and role of sensory dysfunction in children with autism.	Level II *Design* Cross-sectional group comparison 104 people were in the first group, all with the diagnosis of autism, ages 3–56. There were 25 female participants and 79 male participants. The participants were recruited to fill 7 age categories: 3–7, 8–12, 13–17, 18–22, 23–27, 28–32, and 33+. Each category had no fewer than 12 participants. The diagnoses (all of which were given during childhood) were confirmed at the time of the study using *DSM–IV* criteria. 104 gender- and age-matched control participants also participated. All the people in the second group had no history of mental illness or learning, neurological, or developmental disorders. Exclusion criteria were blindness or deafness.	No intervention was used. CARS was used to assess the severity of autism within the group of participants with autism. The Sensory Profile was completed for all participants.	The results indicated that there was a significant difference between groups using the transformed auditory, visual, touch, and oral sensory processing measures. As participants with autism aged, sensory processing responses became more typical, except for low threshold touch, which did not improve significantly. These changes over time were not observed in the control group.	For the control group, some of the Sensory Profiles were completed by a family member, and some were completed by the individual. The caregiver version of the Sensory Profile was given to all participants, even adolescents and adults (some items on the caregiver version may not be appropriate for adolescents and adults), which could account for some of the age differences.
Lin, Cermak, Coster, & Miller (2005)	The objective was to examine the relationship between the length of institutionalization and various aspects of SI in children adopted from Eastern Europe.	Level II *Design* Group comparison 60 school-age children adopted from Eastern European countries to the United States were divided into 2 groups: LIH (>18 mo spent in institutionalization) and SIH (<6 mo spent in institutionalization). This time frame refers to how long the child spent in an institution before being adopted. *LIH:* 12 girls, 18 boys. Mean age = 74.4 mo, range = 51–107 mo.	No intervention was used. Measures were obtained only 1 time to determine differences between groups. *Outcome Measures* • SIPT • Developmental and Sensory Processing Questionnaire	The LIH group scored significantly lower than the SIH group on 5 of the 9 tactile, vestibular, proprioceptive, and visual form and space SIPT tests (Standing and Walking Balance, Kinesthesia, Spatial Visualization, Figure–Ground Perception, Manual Form Perception). The LIH group also scored lower than the SIH group on 3 of the 5 praxis tests (Bilateral Motor Coordination, Sequencing Praxis, Oral Praxis). The LIH group scored lower than the SIH group in 12 of the 17 SIPT tests. In addition, the distribution of scores	The study is confounded by the fact that to have comparable ages between the 2 groups, time spent in adoptive homes was less for those in the LIH group. The SIH group was not randomly selected from a pool of eligible participants, as was the case in the LIH group. Generalizability of the results to children who were not institutionalized in Eastern European countries and the United States is not possible. Moreover, there was no control group in the study.

Author/Year	Study Objectives	Level/Design/Participants	Intervention and Outcome Measures	Results	Study Limitations
		SIH: 14 girls, 16 boys. Mean age = 76.1 mo, range = 48–98 mo. Children were excluded if they had any syndromes, neurological disorders, or primary sensory deficits.		for the SIH was comparable to the normative sample. On the Developmental and Sensory Processing Questionnaire, the LIH group scored significantly higher (more problems) than the SIH group in Touch Seeks, Movement Seeks, Touch Total, Movement Total, Vision, and Audition.	The norms of the SIPT were only for children from the United States, not other countries, so results must be viewed with caution. The Developmental and Sensory Processing Questionnaire lacks reliability and validity evidence and is not norm referenced.
Liss, Saulnier, Fein, & Kinsbourne (2006)	The objective of this study was to examine whether sensory overreactivity can be explained by response to overarousal in a group of children with autism.	Level III *Design* Cross-sectional survey Parent questionnaires were filled out for 222 children who were on the autism spectrum. Parents of 191 children were contacted for follow-up data. Complete data sets were available for 144 children. Diagnoses were confirmed using *DSM–IV* criteria. The mean age of the children was 102.4 mo, and the sample was 79.9% male.	No intervention was used. Parents filled out the following items: • The Sensory Questionnaire, designed for this study, using 60 items from the Sensory Profile • A question about exceptional memory • *DSM–IV* checklist for autism symptoms • Kinsbourne Overfocusing Scale • Vineland Adaptive Behavior Scales	4 stable clusters were derived from the results. Cluster 1 participants (*n* = 17) featured overreactivity to sensory stimuli, perseverative behavior, high overfocusing, and an exceptional memory. Cluster 2 participants (*n* = 36) were relatively high functioning, were not significantly impaired, and exhibited few sensory problems. Cluster 3 participants (*n* = 44) were low functioning with prominent underreactivity and sensory seeking. Cluster 4 participants (*n* = 47) were low on autistic symptoms and high on adaptive functioning and sensory overreactivity, but not as high as Cluster 1 participants on overfocusing, and had an exceptional memory. When a 3-cluster solution is forced, Cluster 4 combines with the Cluster 1, but this combination obscures the overfocusing of Group 1. Cluster 4 members were significantly older than the other clusters.	Study is of good quality.
Martinussen, Hayden, Hogg-Johnson, & Tannock (2005)	The objective was to determine the empirical evidence for deficits in specific modality (spatial vs. verbal) or processing requirements (storage vs. central executive manipulation)	Level I *Design* Meta-analysis 26 studies were included and were published between 1997 and 2003.	No intervention took place. 26 empirical research studies investigating working memory were reviewed using meta-analytic procedures.	Most studies were not confounded by medications. Children with ADHD experience moderate to severe impairment in working memory tasks; this	It was impossible to examine whether comorbid psychiatric disorders or ADHD subtype differences moderated working memory differences, because too few

(Continued)

Appendix C. Evidence Tables

Table C2. Summary of the Evidence Supporting Subtypes of Children With Difficulty Processing and Integrating Sensory Information (cont.)

Author/Year	Study Objectives	Level/Design/Participants	Intervention and Outcome Measures	Results	Study Limitations
	of working memory processes in children with ADHD. Working memory relates to this question because of the differentiation of spatial and verbal working memory skills in children with ADHD.	Studies selected had to include children who were ages 4–18. Children had to have a diagnosis of ADHD. At least 1 of the comparison groups had to consist of normally developing children, and children in both the typically developing group and the ADHD group had to have an IQ of >70.		finding varies according to the modality of the task being used. Large impairments were found in both spatial storage and spatial central executive tasks. More moderate impairments were found in the verbal storage and verbal central executive tasks. Controlling for reading difficulties or language impairments explained a significant amount of variance for the spatial storage domain. However, this finding did not explain a significant amount of variance in the verbal storage or verbal central executive domains.	studies were included that examined these variables. There was variability in diagnostic criteria, and the number of studies within each diagnostic category was small; therefore, this potentially confounding variable could not be analyzed statistically. Publication bias appeared to be present in the spatial storage domain, which may have increased the effect sizes, because unpublished data tend to have smaller effect sizes.
Minshew, Sung, Jones, & Furman (2004)	The purpose of this study was to examine postural control in autism, specifically to determine whether postural abnormalities occur in children with autism and are related to age.	Level II *Design* Group comparison The study used 79 highly functioning people with autism and 61 control participants who were matched to the group with autism on the basis of age and IQ scores. The ages of both groups ranged from 5 to 52. All participants had IQ scores of >70. The participants with autism were excluded if they had any of the following: neurological disorder, genetic disorder, infectious disorder, metabolic disorder, or seizure disorder or were on any medications. Diagnoses of autism were confirmed with an expert clinical evaluation and assessment. The control participants were excluded if they had any of the following: learning or language disability; medical condition requiring regular medication; autism in first-, second-, or third-degree relatives.	No intervention was used. Each participant was tested 1 time. Dynamic posturography was measured using EquiTest. This test included a sensory organization and movement coordination portion. Participants performed under 6 conditions: 1. Fixed platform, eyes open with fixed visual surround 2. Fixed platform, eyes closed 3. Fixed platform, eyes open with sway referenced visual surround 4. Sway referenced platform, eyes open with fixed visual surround 5. Sway referenced platform, eyes closed 6. Sway referenced platform, eyes open with sway referenced visual surround A score of 100 represented no sway, whereas a score of 0 represented a fall.	The people with autism performed significantly worse on all 6 conditions of the sway test. Thus, the people with autism swayed more than control participants, and this was especially true in the conditions in which the sway referenced support surface was used. When looking at the age effects, it was found that development of postural stability was delayed in those people who had autism.	Study is of good quality.

Molloy, Dietrich, & Bhattacharya (2003)	The objective was to measure the postural stability of children with ASD compared with that of children with typical neurological development and to examine the contributions of the visual, vestibular, and somatosensory systems in each group.	Level II *Design* 2-group case–control 8 boys were recruited from a hospital with the criteria being that they had autism or ASD. 8 children matched by age, gender, and race to the children with ASD were in the control group.	This was not an intervention study. Each group was tested once and compared. The AccuSway force platform was used to measure postural sway in 4 conditions that selectively challenge visual, somatosensory, or vestibular input to balance. The Autism Behavior Checklist was given to the parents to complete. Middle-ear pressure, height, weight, foot length, and foot width were all measured because these parameters have been shown in previous studies to covary with postural stability.	The 2 groups did not differ on all of the control variables, including motor abilities. The higher the sway area was, the more at risk the person was for losing balance. For all the conditions in which ≥1 afferent system was modified (visual, somatosensory, vestibular), the children with ASD had a significantly larger sway area than the matched control participants. In all conditions in which visual input was removed, the sway area was significantly greater for children with ASD than for the control participants. Postural stability was not related to symptom severity as measured by the Autism Behavior Checklist test.	The authors did not differentiate in this study between PDD–Not Otherwise Specified and AD. Generalization to children with ASD who have more severe language and cognitive deficits is not possible because the boys in this study were all high functioning. The sample size was small; perhaps there were differences in the control variables between the 2 groups that were not significant because of this lack of power.
Mulligan (1998)	The objective of this study was to evaluate and confirm the 5-factor model of SI dysfunction on the basis of the SIPT. The hypothesized model of factors was as follows: somatosensory processing, bilateral integration and sequencing, somatopraxis, postural ocular movements, visuopraxis.	Level III *Design* Cross-sectional 10,475 existing SIPT test scores were used. They were obtained from 1989 to 1993. Most children in the group had mild disabilities. The entire sample is referred to as the heterogeneous sample. Children with a marked learning disability (*n* = 995) were analyzed as a subgroup.	No intervention was used. The SIPT was administered to all the children.	All 5 patterns of dysfunction were highly correlated with each other. The original hypothesized model had a reasonable fit, but there were weaknesses such as the high correlation between factors. Thus, additional 3-factor, 4-factor, and 5-factor solutions were examined. These revised models eliminated the postural ocular movement pattern and included a praxis pattern in place of the somatopraxis pattern. The 4 first-order factors that were involved with the best model were visuoperceptual deficit, bilateral integration and sequencing deficit, dyspraxia, and somatosensory deficit.	The group of children with learning disabilities may not have been accurately characterized by the therapists conducting the SIPT; thus, this may not have been a homogeneous group. The 4 subtests of the SIPT have weak test-retest reliability.
Mulligan (2000)	The objective of the study was to perform a cluster analysis of children using the scores on the SIPT. This analysis was to explore subgroupings and to examine the 6 profiles currently used in SIPT interpretation.	Level III *Design* Cross-sectional The scores of the SIPT for 1,961 children that were administered 1989–1993 were used in this study. The children were ages	No intervention was used. The SIPT was administered to all the children.	3-, 4-, 5-, and 6- cluster solutions were examined, and the author believed the 5-cluster solution was the best. Although this solution does not indicate specific types of dysfunction, it does indicate the level of severity.	The time window when the tests were administered was quite long (4 yr), which could introduce confounding factors, including history. Only children who had a suspected SI problem

(Continued)

Table C2. Summary of the Evidence Supporting Subtypes of Children With Difficulty Processing and Integrating Sensory Information *(cont.)*

Author/Year	Study Objectives	Level/Design/Participants	Intervention and Outcome Measures	Results	Study Limitations
		4–8 and were primarily White (86%). There were 1,425 boys and 536 girls. Most were receiving special education.		Cluster 1 included 11% of the sample and showed generalized sensory dysfunction and severe dyspraxia. Cluster 2 included 29.6% of the children and was labeled dyspraxia. Z scores were higher than for Cluster 1, although many were still in the dysfunctional range. Cluster 3 included 8.4% of the children and was labeled generalized sensory dysfunction and moderate dyspraxia. Many of the tests were in the dysfunctional range, but not as low as in Cluster 1. Cluster 4 was labeled low-average bilateral integration and sequencing and included 36.6% of the children. This cluster represents children functioning at an average level but with specific difficulties. Cluster 5 was labeled average SI and praxis and included 14.2% of the children. All children in this cluster scored within average range on the SIPT.	(most were receiving special education) were included in the sample, reducing the generalizability to other populations.
Murray, Cermak, & O'Brien (1990)	The objective of the study was to assess the relationship between clumsiness and both visual perception and visual construction (measured by the SIPT) in children with LD.	Level II *Design* Group comparison 2 groups The first group had 21 children; age range was 5 yr 4 mo to 8 yr 7 mo. All children had a diagnosed LD and were receiving special education. This group was further divided into 2 groups on the basis of their scores on the TMI. 12 were classified as clumsy and 9 were classified as nonclumsy. 18 children participated as control participants. Their age range was 5 yr 1 mo to 8 yr 10 mo. None of the children were receiving special education.	No intervention was used. The TMI was given to distribute the children in 2 appropriate groups on the basis of motor ability. The SIPT was administered to all the children.	Both of the groups with LD scored worse than the control group on 4 of the 6 SIPT subtests (Space Visualization, Motor Accuracy, Design Copying, and Constructional Praxis). The clumsy group differed from the nonclumsy group only on the Motor Accuracy and Design Copying tests. There were significant correlations between the score on the TMI and performance on the SIPT on 3 of the 6 subtests (Space Visualization, Motor Accuracy, and Design Copying).	3 children in the control group scored in the mild clumsy range.

Author (Year)	Study Objectives	Level/Design/Participants	Intervention and Outcome Measures	Results	Study Limitations
O'Brien, Cermak, & Murray (1988)	The objective of the study was to investigate the relationship between visual–perceptual and visual–motor deficits and clumsiness in children with LD.	Level II *Design* Group comparison 2 groups The first group had 22 children; age range was 5 yr to 8 yr 10 mo. Each child in this group was diagnosed as having an LD and was receiving special education (16 boys, 6 girls). The group was further broken down into 2 groups using the TMI. 13 were determined to be clumsy, and 9 were determined to be nonclumsy. The second group served as a control and consisted of 22 children without LD. They ranged from 5 yr 6 mo to 8 yr 11 mo (16 boys, 6 girls).	No intervention was used. The following tests were given to all children: • TMI • Developmental Test of Visual–Motor Integration–Revised • Raven's Progressive Matrices • Block Design from the WISC-R • Primary Visual–Motor Test • Rey–Osterrieth Complex Figure Test	Significant differences were found on each measure between the control group and the clumsy group. There were significant correlations between the TMI and Raven's Progressive Matrices (visual–perceptual) and also between the TMI and the Block Design and Rey–Osterrieth Complex Figure Test. There was also a significant correlation found between the TMI and the Primary Visual–Motor Test.	3 children in the control group scored in the mild clumsy range.
O'Riordan & Passetti (2006)	The objective of this study was to assess auditory and tactile discrimination ability in children with autism.	Level II *Design* Group comparison *Experiments 1 and 2:* The first group had 12 children all diagnosed as having high-functioning autism. The mean age was 8 yr 7 mo. The second group consisted of 12 children who were typically developing and served as control participants. Their mean age was 8 yr 7 mo. *Experiment 3:* The group with autism had 13 children, and the control group had 13 children. The mean age for both groups was 10 yr. The rest of the information is the same (e.g., cognitive levels) as Experiments 1 and 2.	No intervention was used. The Raven's Progressive Matrices were used to determine the cognitive ability of the children. *Experiment 1:* The participants heard 2 different tones. 1 of them stayed the same, and the other changed until it became the same frequency as the other tone. The child had to indicate when he or she thought this happened. The time it took to do this was measured. *Experiment 2:* 4 different grades of sandpaper were used. The participant was then presented with pairs of sandpaper and had to tell whether they were the same or different. When the child said the papers were different, he or she had to indicate which paper was rougher. The participant did the task without visual cues (the experimenter also could not see the sandpaper presented).	*Experiment 1:* The children with autism said the tones were the same significantly later in the sequence than did the control participants. This finding indicates they are superior when discriminating between auditory stimuli compared with the performance of the control group. *Experiment 2:* No difference was found between the 2 groups on the ability to discriminate tactile stimuli. *Experiment 3:* There was no difference between the 2 groups in tactile discrimination.	Only children with high-functioning autism were used, so generalization to all children with autism is not possible.

Appendix C. Evidence Tables

(Continued)

Table C2. Summary of the Evidence Supporting Subtypes of Children With Difficulty Processing and Integrating Sensory Information (cont.)

Author/Year	Study Objectives	Level/Design/Participants	Intervention and Outcome Measures	Results	Study Limitations
			Experiment 3: Children had to tell when a string (Von Frey hairs of different diameters) was or was not touching their arm. They had their eyes closed and were looking away.		
Parush, Sohmer, Steinberg, & Kaitz (1997)	The objective of this study was to examine whether ADHD is related to deficits in somatosensory processing.	Level II *Design* Group comparison 2 groups The first group had 49 children; all of them were diagnosed as having ADHD by a professional using *DSM–III–R* criteria. The mean age was 7.7 yr, and each child had normal intelligence. Children also had to be free of medication for ≥1 mo before testing. All the children were boys. The control group, without ADHD, was made up of 49 children who were age- and gender-matched to the first group. In addition, all the children were tested to determine whether they had learning problems. Of the group with ADHD, 84% had learning problems; of the control participants, 8% had learning problems.	No intervention was used. *Outcome Measures* • Touch Inventory for Preschoolers • Texture threshold: Each child's threshold was measured using a custom-made discrimination task • SIPT • The Somatosensory Evoked Potential is a response of the somatosensory pathway. It was evoked by delivering electrical pulses to the median nerve at the wrist. 4 electrodes were placed on the Erb's point, 7th cervical vertebrae, forehead, and the somatosensory cortex. Latencies and amplitudes from the averaged evoked potential were measured.	Touch Inventory for Preschoolers scores were significantly higher for the group with ADHD than for the control group. None of the control participants and 39.5% of the ADHD group were labeled as tactilely defensive from the Touch Inventory for Preschoolers scores. Significant differences were found between the control group and the group with ADHD on all 6 SIPT subtests administered. There was no significant difference between groups on the threshold measure. For the Somatosensory Evoked Potential results, amplitudes of the N13, N20, and P23 were significantly larger for the group with ADHD than were those for the control participants, but there was no significant difference between groups at the periphery (P9 measure).	Study is of good quality.
Pfeiffer, Kinnealey, Reed, & Herzberg (2005)	The objective of the study was to determine whether there are significant relationships between dysfunction in sensory modulation, symptoms of affective disorders, and adaptive behaviors in children and adolescents with AD.	Level III *Design* Correlational The participants were parents of 50 children (42 boys, 8 girls) ages 6–17. All the children had been diagnosed with AD using *DSM–IV* criteria. The children were broken into 2 groups, older (ages 11–17) and younger (ages 6–10). There were 30 children in the younger group and 20 in the older group.	No intervention was used. The following measures were filled out by the parents: • The Sensory Profile measured sensory hypersensitivity and hyposensitivity. • The Adolescent/Adult Sensory Profile was also used. This is usually a self-report, but it was filled out by the parents in this case. • The Adaptive Behavior Assessment System was used to assess typical daily adaptive living skills.	There was a significant relationship between sensory hypersensitivity and anxiety for the entire group and both groups divided by age. Both components of sensory hypersensitivity (sensory sensitivity and sensory avoiding) also had a significant relationship with anxiety. There was a significant relationship between depression and hyporesponsiveness for the whole group and the older group but not for the younger group.	A convenience sample was used in which the children were on different medications and participating in different treatments.

			• The Revised Children's Manifest Anxiety Scale Adapted Parent Version was used to measure the level and nature of anxiety in the children. • The Children's Depression Inventory Adapted Parents Version assessed symptoms of depression.	There was a significant relationship between sensory seeking and symptoms of depression in the whole group and in the older group with symptoms of depression and low registration. A significant relationship was found between symptoms of depression and hypersensitivity in the whole group and younger group but not in the older group. There were no significant relationships between overall adaptive behavior and affective disorders. There were no significant relationships between sensory processing and adaptive behaviors.	
Piek et al. (2004)	The objective of the study was to measure parent report of attention in children with ADHD to determine whether there would be a relationship between motor coordination, attention, and executive functioning.	Level III *Design* Correlational There were 238 participants in the study (117 boys, 121 girls). The mean age was 10.58. The children's verbal IQ had to be >80 to be included in the study. Of the total sample, 28 were identified as being at risk for DCD by scoring <80 on the Neurodevelopmental Index of the McCarron Assessment of Neuromuscular Development. Children who scored ≥100 were put in the control group.	No interventions were used. The WISC–III was used to determine verbal IQ score. The Neurodevelopmental Index of the McCarron Assessment of Neuromuscular Development assessed fine and gross motor skills. The CBCL measured internalizing and externalizing behavior problems in children. The Choice Reaction Time Task assessed visual inspection time. The following computer tasks were used to assess executive functioning: • Go/No-Go assessed motor inhibition • Trail Making/Memory Updating task assessed working memory and behavioral inhibition • Goal Neglect Task	There was a significant relationship between the Neurodevelopmental Index score and inattention. Girls were faster than boys in the Choice Reaction Time Task. Of the 15 measures of executive functioning, the Neurodevelopmental Index correlated with 7 of them. In all cases, better performance on the executive functioning task correlated with higher Neurodevelopmental Index scores. For the Go/No-Go, age was found to be a significant predictor. For the Trail Making/Memory Updating task, Neurodevelopmental Index was a significant predictor of executive functioning once other variables were accounted for. Age and verbal IQ were significant predictors of the Goal Neglect Task. The main effect of group (control vs. those at risk for DCD) was found to be significant.	Study is of good quality.

(Continued)

Appendix C. Evidence Tables   129

Table C2. Summary of the Evidence Supporting Subtypes of Children With Difficulty Processing and Integrating Sensory Information *(cont.)*

Author/Year	Study Objectives	Level/Design/Participants	Intervention and Outcome Measures	Results	Study Limitations
Rinehart et al. (2006)	The objective of this study was to examine movement kinematics in children with high-functioning autism and AD.	Level II *Design* Group comparison 4 groups The first group had 12 children (10 boys, 2 girls). They were all diagnosed using *DSM–IV* criteria as having high-functioning autism. This group was compared with Group 1, a control group matched on age, gender, and IQ. The mean age for both of these groups was 8.1. The third group was made up of 12 children with AD (10 boys, 2 girls). The mean age was 12. This group was compared with another control group selected to be age, gender, and IQ matched to the people from Group 3. The mean age was 11.9.	No intervention was used. The task involved a noninking pen used on a digitizing tablet. There were 3 levels to the task. *Level 1:* Participants had to move the pen quickly toward a target after illumination of the target. *Level 2:* Participants were told where most of the targets would appear (75% vs. 25%). When presented in the unexpected location, they had to inhibit moving to the expected location. *Level 3:* There was an expected side in this condition as well, but the participants had to move to the opposite side of where they saw the target. Errors were measured as mildly, moderately, or severely moving in the wrong direction. Errors were not included in the kinematic analyses. Kinematic measures included preparatory time, movement time, and asymmetry ratio (the shape of the trajectory).	Children with high-functioning autism were slower to prepare their movements than control participants in Levels 1, 2, and 3. The AD group showed similar preparation time as control participants. In movement time, the high-functioning autism group was not affected by expectancy (they did not show faster times when it was to the expected side), but both control groups and the AD group showed this expectancy advantage (they were faster going to the side on which 75% of the targets appeared).	Direct comparison of the group with high-functioning autism and the group with AD was not done because of the age gap. There was a small sample size for all the groups. Because some of the *p* values were nearing significance, it would be helpful to determine whether adding more participants would change these values.
Rogers, Hepburn, & Wehner (2003)	The objective of this study was to examine reports of sensory symptoms in children with DD and to examine the role these symptoms play in the acquisition of adaptive behavior.	Level II *Design* Group comparison 102 children participated in this study and were divided into 4 groups on the basis of diagnosis. The first group had 26 children with autism (mean age = 33.67 mo). The second group had 20 children with fragile X syndrome (mean age = 36.11 mo).	The Mullen Scales of Early Learning were used to determine the mental age of the participants. The Short Sensory Profile was filled out by the parents of all the children to obtain measurement of sensory dysfunction. The Autism Diagnostic Interview–Revised assesses the presence and severity of symptoms of autism.	The children with autism and fragile X had significantly higher scores on the Sensory Profile than did the children with DD and typically developing children. The children with autism had higher scores on the taste/smell category than all the other groups and higher tactile sensitivity and auditory filtering than the children with DD and typically developing children.	The typically developing children did have a significantly higher verbal mental age than did the children with autism. Some of the children with fragile X had autism and some did not.

The third group had 32 children with DD of unknown etiology (mean age = 33.23 mo).

The final group had 24 typically developing children (mean age = 19.5 mo). The control group was younger but matched with other groups on mental age.

The Autism Diagnostic Observation Schedule–Generic elicits autistic behaviors in 4 areas: social interaction, communication, play, and repetitive behaviors.

The VABS reports adaptive behavior scores.

The children with fragile X had higher scores on the low energy/weak muscles than all the other groups and higher scores on tactile sensitivity, underreactive/seeks stimulation, and auditory filtering when compared with the children with DD and typically developing children.

The children with autism and fragile X did not differ from each other but did have significantly higher scores than the children with DD and typically developing children when looking at the Autism Diagnostic Interview–Revised.

The same results were true for the Autism Diagnostic Observation Schedule–Generic.

On the Autism Diagnostic Interview–Revised, the children with autism had higher scores on the repetitive–restrictive behaviors than all the other groups.

Total sensory scores were moderately related to the repetitive–restrictive behaviors on the Autism Diagnostic Observation Schedule–Generic in the children with autism.

Ratio IQ and Autism Diagnostic Interview–Revised total scores were moderately related to sensory symptoms in the children with fragile X.

The Sensory Profile was moderately related to the repetitive–restrictive behaviors in the group with autism.

The standard score on the Mullen Scales of Early Learning was the best predictor of adaptive behavior.

(Continued)

Table C2. Summary of the Evidence Supporting Subtypes of Children With Difficulty Processing and Integrating Sensory Information (*cont.*)

Author/Year	Study Objectives	Level/Design/Participants	Intervention and Outcome Measures	Results	Study Limitations
Rubia, Taylor, Taylor, & Sergeant (1999)	The objective of the study was to investigate temporal organization in children who have high hyperactive behavior.	Level II *Design* Group comparison 2 groups The first group consisted of 11 boys with a mean age of 9.4. All the boys were selected from special education services and scored ≥94th percentile on the attention problems scales of the CBCL or Teacher Rating Form. Exclusion criteria included having a learning disability. The control group was made up of 11 boys with a mean age of 9. They all rated <75th percentile on the CBCL or Teacher Rating Form. None of the participants were on medication. They all scored ≥80 on a full-scale IQ measure.	No intervention was used. The following tasks were completed by all the participants: • *Sensorimotor Anticipation Task*: The participants had to predict by pushing a button when the fourth of 4 stimuli would appear. The interstimulus interval was fixed. • *Free Tapping Task*: The participants had to push a response button 80 times at a freely chosen rhythm. • *Sensorimotor Synchronization Task*: The participants had to coordinate a motor response made with their right finger on a response button to a visual stimulus that appeared at a fixed rate (500, 700, 1,200, 1,800 ms). • *Time Discrimination Task*: 2 visual stimuli appeared on screen, the first always for 5 s and the second for either 3 s or 5 s. The participant had to indicate with a button press whether they were onscreen for the same amount of time or not (right button for same duration or left button for different duration).	The full-scale IQ was significantly different between groups, with the control participants having a higher mean (with the verbal IQ accounting for the differences). *Sensorimotor Anticipation Task*: Anticipation time was not significantly different between the 2 groups. There was a significant group difference for impulsive errors, with the children who were hyperactive making more. There was a significant negative correlation between age and the variability of anticipation time, and number of impulsive errors. There was also a significant correlation between the number of impulsive errors and the scores on the CBCL and Teacher Rating Form. *Free Tapping Task*: There were no significant differences between groups on the mean tapping time. However, children with ADHD had a significantly larger standard deviation than did the control participants. There was a significant correlation between variability of response and age (as age increases, variability decreases) and scores on the CBCL and Teacher Rating Form. *Sensorimotor Synchronization Task*: Contrary to what was expected, the children with ADHD did not show an overall earlier adjustment to respond. However, there was a significant effect in the shortest time interval, in which the children with ADHD had a faster synchronization time. *Time Discrimination Task*: There was no group difference in errors or mean time for decision. However, there was a significant group difference for the variability of decision time.	A small sample size was used. The children differed on IQ scores and thus were not a comparable sample; however, when IQ was used as a covariate, it did not account for a significant amount of variance or change the results.

Sigmundsson, Hansen, & Talcott (2003)	The objective of this study was to examine visual processing in children with DCD using 3 different psychophysical tasks.	Level II *Design* Group comparison 2 groups The first group was made up of 13 children who were tested on the M–ABC and scored the highest (indicating motor problems) out of a sample of 54 children. They were designated as the clumsy group. The mean age was 10.6 (7 girls, 6 boys). The 13 who scored the lowest made up the control group. The mean age was 10.5 (7 girls, 6 boys).	No intervention was used. The M–ABC was given to determine which children had motor problems. 3 visual processing tasks were used: • Measure of global motion processing • Measure of static global pattern processing where the target position was randomized • Measure of static global pattern processing where the target position was fixed	The children who were clumsy had a higher threshold for all 3 of the tasks compared with the control participants. The thresholds for global form sensitivity were highly correlated across all participants. Significant correlations were found between the M–ABC and all 3 tasks. This was in the direction of poor motor skills correlating to lowered visual sensitivity.	The small sample size limits generalizability. IQ was not tested; thus, there may be other differences between the groups than just motor problems. Eye movement control also was not tested in the 2 groups.
Sigmundsson & Hopkins (2005)	The objective of this study was to investigate visual recognition in children with HECP.	Level II *Design* Group comparison 2 groups The first group was made up of the 10 children, from a sample of 80, who scored the highest (indicating motor problems) on the hand–eye coordination tasks on the M–ABC. The mean age was 7.7, and there were 4 girls and 6 boys. The 10 children with the lowest scores made up the control group. The mean age was 8, and there were 6 girls and 4 boys.	No intervention was used. The M–ABC was given to determine which children had motor problems. The visual closure subtest from the Illinois Test of Psycholinguistic Abilities was given to all the children. This test involved the child looking at different scenes. Within each scene, there were partially hidden pictures of the same object. The child had to point out as many as possible.	The children with HECP identified significantly fewer objects than the control participants.	The small sample size limits generalizability. IQ was not tested and could be a confounding variable.
Smits-Engelsman, Wilson, Westenberg, & Duysens (2003)	The objective of this study was to answer the following 3 questions: 1. Are children with DCD/LD slower in their reaction time and movement time on a simple motor task compared with control children? 2. Are children with DCD/LD more sensitive to increased information load? 3. Do differences in movement time and accuracy between children with DCD/LD and control children increase or decrease depending on control mode?	Level II *Design* Group comparison From each of the 4 grades in Dutch schools for children with learning disabilities, 8 children were selected to participate ($n = 32$). They had no known movement disorder caused by medical diagnosis or physical handicap. The mean age was 11.3 (16 boys, 16 girls). All were classified as having DCD by DSM–IV criteria.	No intervention was used. The following measures were given to the children for classification purposes: • M–ABC • Concise Assessment Method for Children's Handwriting • WISC–R A graphical aiming task was used experimentally. The children had to draw a line between 2 targets using 2 movement directions (e.g., from top left to bottom right). 3 target sizes were used.	The children with DCD/LD moved faster but had a larger spread, which led to less accuracy in the target endpoint. They also used greater and more variable pressure. The children with DCD/LD made twice as many errors in the Cyclic Aiming Movement Regimen. The children with DCD/LD had a larger increase in endpoint spread in the 8-mm condition when compared with the control participants.	The current results do not totally rule out a feedback-processing deficit, and the results must be interpreted with caution.

(Continued)

Appendix C. Evidence Tables

Table C2. Summary of the Evidence Supporting Subtypes of Children With Difficulty Processing and Integrating Sensory Information (cont.)

Author/Year	Study Objectives	Level/Design/Participants	Intervention and Outcome Measures	Results	Study Limitations
		There was also a group of age- and gender-matched children without DCD ($n = 32$, mean age = 11.2).	Participants performed this task in 2 different movement regimens: 1. Discrete Aiming Movement Regimen (start on acoustic signal, reverse on next acoustic signal) 2. Cyclical Aiming Movement Regimen (start and end with 1 acoustic signal). All data were recorded using a digitizer tablet.	The difference in time between the Cyclic and Discrete Aiming Movement Regimen was larger for the children with DCD/LD. The children with DCD/LD moved faster when responding to the tone in starting movement in the Discrete Aiming Movement Regimen.	
Snow, Blondis, Accardo, & Cunningham (1993)	The objective of this study was to examine performance on motor and sensory tasks in children who were academically average and academically disabled.	Level II *Design* Group comparison/longitudinal 2 groups Each group was seen on 3 separate occasions (roughly 1 yr apart). The first group was made up of 17 children who were all identified as academically disabled. There were 12 boys and 5 girls in this group. 9 of these children were formally identified as having LD, and 8 were receiving remedial instruction in subjects such as reading or math. The mean age of participants in Session 1 was 73.88 mo; for Session 2, 84.76 mo; and for Session 3, 97.71 mo. The second group was made up of 28 children who acted as control participants (20 boys, 8 girls). The mean age of participants in Session 1 was 74.75 mo; for Session 2, 86.25 mo; and for Session 3, 99.39 mo.	No intervention was used. The following tasks were given to each child: • *Stereognosis*: The child had to identify 5 familiar objects (e.g., penny) with eyes open and closed. • *Graphesthesia*: The child was shown drawings (e.g., a circle). He or she then closed his or her eyes and had the form drawn in his or her palm and had to identify it. • *Motor coordination*: The child engaged in a hand pronation/supination task. • *Associated movements*: The child had to touch each finger in his or her hand with the thumb in succession. • *Motor slowness*: The hand pronation/supination, finger touching, and a heel–toe alternation task were timed.	Developmental trends in which children in both groups performed better over time were seen for most variables. On the graphesthesia task, there was a significant group and time effect. A significant group and time effect was found for motor coordination. There was also a significant Group × Time interaction. There was considerable developmental improvement for the group with academic disabilities. Both the group main effect and Group × Time interaction were significant for associated movements. In motor slowness, a significant group main effect was found, as was a significant Group × Time interaction, meaning that the group with academic disabilities got better at this task as they aged.	Because of the longitudinal nature of the study, attrition was a factor. There was a small sample size.
Stoodley, Fawcett, Nicolson, & Stein (2005)	The objective was to investigate standing balance in children with dyslexia.	Level II *Design* Group comparison 16 children with developmental dyslexia (11 boys, 5 girls). The average age was 11 yr 4 mo.	No intervention was used. All participants were tested 1 time. To measure verbal and nonverbal cognitive ability and verbal short-term memory, the WISC-R was used with a portion of the	The only cognitive measure that showed significant difference between the groups was the digit span (dyslexia group scored lower than the control group). There were significant group	There was a significant difference in the ages of the 2 groups. Relatively small sample size limits generalizability.

		19 children were in the control group (11 boys, 8 girls). The average age was 9 yr 4 mo. All the children were right-handed.	children. For the rest of the children, the British Abilities Scales II were used. To measure orthographic and phonological literacy abilities, the Orson Orthographic Test, a word–pseudohomophone discrimination task, and a phonological test were used. It presented 3 words, and the child had to decide which sounded like a real word. To measure balance, the Polhemus tracking system was used. The child was asked to balance as best as he or she could in the following conditions: • Right foot, eyes open • Right foot, eyes closed • Left foot, eyes open • Left foot, eyes closed	differences in the orthographic and phonological tasks, in which the children with dyslexia performed more errors on both tasks. The group with dyslexia performed significantly worse in the balancing task in the right-foot and left-foot eyes-open tasks. The children with dyslexia also dropped their foot significantly more than the control group in the eyes-closed balance tasks; however, there was no significant difference on the balance score between groups for the eyes-closed task. In both the control group and the group of children who had dyslexia, balancing ability significantly related to cognitive ability. Literacy and balance abilities were related only in the dyslexia group, not in the control group.	
Tecchio et al. (2003)	The objective of this study was to examine initial stages of auditory sensory processing through MEG recording of the mismatch field in children at the lower-functioning end of the autistic spectrum.	Level II *Design* Group comparison 14 people who met the *DSM–IV* criteria for autism participated in this study (11 male, 3 female). The age range was 8 to 32 ($M = 16$). 10 age- and gender-matched people also participated as control participants.	No intervention was used. The Adaptive Behavior Inventory yields an Adaptive Behavior Quotient, which assesses adaptive behavior. CARS was given to measure the severity of autism. An acoustic oddball paradigm was used with all participants, in which deviant stimuli were randomly interspersed with standard stimuli. They heard these tones while MEG recordings were being taken.	The Adaptive Behavior Quotient placed all the participants with autism in the intellectually disabled range compared with the control participants. All the participants with autism were moderately to severely impaired in verbal communication. The localization of the sources of the brain response occurring at approximately 100 ms showed a significantly deeper position for the participants with autism than for the control participants. The mismatch field total power was significantly lower in the participants with autism than in the control participants.	Small sample size limits generalizability. The participants with autism were suffering from other diagnoses that could have affected the results (e.g., seizures).

(Continued)

Table C2. Summary of the Evidence Supporting Subtypes of Children With Difficulty Processing and Integrating Sensory Information (cont.)

Author/Year	Study Objectives	Level/Design/Participants	Intervention and Outcome Measures	Results	Study Limitations
Tervo, Azuma, Fogas, & Fiechtner (2002)	The purpose of the study was to identify group differences between children who have ADHD–MD and those who have only ADHD and to determine the responsiveness to medication (methylphenidate) of the ADHD–MD group.	Level I *Design* Triple-blind, placebo-controlled crossover study A drug protocol was randomly assigned to each participant. 22 children were identified as having ADHD–MD (19 boys, 3 girls). All of the children in this group were classified as having severe motor problems and "soft neurological signs." 41 children were identified as having only ADHD (30 boys, 11 girls).	This was an intervention study evaluating the effects of medication (methylphenidate). *Outcome Measures* The treatment effects were measured using the Abbreviated Symptom Questionnaire for Parents and Teachers. The Side Effects Rating Scale measure commonly reported stimulant medication side effects. CBCL was used to measure behavioral problems assessed by caregivers. The Teacher Report Form measured behavioral problems according to the child's teacher. Conners' Parent Rating Scale assessed behavior on 5 domains and the Hyperactivity Index. Conners' Teacher Rating Scale is similar to Conners' Parent Rating Scale but for teachers. Child Attention Problems Rating Scale has an Inattention and Hyperactivity scale. These were used to sort the children into subgroups. The Home Situations Questionnaire measures the pervasiveness of child behavior problems across home situations. The School Situations Questionnaire rates the pervasiveness of child behavior problems in school settings. The Selective Motor Functioning Checklist was used to measure motor functioning.	Parents reported that children with ADHD–MD were more likely to have selective motor functioning problems (including falling; accident prone; less active in sports; tiring quickly; and having difficulty with jumping, skipping, and hopping). There was no association between having ADHD–MD and receiving special education (41 children with ADHD received it and 10 children with ADHD–MD received it). The ADHD–MD group had more severe problems with inattention and overactivity. Children with ADHD–MD had more extreme social problems, thought problems, and attention problems than did the group with ADHD. Parents and teachers reported that children with ADHD–MD had more severe and pervasive problems at home and at school than did the children with ADHD. Results of the medication trial show that both groups had a significant linear response to the medication. Results also showed that the medication was equally effective for both groups.	Before comparison with other studies can occur, more standardization needs to occur with regard to the neurological conditions present in addition to ADHD–MD. The study sample was small, so the lack of significant effects found in some of the analyses of variance could be caused by this lack of power.

| Toplak & Tannock (2005) | The objective was to investigate time perception performance with auditory and visual stimuli in children with and without ADHD. | Level II

Design
Group comparison
2 groups

The first group consisted of 46 adolescents (87% boys) who all were diagnosed as having ADHD. The second group was 44 adolescents (45.5% boys) with no disabilities. The mean age for both groups was 15.5. | No intervention was used. All participants were tested 1 time. To confirm the ADHD diagnosis, the Schedule for Affective Disorders and Schizophrenia for School Age Children Present and Lifetime Versions and Conners' Rating Scale were used to assess all the children in the clinical group.

The Wechsler Abbreviated Scale of Intelligence gave a measure of intelligence.

The WRAT–3, the Comprehensive Test for Phonological Processing, and the Test of Word Reading Efficiency were used to assess reading skills.

The Clinical Evaluation of Language Fundamentals was used to assess oral language ability.

The outcome measures of duration discrimination tasks also were administered. These included a visual and auditory task with 2 different interval lengths (200 and 1,000 ms). 2 control tasks also were administered (size and frequency discrimination).

Outcome measures for working memory and memory span included the digit span and spatial span from the WISC–III. | There was a significant effect of duration, meaning that both groups showed higher thresholds in the longer interval than in the shorter.

The people with ADHD displayed significantly higher thresholds in the duration discrimination tasks.

The lack of group differences found for the control tasks between the control group and the group with ADHD lends evidence to the notion that group differences on the duration discrimination task are not caused by general perceptual skills or a lack in response demands but actual time perception difficulties.

Visual–spatial memory was significantly associated with visual and auditory duration at the 1,000-ms interval for the group with ADHD. In addition, auditory memory was significantly associated with auditory duration threshold at the 1,000-ms interval for the control group. There were differences between the groups in auditory span memory, reading ability, and language ability. | Some of the children in the ADHD group were on medication; others were not. |

(Continued)

Table C2. Summary of the Evidence Supporting Subtypes of Children With Difficulty Processing and Integrating Sensory Information (cont.)

Author/Year	Study Objectives	Level/Design/Participants	Intervention and Outcome Measures	Results	Study Limitations
Van Waelvelde, De Weerdt, De Cock, & Smits-Engelsman (2004)	The objective of this study was to explore the relationship between perceptual tasks, perceptual–motor tasks, and overall motor ability in children with DCD and to examine the association with 3 specific motor tasks: tracing, jumping, and ball catching.	Level II *Design* Group comparison 2 groups The first group was made up of 36 children (22 boys, 14 girls; ages 9 and 10). They had to have an IQ >70. All scored <5th percentile on the M-ABC. The second group was made up of age and gender-matched control participants (n = 36; mean age = 10 yr, 1 mo), all of whom scored >15th percentile on the M-ABC.	No intervention was used. The M–ABC was used to determine which children had DCD. Timing of a response to a visual stimulus was measured. The children were instructed to click a mouse button when a moving ball (on screen) reached a target zone. The speed of the ball varied. The children performed a ball-catching task in which they had to catch a ball that was bounced to them as well as tossed. They had to catch with 2 hands and with 1 hand. The jumping item from the KTK also was used. They had to jump from side to side over a little beam as many times as they could in 15 s (KTK jump). The VMI was used, which consists of 27 geometric figures that have to be copied to paper (VMI copy). The supplemental VMI tracing task also was administered.	The children with DCD performed significantly worse than the control participants on all tasks except the systematic error of the visual timing task. In the group of children with DCD, visual timing was significantly related to the ball-catching task. The VMI copy task was significantly correlated to the M–ABC and the VMI tracing task.	A confounding factor is that the children in the DCD group had a lower mean IQ than the control group, and the IQ score was not used as a covariate in the analyses.
Van Waelvelde et al. (2006)	The objective was to examine whether children with DCD performed more poorly than control participants on the RMT, to examine whether children with DCD responded differently when sensory information was omitted when compared with control participants, and to examine whether deficits in movement parameterization were associated with movement and drawing.	Level II *Design* Comparison of 2 groups 36 children with DCD (mean age = 10) and an IQ of ≥70 were included. They had no PDD and no medical diagnosis that would interfere with their motor development. Only children who scored <5th percentile on the M-ABC were included in the study. 36 age- and gender-matched control participants (mean age = 10 yr, 1 mo). Only children who scored >15th percentile on the M-ABC were included in the control group.	This was not an intervention study. Each group was tested once and compared. The M–ABC is an identification and evaluation tool used with children who have mild to moderate motor impairment. 1 item from the KTK was used. This was a jumping test. The Motor Coordination test, a supplement of the VMI, was used. This was a drawing test. The RMT evaluates accuracy and stability in time and space, as well as fluency of rhythmic movements of the arm.	Children with DCD performed significantly worse on the M–ABC, KTK jump, and tracing test than the control participants. *Results for the RMT* Children with DCD were significantly less accurate in time and space and displayed larger variability when compared with the control group. When the audible signal was eliminated, both groups performed similarly. However, when vision was withdrawn, the children with DCD had more significant disturbances than the control group. There was a significant correlation between both the drawing task and the jumping task with several aspects of the RMT.	Several of the children in the DCD group had other DD that could have been a confounding factor in the results.

Vernazza-Martin et al. (2005)	The objective of the article was to address the following 3 questions: 1. Are gait parameters modified in children with autism? 2. Is equilibrium control affected in children with autism? 3. Is locomotion adjusted to the experimenter-imposed goal?	Level II *Design* Group comparison 9 children who were classified as autistic using *DSM–IV* guidelines participated in the study. Children who had Rett syndrome, AD, or disintegrative disorders of childhood were excluded from this sample. 6 typically developing children participated in the study. All the children were between the ages of 4 and 6.	No intervention was used. All participants were tested 1 time. A commercially available automatic motion analyzer system was used to perform kinematic gait analysis. The children wore a body suit with markers at specific locations on their feet, hip, and shoulder and behind the ear. Cameras recorded both the markers and the entire scene. The child was asked to walk a specified distance while being recorded. Trials ranged from 4 to 14 depending on the ability of the child and the acquired data. The following parameters were measured: • Stride duration, step length, gait velocity, cadence, swing, and stance period • The *SD* of the absolute head, shoulder, and pelvis angles • The stabilization of a given segment either on the external space or the underlying anatomical segment • Sacrum trajectory in the sagittal plane • Mean distance between the last sacrum positions and the center of the door • Mean orientation of the trajectory to the door	None of the gait parameters except step length were significantly different between the 2 groups, with the children who had autism taking shorter steps. When looking at the absolute angular dispersion of the head, it was shown that the children with autism oscillated their head and trunk segments in a more irregular manner than the typically developing children. The children with autism displayed more oscillations of the head in 3 planes, of the shoulder in the horizontal and frontal planes, of the pelvis in the horizontal plane, and of the trunk in the sagittal plane. These results suggest that the children with autism had less stability of the head, shoulder, pelvis, and trunk while walking compared with the control group. Children with autism also did not perform the task completely or as directly as the children in the control group.	Small sample size limits generalizability.

(Continued)

Table C2. Summary of the Evidence Supporting Subtypes of Children With Difficulty Processing and Integrating Sensory Information (cont.)

Author/Year	Study Objectives	Level/Design/Participants	Intervention and Outcome Measures	Results	Study Limitations
Vickers, Rodrigues, & Brown (2002)	The objective was to compare motor coordination in adolescents with ADHD to motor coordination in adolescents without disorders using kinematic analysis.	Level II *Design* Group comparison 8 boys (mean age = 14.3, range = 13–16) were selected from a sample of 43 respondents on the basis of a screening interview using the ADHD Clinical Questionnaire and confirmed diagnosis of ADHD. The children with ADHD were tested twice, 1 time while taking their ADHD medication (ADHD–On), and another time while off their medication for ≥48 hr (ADHD–Off). The control group consisted of 7 boys age matched (mean age = 14.9, range = 14–16). All the participants were screened for learning disabilities, anxiety disorders, reading disabilities, and the use of other medications.	No interventions were used. The control group was tested once, and the ADHD group was tested twice, once on medication and once off medication. A vision in action (virtual reality) system was used to measure eye movements and duration, arm movements and duration, and velocity during a table tennis activity. There were 2 conditions in this task: The long-duration precue, in which the cue light lit up 2 s before the serve, and the short-duration early cue, in which the cue light lit up 350 ms after the ball was served.	The children in the control group were significantly more accurate than both the ADHD–On and ADHD–Off groups. No significant differences were found in accuracy between the ADHD–On and ADHD–Off groups. The children in the control group had significantly lower gaze frequency and quiet eye duration than the children in the ADHD–Off group. The ADHD–Off group was late in responding to the ball in the long-duration condition. In terms of arm velocities, the ADHD–On group tended to overhit the ball and the ADHD–Off group tended to underhit the ball. The arm movements in both of the ADHD groups were normal in the short-duration early-cue condition but impaired in the long-duration precue condition.	The sample size was small, which limits generalizability. The age range was limited. 3 of the children in the control group played competitive badminton, which required similar skills to table tennis. This experience could make them more adept with these types of skills than the typical child, therefore confounding the results of the study, especially because of the small sample size. 2 of the participants had been off medications for an extended period of time; this condition was different from the other children in the ADHD–Off group, who had been off medications for approximately 48 hr. This difference could lead to error in the results.
Watling, Deitz, & White (2001)	The objective of the study was to compare factor score patterns derived from the Sensory Profile in children with and without autism.	Level II *Design* Group comparison 2 groups The first group was made up of 40 children who had either autism or PDD. Their age ranged from 3 yr to 6 yr 11 mo. There were 7 boys to every 1 girl. The 40 control participants were age- and gender-matched to the group with autism. They all had no medical conditions.	No intervention was used. Each parent filled out the Sensory Profile for their child.	Score differences between the 2 groups were significant on 8 of the 10 factors: Sensory Seeking, Emotionally Reactive, Low Endurance/Tone, Oral Sensitivity, Inattention/Distractibility, Poor Registration, Fine Motor/Perceptual, and Other. The children with autism tended to have scores that were more variable across the range of scores than did the control participants.	Small sample size limits generalizability. Only White children from 1 region of the country were used, so generalizability is limited.

Author/Year	Study Objectives	Level/Design/Participants	Intervention and Outcome Measures	Results	Study Limitations
P. H. Wilson, Maruff, Ives, & Currie (2001)	The objective of the study was to investigate motor imagery in children with DCD, emphasizing kinesthetic imagery.	Level II *Design* Group comparison The first group consisted of 20 children who scored <15th percentile on the M–ABC and were found to have DCD. There were 12 boys and 8 girls (mean age = 119.3 mo). They also met the *DSM–IV* criteria for DCD. A control group, matched on age (M = 120.3 mo), was selected from the same schools and scored >20th percentile on the M–ABC. *Exclusion Criteria* • Current or past history of neurological disease. • Psychiatric disorders (including ADHD) • IQ < 80	WISC–III was used to assess IQ. A visually guided pointing task measured movement durations for real and imagined movements. For real trials, 1 hand movement consisted of a hand motion from the far side of a vertical line to touch a target, and then back. Participants did this movement 5 times and were timed. The imagined condition was the same, but participants kept their hand in the same spot and with eyes open imagined how long it would take. A load condition also was examined by adding a 200-g weight to the top of the pencil. The praxis imagery questionnaire was given to assess different aspects of praxis imagery.	The overall duration was slower for real and imagined movements for the children with DCD than for the control group. Movements were slower in the load conditions than in the no-load conditions. For the control group, there was no difference between the duration of real and imagined movements under the no-load condition, but the duration was significantly slower than real movements under the load condition. In the children with DCD, imagined movements were performed faster than real movements in both the load and the no-load conditions. In the control group, the durations of real and imagined movements were highly correlated under the load and no-load conditions. This finding was not true for the children with DCD. On the praxis imagery questionnaire, the children with DCD only performed significantly worse on 1 subscale (kinesthetic) than the control participants. There was more variability in the children with DCD when performing the real movements than in the control participants.	Study is of good quality.

(Continued)

Table C2. Summary of the Evidence Supporting Subtypes of Children With Difficulty Processing and Integrating Sensory Information (cont.)

Author/Year	Study Objectives	Level/Design/Participants	Intervention and Outcome Measures	Results	Study Limitations
P. H. Wilson & McKenzie (1998)	The objective of the study was to synthesize findings through meta-analysis regarding children with motor impairments (DCD) on perceptual and motor measures of information processing.	Level I *Design* Meta-analysis Data were collected from 50 studies from 1963 to 1996 that looked at clumsy and nonclumsy children on measures of perceptual and motor control information processing. The 50 studies yielded 374 effect sizes and included 983 DCD and 987 control participants ages 5–16. *Inclusion Criteria* • Comparison between a control group and a group meeting the minimum requirements for DCD, using measures of information processing • Information given was enough to calculate effect size • The children in the DCD group had no neurological disorders and no physical or sensory impairments and had normal IQ	Effect sizes were calculated for all group comparisons using the correlation coefficient r, with $r = .1$ = small effect size, $r = .3$ = moderate effect size, and $r = .5$ = large effect size. Studies were coded on the basis of the following areas: *Visual Processing* • Ophthalmic factors • Visuoperceptual/visuospatial • Complex visuospatial (item score) with some motor involvement • Complex visuospatial (scale score) • Visuospatial memory *Other Perceptual Processing* • Kinesthetic perception (limb movement and position) • Cross-modal perception *Motor Control: Motor Planning and Execution* • Chronometric (reaction time, movement time, accuracy, dwell time) • Kinematics: Topography of movement (initiation time, trajectory, accuracy, variability) • Motor programming (rotary pursuit, movement time, timing variability, dwell time, accuracy) *General Intelligence* • Wechsler scales *Motor Skill* • Motor screening (total score)	The overall effect size at the group level was moderate, indicating the groups could be discriminated between. With the more recent publications, the group differences on outcome measures decreased. On all measures, the DCD group performed at an inferior level compared with the control group. Complex visuospatial tasks involving motor components performance discriminated the most between groups: overall effect size = .55. Visuospatial tasks without motor components had an effect size of .43. Kinesthetic perception (effect size = .40) and cross-modal perception (effect size = .34) all discriminated between groups but to a lesser degree.	Only published studies were included in this analysis. This situation usually leads to larger effect sizes than in unpublished studies. A meta-analysis cannot control for confounding factors in the studies reviewed.
Yochman, Ornoy, & Parush (2006)	The purpose of this study was to compare the sensory, motor, language, and intellectual abilities of children with and without ADHD. In addition, this study aimed at	Level II *Design* Group comparison 2 groups	No intervention was used. All participants were tested once. *Outcome Measures* The Miller Assessment for Preschoolers was given to	The results show that the children with ADHD scored lower than the typically developing children on all measures.	These findings are confined to just 1 specific geographic region (Jerusalem), so the findings lack generalizability outside this area.

	identifying which measures can predict group classification of children with and without ADHD.	The first group was 49 children with ADHD (39 boys, 10 girls; mean age = 4 yr 7 mo, range = 3 yr 10 mo–6 yr). To be included in this group, children had to fulfill several requirements. They had to score ≥1.5 SD below the mean on the hyperactivity or aggressive subscales of the PBQ. They also underwent a physical and neurological examination by a physician to verify the diagnosis of ADHD and exclude children with physical or neurological deficits. They also had to have normal intelligence, which was measure by the WPPSI. The comparison group consisted of 48 children without physical or neurological deficits (38 boys, 10 girls; mean age = 4 yr 8 mo, range = 3 yr 11 mo–6 yr). This group had to score within normal range on all scales of the PBQ and have normal intelligence according to the WPPSI.	measure sensory, motor, and cognitive skills. The VMI was given to evaluate visual and motor integration. The Reynell Developmental Language scale was used to measure expressive- and receptive-language skills. The Sensory Profile consists of scales, rated by parents, to assess sensory events in daily life.	High percentages were found in several deficits for children with ADHD, compared with the typically developing children, when looking at each of the measures. Children with ADHD had significantly more co-occurring deficits (scoring low on more than 1 of the measures), whereas co-occurring deficits were rare in the comparison group. A logistic regression analysis indicated that the significant predictors of group membership were the WPPSI verbal IQ, the Miller Assessment for Preschoolers coordination, and the Sensory Profile.	The researchers needed to approach a large number of potential participants to get an appropriate sample size. The deficits found in the children who had ADHD may have been related to test-taking difficulties.
Yochman, Parush, & Ornoy (2004)	The objective of the study was to compare parents' perceptions of the responses of their preschool children to sensory events in daily life. This study examined children with and without ADHD.	Level II *Design* Matched group comparison 2 groups The first group consisted of 48 children (39 boys, 9 girls) who had ADHD. The ages ranged from 4 to 6 (M = 4.7). Selection criteria for the children who had ADHD were as follows: • A score >1.5 SDs above the mean on the hyperactivity or aggressive factors on both the teacher's and parent's PBQ • Classification of ADHD by a neuropediatrician	No intervention was used. The following measurement tools were used for sample selection purposes: • PBQ • WPPSI The Sensory Profile was filled out by all the parents to obtain measures of the child's response to sensory events that occur in daily life.	Scores for the group with ADHD were significantly lower than those for the control group on 6 of the 9 factors of the Sensory Profile (sensation seeking, emotionally reactive, oral sensory sensitivity, inattention/distractibility, sedentary, and fine motor/perceptual). The 3 factors that were not different included low endurance–tone, poor registration, and sensory sensitivity. Significant differences were found between the groups on 11 of the 14 section scores, including sensation seeking, emotionally reactive, low endurance/tone, oral sensory	The generalizability of the sample is limited because of the low response rate and because it was taken from only 1 geographic region. The results could be biased because all the data were based on parents' reports.

(Continued)

Table C2. Summary of the Evidence Supporting Subtypes of Children With Difficulty Processing and Integrating Sensory Information (cont.)

Author/Year	Study Objectives	Level/Design/Participants	Intervention and Outcome Measures	Results	Study Limitations
		• Normal intelligence measured by the WPPSI The second group consisted of 46 typically developing children who were matched to Group 1 in age, gender, and parent socioeconomic status. The mean age was 4.8.		sensitivity, inattention/distractibility, poor registration, sensory sensitivity, sedentary, and fine motor/perceptual. Those relating to sensory processing are auditory, visual, touch, multisensory, and oral sensory processing. Those in the modulation section that were significantly different were body position and movement, activity level, and visual–emotional activity. All 3 subsections in the behavior and emotional responses section were significantly different (social–emotional, behavior, and thresholds for response). The 3 subsections that were not significantly different between the groups were vestibular (sensory section), endurance/tone, and emotional responses (both in the modulation section). A correlation between the Sensory Profile and the PBQ indicated that the more deficits in sensory processing there were, the more hyperactive the child's behavior would be.	
Zoia, Pelamatti, Cuttini, Casotto, & Scabar (2002)	This study had 3 objectives: 1. To examine the extent to which gesture performance depends on input modality 2. To examine which input modalities facilitate gesture performance at different ages 3. To examine whether gestural development patterns differ in children with and without DCD.	Level II *Design* Group comparison 35 children with DCD participated in the study (29 boys, 6 girls), determined by performance on the M–ABC <5th percentile. 105 typically developing children participated in the study as a control group (94 boys, 11 girls). All the children were ages 5–10. They were further broken down into age groups: 5–6, 7–8, and 9–10.	No intervention was used. All participants were tested 1 time. The M–ABC was given to determine into which group the children would fall. Raven's Colored Progressive Matrices test was used to rule out any cognitive deficit. The Test of Reception of Grammar was used to make sure all the children understood verbal commands. The transitive gestural task consisted of 17 items in which participants had to perform common gestures like brushing	The differences between the 2 groups were significant in all conditions except in the 5–6 age group in the imitation modality and in the 9–10 age group in the visual modality. Significant interactions were found between age and modality and group and modality. In every modality, performance increased significantly with age. The children with DCD were significantly less likely to correctly perform the gestures than were the control participants.	Study is of good quality.

All the children were given the M–ABC to determine which group they would be in. To be in the DCD group, the child had to score <5th percentile.

Both groups were determined to have no cognitive deficits and to be able to understand verbal directions.

their teeth. Each task was done in 4 different modalities:
1. Imitation, in which the reproduction of the gesture was carried out by the researcher
2. Visual + Tactile, in which the real use of objects was used
3. Visual, in which the child was asked to mime the use of a seen object
4. Verbal, in which the child was asked to perform the gesture in response to a verbal command

Each gesture was then evaluated and given a 1 if performed correctly or a 0 if not.

With the exception of the verbal modality, the difference between the groups lessened as the children got older. For Visual + Tactile and verbal modalities, the 2 groups were significantly different at each age, whereas with the imitation and visual modalities, there was no significant difference between the groups in the older age category. For each age group, and with both groups, the Visual + Tactile and imitation modalities resulted in better performance.

Note. AD = Asperger disorder; ADHD = attention deficit hyperactivity disorder; ADHD–MD = ADHD with motor disorder; ADLs = activities of daily living; ASD = autism spectrum disorder; BOTMP = Bruininks–Oseretsky Test of Motor Proficiency; CARS = Childhood Autism Rating Scale; CBCL = Child Behavior Checklist; COP = center of pressure; DCD = developmental coordination disorder; DD = developmental disabilities or delays; DSM–III–R = *Diagnostic and Statistical Manual of Mental Disorders*, 3rd ed., rev.; DSM–IV = *Diagnostic and Statistical Manual of Mental Disorders*, 4th ed.; EMG = electromyography; HECP = hand–eye coordination problems; KAT = kinesthetic acuity test; KTK = *Körperkoordinationstest für Kinder*; LD = learning disabilities or disorders; M–ABC = Movement Assessment Battery for Children; MEG = magnetoencephalography; ML = movement length; PBQ = Preschool Behavior Questionnaire; PDD = pervasive developmental disorder; RMT = Rhythmic Movement Test; *SD* = standard deviation; SEQ = Sensory Experiences Questionnaire; SI = sensory integration; SIAPA–CV = Structured Interview for Assessing Perceptual Anomalies–Child Version; SIPT = Sensory Integration and Praxis Test; TDDT–R = Tactile Defensiveness and Discrimination Test–Revised; TMI = Test of Motor Impairment; VABS = Vineland Adaptive Behavior Scales; VMI = Beery–Buktenica Developmental Test of Visual–Motor Integration; WISC–III = Wechsler Intelligence Scale for Children, 3rd ed.; WISC–R = Wechsler Intelligence Scale for Children–Revised; WPPSI = Wechsler Preschool and Primary Scale of Intelligence; WRAT = Wide Range Achievement Test.

This table is a product of AOTA's Evidence-Based Practice Project and the *American Journal of Occupational Therapy*. Copyright © 2010 by the American Occupational Therapy Association. May be freely reproduced for personal use in clinical or educational settings as long as the source is cited. All other uses require written permission from the American Occupational Therapy Association. To apply, visit www.copyright.com.

From Davies, P. L., & Tucker, R. (2010). Evidence review to investigate the support for subtypes of children with difficulty processing and integrating sensory information (Suppl. Table 1). *American Journal of Occupational Therapy, 64,* 391–402. doi: 10.5014/ajot.2010.09070

Table C3, Part I. Evidence for Functional Performance Difficulties in Children and Adolescents With Difficulty Processing and Integrating Sensory Information: Play–Leisure and Social Participation

Author/Year	Study Objectives	Level/Design/Participants	Intervention and Outcome Measures	Results	Study Limitations
Bieberich & Morgan (2004)	The objective was to compare children with autism and children with Down syndrome on dimensions of cognitive function, self-regulation, and affective expression during play.	Level II Cohort design *Participants* 14 children with autism and 15 children with Down syndrome	Nonintervention; observational study *Outcome Measures* • Peabody Picture Vocabulary Test–Revised • CARS • Minnesota Preschool Affect Rating Scales • Play observation	The patterns of ratings within each group were similar from the first observation to the second observation, with the autism group showing more deviant ratings on measures of self-regulation and affective sharing. From the first to second time, children with autism showed relatively high stability for the self-regulation factor but less stability than children with Down syndrome for all 3 factors of cognitive function, self-regulation, and dimensions of affective expression.	The sample size for each group was small. The study did not include a control group of normally developing children matched for mental age. The study examined self-regulation and affective expression in an observational laboratory setting that may have elicited responses that differ from those in a more naturalistic setting.
Cairney et al. (2005)	The objective was to study a theoretical model determining whether there is a link between DCD and reduced physical activity, with generalized self-efficacy as a mediating influence.	Level III Nonrandomized cross-sectional design *Participants* 564 children in grades 4–8	Nonintervention; observational study *Outcome Measures* • Bruininks–Oseretsky Test of Motor Proficiency, short form • Children's Self-Perceptions Toward Physical Activity • Participation Questionnaire	7.5% of the study population met the requirements for probable DCD. 28% of the variance in children's activity level was predicted by both generalized self-efficacy and DCD.	The study was unable to actually test causal ordering between variables of self-efficacy and DCD. Data were not derived from a random sample of students. Many factors are involved in a child's play other than those examined in this study.
Channon, Charman, Heap, Crawford, & Rios (2001)	The objective of the study was to compare adolescents with Asperger syndrome with typically developing adolescents on a novel problem-solving task that presented videotaped scenarios in real-life-type social contexts.	Level II Case-control design *Participants* 2 groups, 15 adolescents and young adults with Asperger syndrome and 15 gender-matched control participants	Nonintervention; observational study *Outcome Measures* • Predicaments problem-solving task followed viewing of a real-life videotaped scenario or story of the scenario • Dysexecutive Questionnaire	The Asperger group was impaired in several aspects of problem solving, including recounting the pertinent facts, generating possible high-quality problem solutions, and selecting optimal and preferred solutions. This group's solutions differed most from those of the typically developing group in social appropriateness.	It cannot be taken for granted that tasks of the nature used in this research study predict real-life problem-solving behavior in similar situations.

Cummins, Piek, & Dyck (2005)	The objective was to assess whether children with motor coordination problems have difficulty with empathetic abilities and to determine whether there is a significant relationship between motor coordination problems, visual–spatial processing, and social behavior.	Level II Case–control design *Participants* 2 groups: 39 children with probable DCD and 39 children in the control group	Nonintervention; observational study *Outcome Measures* • McCarron Assessment of Neuro-Muscular Development • Neuromuscular Development Index • WISC-III • Emotional Recognition Scale • CBCL	The movement difficulty group scored significantly lower than the control group on the measures of ability to recognize facial emotion cues and 1 measure of emotional understanding. When other variables were accounted for, the Neuromuscular Development Index was a significant predictor of social problems.	Assessment of social skills and empathetic abilities took place in a clinical setting rather than a natural setting.
Downs & Smith (2004)	The objective was to examine, in children with autism, whether problems exhibiting cooperative social behavior reflect global developmental delays or autism-specific deficits.	Level II Case–control design *Participants* 3 groups: 10 children with autism who had average IQ, 16 children with ADHD and ODD, and 10 typically developing children	Nonintervention; observational study *Outcome Measures* • Social Orientation Choice Card • Questions developed by Howlin, Baron-Cohen, and Hadwin to determine level of emotional understanding • Prisoner's dilemma game • Behavioral Development Questionnaire	In cooperative behavior, level of emotional understanding, and aloof behavior, the autism group outperformed the ADHD/ODD group and did not differ significantly from typically developing children. However, the autism group showed worse emotion recognition and more active but odd behavior than the other groups.	This was a small, all-male sample that yielded low statistical power and limited the generalizability of the results. Lack of differences in social value orientation and cooperative behavior found between the children with autism and the children in the nonclinical group may have resulted from random responding because of poor comprehension of the Social Orientation Choice Card or the prisoner's dilemma task.
Dziuk et al. (2007)	The objective was to understand the relationship between dyspraxia and motor skill development in children with autism and to determine whether dyspraxia observed in children with autism can be accounted for by problems with motor skills.	Level II Case–control design *Participants* 94 participants, ages 8–14: 47 high-functioning children with ASD diagnosis and 47 typically developing children	Nonintervention; observational study *Outcome Measures* • WISC-III • WISC-IV • Florida Apraxia Screening Test (Revised), adapted for children • Physical and Neurological Assessment of Subtle Signs • ADOS	After controlling for age and IQ, basic motor skill was a significant predictor of performance on praxis examination. The ASD group continued to show significantly poorer praxis than control participants after accounting for basic motor skill. Praxis performance was a strong predictor of the defining features of autism, measured using the ADOS, and this correlation remained significant after accounting for basic motor skill.	The praxis examination was adapted for children from an adult apraxia battery. The age range of the children was limited to 8–14. This limitation allowed for a more homogeneous group to evaluate. However, a broader age range would evaluate dyspraxia more comprehensively throughout childhood and adolescence. The amount of

(Continued)

Table C3, Part I. Evidence for Functional Performance Difficulties in Children and Adolescents With Difficulty Processing and Integrating Sensory Information: Play–Leisure and Social Participation (*cont.*)

Author/Year	Study Objectives	Level/Design/Participants	Intervention and Outcome Measures	Results	Study Limitations
					experience the children had in performing these complex gestures is difficult to ascertain. Their individual experiences contribute to their ability to perform meaningful gestures, which could increase their number of correctly performed gestures.
Hilton, Graver, & LaVesser (2007)	This study examined the relationship between social competence and sensory processing in children with high-functioning ASD.	Level III *Participants* 36 participants, ages 6–10, with high-functioning ASD	Nonintervention; observational study *Outcome Measures* • Social Responsiveness Scale • Sensory Profile	All the relationships between the Social Responsiveness Scale t scores and the Sensory Profile quadrant scores were statistically significant. The quadrants of sensation seeking and low registration had a moderately negative correlation, whereas the quadrants of sensory sensitivity and sensation avoiding had strongly negative correlations.	The use of questionnaire-format assessments was a limitation. The accuracy of these assessments is based on a parent's ability to understand and answer the questions accurately. Participants used were a convenience sample, recruited from a limited section of the country with limited ethnic diversity.
Jackson et al. (2003)	The objective was to examine play and language interactions in children with autism in social initiation and responsiveness, focusing on quality of sustained interactions between children with autism and other children and adults in a natural setting.	Level III Nonrandomized cross-sectional design *Participants* 33 participants: 19 children with autism and 14 children with intellectual disabilities	Nonintervention; observational study *Outcome Measure* Social Behavior Coding Scheme	Children with autism produced fewer positive responses and more "no responses" than children with intellectual disabilities. Both groups were more likely to make positive responses to adults and not to respond to other children. Moreover, although the frequency of conversations was not different for the 2 groups, children with autism were significantly less likely to engage in sustained play compared with children with intellectual disabilities.	The study used a small sample size. Peers were all from special education classrooms, so findings cannot be generalized to interactions with typically developing children. Because of the nature of the coding used in the current study, it was not possible to determine whether conversations were need-oriented or scripted/learned.

Author/Year	Study Objectives	Level/Design/Participants	Intervention and Outcome Measures	Results	Study Limitations
Lloyd, Reid, & Bouffard (2006)	The objective was to examine the domain-specific self-regulatory skills of boys with DCD.	Level II Case–control design *Participants* 10 boys with DCD and 10 boys without DCD	*Intervention* Participants were taught to think aloud guided by Zimmerman's (2000) social cognitive model of self-regulation. *Outcome Measures* • Sport-specific problem-solving task (hockey shot) • Educational problem-solving task (peg solitaire) • Coding verbalizations developed under 5 categories: goals, knowledge, emotion, monitoring, and evaluation	The quantity of verbalization was similar in both groups, but differences were found in verbalization quality. Results indicated that boys with DCD had emotional and planning differences on the hockey task, but only planning differences were evident on the peg solitaire task.	The small sample size limits generalizability to other populations.
Macintosh & Dissanayake (2006)	The objective was to determine the differences and similarities in the social skills and behavior problems of children with high-functioning autism and Asperger disorder, from both their parents' and teachers' perspectives, relative to each other and also to their typically developing peers.	Level II Nonrandomized case–control design *Participants* 3 groups: 20 children with high-functioning autism, 19 children with Asperger disorder, and 17 typically developing children, matched on chronological and mental age	*Outcome Measure* Social Skills Rating System	The children with high-functioning autism and Asperger disorder were not differentiated on any social skill or problem behavior on the basis of either teacher or parent report. However, both children with autism and those with Asperger disorder demonstrated significant social skill deficits and problem behaviors on the Social Skills Rating System relative to the typically developing children and an original standardization sample of "nonhandicapped" male primary school children.	The sample size was small, which can make it difficult to generalize the study to a larger population.
Molloy, Dietrich, & Bhattacharya (2003)	The objective was to measure the postural stability of children with ASD compared with children with typical neurodevelopment and to measure the relative contributions of the visual, somatosensory, and vestibular afferent systems in each group.	Level II Case–control design *Participants* 2 groups: 8 boys with ASD (without gross motor abnormalities) and 8 age-, race-, and gender-matched control participants	Nonintervention; observational study *Outcome Measure* Postural sway measurements were performed using the AccuSwayPLUS force platform.	Children with ASD had significantly larger sway areas under all test conditions in which afferent input was modified. The children with ASD appeared to rely most on the visual cues to reduce sway and maintain balance. Under conditions in which vision was occluded, the children with ASD had a significantly greater increase in their sway area, compared with	The small sample size limits how generalizable the study is to the population.

(Continued)

Appendix C. Evidence Tables

Table C3, Part I. Evidence for Functional Performance Difficulties in Children and Adolescents With Difficulty Processing and Integrating Sensory Information: Play–Leisure and Social Participation *(cont.)*

Author/Year	Study Objectives	Level/Design/Participants	Intervention and Outcome Measures	Results	Study Limitations
				the control participants, regardless whether somatosensory input was also modified. For the high-functioning boys with ASD, postural sway testing provided evidence for a deficit in the integration of information from the visual, somatosensory, and vestibular afferent systems.	
Orsmond, Krauss, & Seltzer (2004)	The objective was to investigate peer relationships and participation in social and recreational activities among adolescents and adults with autism who live at home.	Level III Nonrandomized cross-sectional design *Participants* 235 adolescents and adults ages 10–47	Nonintervention; observational study *Outcome Measures* • Autism Diagnostic Interview–Revised • Social and recreation activities reported on through a modified version of a measure developed for the National Survey of Families and Households • Revised ADL Index • Inventory for Client and Agency Planning • Environmental factors	Having peer relationships was predicted by individual characteristics (younger age and less impairment in social interaction skills) but not by characteristics of the environment. Greater participation in social and recreational activities was predicted by characteristics of the individual with autism (greater functional independence, less impairment in social interaction skills, higher levels of internalizing behaviors) and characteristics of the environment (greater maternal participation in social and recreational activities, greater number of services received, and inclusion in integrated settings while in school).	Participants were volunteers and may not be representative of the full population of adolescents and adults with autism. All sample members in the analysis coresided with their parent(s), and thus the peer relationships and social activities of people with autism who reside in other community or institutional settings may differ from these results. All data were obtained from the mothers. The sample members may have had peer relationships in school or work with which the mother was less familiar.
Poulsen, Ziviani, Cuskelly, & Smith (2007)	The objective was to examine the impact of leisure occupational performance patterns and contexts on the perceptions of loneliness in boys with DCD.	Level II Case-control design *Participants* 2 groups: 60 boys with DCD and 113 boys without DCD, ages 10–13, matched for grade level, chronological age, and socioeconomic status	Nonintervention; observational study *Outcome Measures* • M-ABC • Loneliness and Social Dissatisfaction Questionnaire	Boys with DCD recorded significantly higher loneliness and lower participation rates in all group physical activities, whether structured (e.g., team sports) or unstructured (e.g., informal outdoor play) than boys without DCD. An inverse relationship between physical coordination ability and loneliness was mediated by participation in team sports. Childhood physical coordination difficulties were significantly associated with loneliness.	Because the study was cross-sectional, experimental manipulation of the mediatory variable, team sports participation, was not possible. The sample was not representative of the population. It was difficult to determine whether children were lonely before the team sports, or if their inability to participate in team sports resulted in their loneliness.

Rinehart et al. (2006)	The objective was to investigate movement kinematics—that is, movement preparation, movement execution, and the shape of the movement trajectory (time spent in accelerative vs. decelerative phases) in children with high-functioning autism and Asperger disorder using a kinematic paradigm similar to that used in previous motor investigations of patients with neurodegenerative disorders—and to examine the impact of an executive load on movement kinematics by including expectancy and inhibitory components.	Level II Case–control design *Participants* 12 people with high-functioning autism as well as 12 control participants matched on age, gender, and full-scale IQ. In addition, 12 people with Asperger disorder and another 12 control participants were recruited and matched according to age, sex, and full-scale IQ.	Nonintervention; observational study *Outcome Measure* WACOM SD420 digitizing tablet	Results indicated that high-functioning autism is more consistently associated with impaired motoric preparation and initiation than it is with Asperger disorder. Data also suggest that this dissociation is not necessarily underpinned by greater executive dysfunction vulnerability in autism relative to Asperger disorder.	It would have been desirable to directly compare high-functioning autism and Asperger disorder groups. This was not possible in view of the developmentally critical age gap between groups. The small sample size is likely to be responsible for the inconsistent between-task findings.
Smyth & Anderson (2000)	The objective was to determine whether children with poor coordination were fully involved across the range of play activities or spent time by themselves or in very small groups, whether they engaged in social but not physical play and whether this situation changed with age, and whether they engaged in skill mastery that could be physical but not social.	Level II Case–control design *Participants* 2 groups: 55 children assigned to a DCD group and 55 assigned to a control group on the basis of their scores on the M–ABC	Nonintervention; observational study *Outcome Measures* Play and social skills were coded using a coding scheme developed in 2 schools that were not part of the main study.	Children in the DCD group spent more time alone, were onlookers more often, and played formal games in large groups less often if they were boys and informal games in large groups less often if they were girls. Social fantasy play did not differentiate between the two groups, but social physical play did, particularly in the older age groups. Play performance in the DCD group was more variable, with some boys taking an active part in team games, whereas others never took part in them.	It was difficult to determine whether children initially did not participate in group playground games or whether they did not participate because they had been excluded in the past. The coding scheme developed to measure play and social skills had not had formal reliability (with the exception of interrater reliability) and validity measures performed on it.
Vernazza-Martin et al. (2005)	The objective was to examine postural anticipation and multijoint coordination during locomotion in healthy and autistic children.	Level II Case–control design *Participants* 2 groups: 9 children meeting DSM–IV criteria for autism and 6 typically developing children, ages 4–6	Nonintervention; observational study *Outcome Measure* Kinematic gait analysis was performed using a commercially available automatic motion analyzer (ELITE system).	A kinematic analysis of gait indicates that rather than gait parameters or balance control, the main components affected in autistic children during locomotion are the goal of the action, the orientation toward this goal, and the definition of the trajectory, probably because of an impairment of movement planning.	The small sample size limits generalizability.

(Continued)

Table C3, Part I. Evidence for Functional Performance Difficulties in Children and Adolescents With Difficulty Processing and Integrating Sensory Information: Play–Leisure and Social Participation (cont.)

Author/Year	Study Objectives	Level/Design/Participants	Intervention and Outcome Measures	Results	Study Limitations
E. Williams, Reddy, & Costall (2001)	The objective was to examine functional play in children with autism using a refined analysis of such play, subtyping the functional acts into various categories in terms of the developmental progression suggested by research with typical infants.	Level II Nonrandomized case–control design *Participants* 3 groups: 15 children with autism, 15 typically developing infants, and 15 children with Down syndrome	Nonintervention; observational study *Outcome Measure* Play behaviors (rated for duration, frequency, diversity, and integration)	Although there were no group differences in overall measures of the proportion of total play time spent in functional play and in the number of functional acts performed, a closer analysis of the composition of this play did reveal striking qualitative differences. The functional play of the autism group was less elaborated, less varied, and less integrated than that of the control participants.	The small sample size decreases generalizability to the population. Groups were matched only on the basis of general development age from the Bayley Scales of Infant Development, not gender or chronological age.

Note. ADHD = attention deficit hyperactivity disorder; ADLs = activities of daily living; ADOS = Autism Diagnostic Observation Schedule; ASD = autism spectrum disorder; CARS = Childhood Autism Rating Scale; CBCL = Child Behavior Checklist; DCD = developmental coordination disorder; *DSM–IV* = *Diagnostic and Statistical Manual of Mental Disorders, 4th Edition*; M–ABC = Movement Assessment Battery for Children; ODD = oppositional defiant disorder; WISC = Wechsler Intelligence Scale for Children.

This table is a product of AOTA's Evidence-Based Practice Project and the *American Journal of Occupational Therapy*. Copyright © 2010 by the American Occupational Therapy Association. May be freely reproduced for personal use in clinical or educational settings as long as the source is cited. All other uses require written permission from the American Occupational Therapy Association. To apply, visit www.copyright.com.

From Koenig, K. P., & Rudney, S. G. (2010). Performance challenges for children and adolescents with difficulty processing and integrating sensory information: A systematic review (Suppl. Table 1). *American Journal of Occupational Therapy, 64,* 430–442. doi: 10.5014/ajot.2010.09073

Table C3, Part II. Evidence for Functional Performance Difficulties in Children and Adolescents With Difficulty Processing and Integrating Sensory Information: ADLs and IADLs

Author/Year	Study Objectives	Level/Design/Participants	Intervention and Outcome Measures	Results	Study Limitations
Case-Smith (1995)	The objective was to investigate the relationships among sensorimotor components; standardized measures of fine motor skills; and functional performance in self-care, mobility, and social interaction as well as to examine which sensorimotor components and fine motor skills were predictors of functional performance.	Level III Nonrandomized cross-sectional design *Participants* 30 preschool children with motor delays	Nonintervention; observational study *Outcome Measures* • Motor Assessment Outcomes Model (including tests of in-hand manipulation, tactile defensiveness, stereognosis, grasping strength, and fine motor skill) • PEDI	Significant correlations were found among sensorimotor components and discrete fine motor skills as measured on standardized observational tests. Few correlations emerged between foundational components of fine motor skill and functional performance in self-care, mobility, and social function.	The small sample size and narrow age range limited generalizability. Focus was on only 1 aspect of motor function. Sensorimotor components selected for analysis do not represent all of the components that contribute to a child's fine motor skills.

Honomichl, Goodlin-Jones, Burnham, Gaylor, & Anders (2002)	The objective was to examine sleep patterns in children with PDDs.	Level III Nonrandomized cross-sectional design *Participants* 100 children with PDDs, ages 2–11	Nonintervention; observational study *Outcome Measures* • Sleep diary • CSHQ • Parenting Events Questionnaire	Before data collection, slightly more than half of the parents, when queried, reported a sleep problem in their child. Subsequent diary and CSHQ reports confirmed more fragmented sleep in those children who were described by their parents as having a sleep problem compared with those without a designated problem. Children with PDD, regardless of parental perception of problematic sleep, all exhibited longer sleep onset times and greater fragmentation of sleep than that reported for age-matched community norms.	It is possible that a higher proportion of parents who were concerned that their child might have a sleep problem chose to participate in the study.
Linderman & Stewart (1999)	The objective was to explore the effects of SI-based occupational therapy provided in an outpatient clinic on the functional behaviors of 2 young children with PDD at home.	Level VI Single-subject (2 cases), pretest–posttest design *Participants* 2 participants, both age 3 and boys, with a diagnosis of PDD who had not previously received a consistent program of SI-based occupational therapy	*Intervention* Intervention was SI-based, but for review, only performance measures were used. *Outcome Measure* Adapted version of Cook's Revised Functional Behavior Assessment for Children With Sensory Integrative Dysfunction	Both boys displayed significant improvements in the areas of social interaction, approach to new activities, response to holding or hugging, and response to movement. Decreases were noted in the frequency and duration of disruptive behaviors (e.g., high activity levels, aggressive behaviors), and an increase in functional behaviors, such as spontaneous speech, purposeful play, and attention to activities and conversation, was observed.	Single-subject design makes it difficult to generalize the results to other populations. Concurrent interventions that were not part of this study, such as speech therapy, preschool, vitamins, and the like, may have confounded the results.
Mandich, Polatajko, & Rodger (2003)	The objective was to explore the effect of DCD on participation in the typical activities of childhood and the importance of this participation for children with DCD from the perspective of the parent.	Qualitative study *Participants* 12 participants	Interviews were conducted with parents of children with DCD who attended a clinic specializing in using the Cognitive Orientation to Daily Occupational Performance approach.	Interviews revealed that difficulty in everyday activities had serious negative effects for the children. Intervention focused on enablement at the activity and participation level was found to have a significant positive impact on the children's quality of life. Emerging themes included that performance competency played an important role in being accepted by peers and being able "to be part of the group." Parents reported that successful participation built confidence in their children and allowed them to try other new activities.	The study was qualitative; therefore, the findings warrant further investigation, but it is difficult to generalize them to other populations.

(Continued)

Table C3, Part II. Evidence for Functional Performance Difficulties in Children and Adolescents With Difficulty Processing and Integrating Sensory Information: ADLs and IADLs *(cont.)*

Author/Year	Study Objectives	Level/Design/Participants	Intervention and Outcome Measures	Results	Study Limitations
Reeves (1998)	The objective was to explore the use of a sensory integration frame of reference in the evaluation and treatment of a child with delays in fine motor skills; low frustration level; poor eating behavior; low self-esteem; unusual fears; and increased sensitivity to tactile, visual, and auditory stimuli.	Level VI Single-case design (1 case) *Participant* Participant was a 6-yr-old boy with delays in fine motor skills; low frustration level; poor eating behavior; low self-esteem; unusual fears; and increased sensitivity to tactile, visual, and auditory stimuli.	*Intervention* 9 months of occupational therapy intervention using an SI approach for 1 hr 1×/wk *Outcome Measure* Measurement of goals set after evaluation related to self-esteem, self-help, gross motor, fine motor, and oral–motor skills	Improvement was observed in all of the areas of concern, including goals that the child had set for himself related to riding a bike and tying his shoes.	Single-subject design makes it difficult to generalize results to other populations.
S. Reynolds & Lane (2008)	The objective was to present case study reports that identify and describe a set of children who exhibited behaviors of sensory overresponsivity and had no other co-occurring neurological or psychological diagnoses.	Level V Case reports (3 cases) *Participants* 3 children—an 11-yr-old boy, an 8-yr-old boy, and a 12-yr-old girl—who presented with a profile of sensory overresponsivity without a co-occurring diagnosis	Nonintervention; observational study *Outcome Measures* • Sensory Over-responsivity Inventory (SensOR) • Parent Interview The following assessments were used to rule out the presence of additional diagnoses typically associated with sensory processing disorders: • CARS • Child Symptom Inventory–4	3 case studies provide preliminary support for the existence of sensory overresponsiveness in the absence of other diagnostic classifications. Overresponsivity to tactile stimulation was a consistent area of deficit that affected family routines and ADLs.	Case reports are difficult to generalize to other populations.
Rodger et al. (2003)	The objective was to examine the motor and functional skills of children with DCD.	Level III Nonrandomized cross-sectional design *Participants* 20 children with DCD (8 boys, 12 girls, ages 4–8)	Nonintervention; observational study *Outcome Measures* • Neurodevelopmental Physiotherapy Assessment • PEDI • PDMS (fine motor portion) • VMI • Test of Legible Handwriting • Handwriting Speed Test • Videotaped sample of cutting using scissors • Pictorial Scale of Perceived Competence and Social Acceptance	The children with DCD performed at the lower end of the normal range on the PDMS. Their performance on the VMI was within the average range. Videotaped observations of the children's handwriting and cutting indicated that 29% were left-handed and that a large proportion of all children used unusual pencil grasp patterns and immature prehension of scissors. The participants rated themselves toward the more competent and accepted end of the Pictorial Scale of Perceived Competence and Social Acceptance over the dimensions of physical and cognitive competence and peer and maternal acceptance.	This study was a pilot investigation, which by nature has a small sample size and limited generalizability to other populations.

Author/Year	Study Objectives	Level/Design/Participants	Intervention and Outcome Measures	Results	Study Limitations
				The PEDI revealed generally average performance on social and mobility function; however, self-care function was below the average range for their age.	
Schreck, Williams, & Smith (2004)	The objective was to explore differences in eating behavior in children with autism and typically developing children.	Level II Case–control design *Participants* 2 groups: 138 children with autism and 298 children in the control group, ages 5–12	Nonintervention; observational study *Outcome Measures* • Children's Eating Behavior Inventory • Food Preference Inventory • Gilliam Autism Rating Scale • Personal History Form (date of birth, weight, height, and gender)	Results indicated that the children with autism had significantly more feeding problems and ate a significantly narrower range of foods than the children without autism.	The selection process for the families of children with autism could have skewed results. The sample of children also could have been restricted because of the chosen target age group. Use of parental report of foods eaten by children may have created less accurate results than method of actual presentation of foods.
B. P. White, Mulligan, Merrill, & Wright (2007)	The objective was to determine whether children with possible sensory processing deficits, as measured by the Sensory Profile, performed less well on an occupational performance measure than children with typical Sensory Profile scores.	Level III Nonrandomized cross-sectional design *Participants* 68 children divided into 2 groups on the basis of their scores on the Sensory Profile	Nonintervention; observational study *Outcome Measures* • AMPS • Sensory Profile	There were significant differences between groups on the AMPS ADLs Motor and ADLs Process measures; the children with atypical Sensory Profile scores showed increased functional difficulties. Correlations revealed significant relationships among the measures.	A small convenience sample of primarily White children was used; as a result, the sample may not adequately represent the population of children with and without sensory processing dysfunction. Because there is no definitive diagnostic cutoff on the Sensory Profile that determines whether a child has sensory processing deficits, the categorization of the children as *typical* or *atypical* sensory processors was made on the basis of clinical judgment of the child's Sensory Profile scores.

Note. ADLs = activities of daily living; AMPS = Assessment of Motor and Process Skills; CARS = Childhood Autism Rating Scale; CSHQ = Children's Sleep Habit Questionnaire; DCD = developmental coordination disorder; PDD = pervasive developmental disorder; PDMS = Peabody Developmental Motor Scale; PEDI = Pediatric Evaluation of Disability Inventory; SI = sensory integration; VMI = Developmental Test of Visual–Motor Integration.

This table is a product of AOTA's Evidence-Based Practice Project and the *American Journal of Occupational Therapy*. Copyright © 2010 by the American Occupational Therapy Association. May be freely reproduced for personal use in clinical or educational settings as long as the source is cited. All other uses require written permission from the American Occupational Therapy Association. To apply, visit www.copyright.com.

From Koenig, K. P., & Rudney, S. G. (2010). Performance challenges for children and adolescents with difficulty processing and integrating sensory information: A systematic review (Suppl. Table 2). *American Journal of Occupational Therapy, 64,* 430–442. doi: 10.5014/ajot.2010.09073

Table C3, Part III. Evidence for Functional Performance Difficulties in Children and Adolescents With Difficulty Processing and Integrating Sensory Information: Rest and Sleep

Author/Year	Study Objectives	Level/Design/Participants	Intervention and Outcome Measures	Results	Study Limitations
Allik, Larsson, & Smedje (2006)	The objective was to examine sleep patterns of school-age children with high-functioning autism and Asperger disorder.	Level II Case–control design *Participants* 2 groups: 32 school-age children with Asperger syndrome and high-functioning autism were compared with 32 typically developing age- and gender-matched children.	Nonintervention; observational study *Outcome Measures* • Parent-reported sleep problems • Child sleep diary • Actigraphy (The actigraph used in the study was a self-contained minicomputer the size of a wristwatch that was worn on the child's non-dominant arm and recorded all movements exceeding the 0.05-g threshold and translated the movements into electrical signals.) • High-Functioning Autism Spectrum Screening Questionnaire	Parents of children with Asperger syndrome and high-functioning autism more commonly reported that their children had difficulty falling asleep. 1 wk of sleep recording with diary and actigraphy confirmed that children in the Asperger syndrome and high-functioning autism group spent a longer time awake in bed before falling asleep than children in the control group. This situation was possibly because the children in the Asperger syndrome and high-functioning autism group had earlier bedtimes than their matched peers. The sleep patterns of children with Asperger syndrome and high-functioning autism did not differ significantly from each other.	It is unknown whether the sample of children with PDD was representative of children with Asperger syndrome and high-functioning autism in general. There is a possibility that families that have children with PDD and disturbed sleep were more likely to accept the offer to participate in the study. Exclusion criteria resulted in the selection of healthy and nonmedicated children. Severely sleep-disturbed children who received medication for sleep problems may have been excluded from the sample. Study had a 1-wk observation period, which is possibly an insufficiently representative period of time. The need for at least 14 days of sleep diary recording to obtain valuable information has been emphasized in the literature. Focus was on the basic aspects of nighttime sleep and did not take into account the possibility of daytime napping.
Honomichl, Goodlin-Jones, Burnham, Gaylor, & Anders (2002)	The objective was to examine sleep patterns in children with PDD.	Level III Nonrandomized, cross-sectional design *Participants* 100 children with PDD, ages 2–11	Nonintervention, observational study *Outcome Measures* • Sleep diary • CSHQ • Parenting Events Questionnaire	Before data collection, slightly more than half of the parents, when queried, reported a sleep problem in their child. Subsequent sleep diary and CSHQ reports confirmed more fragmented sleep in those children who were described by their parents as	It is possible that a higher proportion of parents who were concerned that their child might have a sleep problem chose to participate in the study.

Study	Objective	Level/Design/Participants	Intervention and Outcome Measures	Results	Study Limitations
Shochat, Tzischinsky, & Engel-Yeger (2009)	The objective was to explore the relationship between sleep habits, behavior, and sensory processing.	Level III Nonrandomized, cross-sectional design *Participants* 51 typically developing school-children (mean age = 8.6)	Nonintervention: observational study *Outcome Measures* • CSHQ • Short Sensory Profile • Conners' Global Index from the Conners' Parent Rating Scale	having a sleep problem compared with those without a designated problem. Children with PDD, regardless of parental perception of problematic sleep, all exhibited longer sleep onset times and greater fragmentation of sleep than that reported for age-matched community norms. Significant relationships between sensory processing, sleep, and behavior were found. The relationship between sleep and behavior was not as strong when sensory processing abilities were controlled for, indicating that sensory processing may contribute more to sleep disturbances, especially in the areas of tactile sensitivity. Tactile sensitivity was also a predictor of behavior as measured by Conners' Global Index. Underresponsive or seeks sensation was a predictor of behavior as well, indicating links to arousal that may affect day and night sleep and behavior.	The small sample size and reliance only on parent report of sensory processing, behavior, and sleep habits limited this study.

Note. CSHQ = Children's Sleep Habit Questionnaire; PDD = pervasive developmental disorder.

This table is a product of AOTA's Evidence-Based Practice Project and the *American Journal of Occupational Therapy.* Copyright © 2010 by the American Occupational Therapy Association. May be freely reproduced for personal use in clinical or educational settings as long as the source is cited. All other uses require written permission from the American Occupational Therapy Association. To apply, visit www.copyright.com.

From Koenig, K. P., & Rudney, S. G. (2010). Performance challenges for children and adolescents with difficulty processing and integrating sensory information: A systematic review (Suppl. Table 3). *American Journal of Occupational Therapy, 64,* 430–442. doi: 10.5014/ajot.2010.09073

Table C3, Part IV. Evidence for Functional Performance Difficulties in Children and Adolescents With Difficulty Processing and Integrating Sensory Information: Education and Work

Author/Year	Study Objectives	Level/Design/Participants	Intervention and Outcome Measures	Results	Study Limitations
Baranek et al. (2002)	The objective was to examine sensory processing and its relationship to occupational performance in children with fragile X syndrome.	Level III Nonrandomized, cross-sectional design *Participants* 1 group, 15 boys with full-mutation fragile X syndrome, ages 53–123 mo	Nonintervention; observational study *Outcome Measures* Occupational performance measures: • School Function Assessment • Vineland Adaptive Behavior Scales • Sensory Profile Caregiver Questionnaire • Tactile Defensiveness and Discrimination Test–Revised • Sensory Approach–Avoidance Rating	Several significant correlations were found, independent of effects of age and IQ. Avoidance of sensory experiences (internally controlled) was associated with lower levels of participation in school, self-care, and play. Aversion to touch from externally controlled sources was associated with a trend toward greater independence in self-care.	Replication studies with larger samples of children with fragile X syndrome, as well as children with other developmental disorders, are needed to determine the generalizability of these findings. Further research also needs to address the limitations inherent in some measures developed for this study.
Baranek, David, Poe, Stone, & Watson (2006)	The objective was to describe a new caregiver report assessment, the Sensory Experiences Questionnaire, and to explain the nature of sensory patterns of hyper- and hyporesponsiveness, their prevalence, and developmental correlates in children with ASDs compared with typically developing children.	Level II Case-control design *Participants* 258 children, ages 5–80 mo, collected using convenience-sampling methods Sample included 56 participants identified as having autism, 24 participants with other PDDs, 33 participants with developmental disabilities/mental retardation, and 35 with other developmental delays compared with 110 typically developing children.	Nonintervention; observational study *Outcome Measure* Sensory Experiences Questionnaire	Prevalence of sensory symptoms for the autism group was found to be 69%, and sensory symptoms were found to be inversely related to mental age. The autism group had significantly higher symptoms than either the typically developing or developmental delays groups and presented with a unique pattern of response to sensory stimuli and hyporesponsiveness in both social and nonsocial contexts. A similar pattern of hyperresponsiveness was seen in the autism and developmental delays groups was significantly greater in both clinical groups than in the typically developing group.	Although findings demonstrate adequate psychometrics to support using the Sensory Experiences Questionnaire for its intended purpose, further validation is needed. Cross-sectional data provide some understanding of the developmental nature of sensory features in young children, but longitudinal measures would provide more robust conclusions. The subjective nature of parent report data may also be construed as a methodological limitation.
Dewey, Kaplan, Crawford, & Wilson (2002)	This study investigated the problems of attention, learning, and psychosocial adjustment evidenced by children with DCD.	Level II Case-control design *Participants* 45 children identified with DCD, 51 children identified as being suspect for DCD, and 78 comparison children without	Nonintervention; observational study *Outcome Measures* • Attention Problems subscale of the CBCL • Hyperactivity Index from the Abbreviated Symptom Questionnaire	Results revealed that children with DCD and children suspect for DCD obtained significantly poorer scores on measures of attention and learning (reading, writing, and spelling) than the comparison children. Children with DCD and those suspected	Sample may be biased because the sample of children with DCD was ascertained from a large sample of children, which included typically developing children and children with attention and learning

Author	Study Objectives	Level/Design/Participants	Intervention and Outcome Measures	Results	Study Limitations
		motor problems on standardized tests of motor function	• Parent form of the CBCL • Woodcock–Johnson Psychoeducational Battery–Revised	for DCD also were found to display a relatively high level of social problems and a relatively high level of somatic complaints, according to parent report.	problems. No child was specifically referred because of motor skill difficulties.
Dunbar (1999)	The objective was to examine the relationships between a child's sensory processing skills and his or her home and school environments.	Level V Case study design *Participants* 3-yr-old girl exhibiting difficulty in occupational performance in her home and preschool contexts	Intervention but for review only focused on performance measures *Outcome Measures* • Sensory history • DeGangi–Berk Test of Sensory Integration • Early Inventory Developmental Profile	Child made gains as evidenced by increase in scores on the DeGangi–Berk Test of Sensory Integration, as well as specific improvements related to occupational performance that had meaning for her family (ability to engage in tabletop play activities, cessation of head banging, diminishment of tantrums, and sleeping through the night).	Generalizability is limited because of case study model.
Hauck & Dewey (2001)	The objective was to examine 3 theories (developmental lag, bilateral dysfunction, poor motor skills) that have been proposed to explain the high rates of ambiguous hand preference in young children with autism.	Level II Case–control design *Participants* 3 groups: 20 children with autism matched with 20 children with developmental delays and 20 typically developing children	Nonintervention; observation study *Outcome Measures* • Hand Preference Demonstration Test • Bayley Scales of Infant Development–2nd Edition or the Stanford–Binet Intelligence Scale–4th Edition • Battelle Developmental Inventory–Motor Domain	Study indicated that the lack of development of a hand preference in children with autism was not a direct function of their cognitive delay (developmental lag hypothesis), because children with developmental delays showed a dissimilar pattern of hand preference. Lack of a definite hand preference in children with autism was also not caused by a lack of motor skill development (poor motor skills hypothesis), because the children with developmental delays displayed similar levels of gross and fine motor skills without the accompanying lack of a definite hand preference. The bilateral brain dysfunction hypothesis was supported by the finding that children with autism with a definite hand preference displayed better performance on motor, language, and cognitive tasks than children with autism who did not display a definite hand preference.	Small sample size reduced generalizability. The population used in the study was young, and participants may not have naturally developed a hand preference at this point. Variability in how hand preference is classified made it difficult to draw definitive conclusions about the left-handedness rates in autism.

(Continued)

Table C3, Part IV. Evidence for Functional Performance Difficulties in Children and Adolescents With Difficulty Processing and Integrating Sensory Information: Education and Work *(cont.)*

Author/Year	Study Objectives	Level/Design/Participants	Intervention and Outcome Measures	Results	Study Limitations
Parham (1998)	The objective was to investigate the relationship of SI development to school achievement.	Level II Multivariate longitudinal case–control study *Participants* 2 groups: 32 randomly selected school-identified children with learning disabilities and 35 randomly selected children without learning disabilities, ages 6–8	Nonintervention; observational study *Outcome Measures* • Sensory Integration and Praxis Tests • Kaufman Assessment Battery for Children	SI factors were strongly related to arithmetic achievement at younger ages; the strength of this association declined with age. The reverse pattern was found for reading: SI was not significantly related to concurrent reading achievement at younger ages but was related to it at later ages. An unexpected finding was the strength of the relationship of the SI factors, particularly praxis, to arithmetic achievement.	Language-related and verbal ability measures were eliminated. Arithmetic measure consisted only of orally administered problems.
Rogers, Hepburn, & Wehner (2003)	The objective was to examine how early and how well sensory symptoms differentiate autism from other developmental disorders by using various tools to examine the relationship of sensory symptoms with intellectual ability, age, severity of autism, and severity of specific symptom clusters associated with autism and to investigate how these sensory symptoms may contribute to the acquisition of adaptive behavior in young children.	Level II Case–control design *Participants* 4 groups totaling 102 participants: 26 children with autism, 20 children with fragile X syndrome, 32 children with developmental disabilities of mixed etiology, and 24 typically developing children, ages 21–50 mo	Nonintervention; observational study *Outcome Measures* • Short Sensory Profile • Autism Diagnostic Interview–Revised • ADOS–Generic • Mullen Scales of Early Learning • Vineland Scales of Adaptive Behavior, Interview Edition	Differences were detected between the groups for tactile sensitivity, taste/smell sensitivity, underreactive/seeks stimulation, auditory filtering, and low energy/weak muscles. Children with fragile X syndrome and children with autism had significantly more sensory symptoms than the 2 comparison groups. Both groups were more impaired than the developmentally delayed and typically developing children in tactile sensitivity and auditory filtering. Children with autism were more abnormal in response to taste and smell than all other groups. Children with fragile X syndrome were more impaired than all other groups in low energy/weak muscles. A significant correlation was found between parent report of sensory symptoms using the Short Sensory Profile and clinician observation of repetitive-restricted behavior symptoms on the ADOS for the group with autism. Finally, abnormal sensory reactivity had a significant relationship with adaptive behavior.	A real understanding of sensory symptoms in autism and other disorders will require not only behavior observation and reports but also psychophysiological responses to sensory stimuli.

Note. ADOS = Autism Diagnostic Observation Schedule; ASD = autism spectrum disorder; CBCL = Child Behavior Checklist; DCD = developmental coordination disorder; PDD = pervasive developmental disorder; SI = sensory integration.

This table is a product of AOTA's Evidence-Based Practice Project and the *American Journal of Occupational Therapy.* Copyright © 2010 by the American Occupational Therapy Association. May be freely reproduced for personal use in clinical or educational settings as long as the source is cited. All other uses require written permission from the American Occupational Therapy Association. To apply, visit www.copyright.com.
From Koenig, K. P., & Rudney, S. G. (2010). Performance challenges for children and adolescents with difficulty processing and integrating sensory information: A systematic review (Suppl. Table 4). *American Journal of Occupational Therapy, 64,* 430–442. doi: 10.5014/ajot.2010.09073

Table C4. Summary of the Evidence of the Effectiveness of Occupational Therapy Interventions Using a Sensory Integration Approach for Children and Adolescents

Author/Year	Study Objectives	Level/Design/Participants	Intervention and Outcome Measures	Results	Study Limitations
Allen & Donald (1995)	The objective was to examine the effect of occupational therapy using an SI approach on motor proficiency of children with motor learning difficulties.	Level IV AB design, case series *Participants* $N = 5$ boys; ages 5–11 *Inclusion:* • Medical referral for motor or learning problems • No medical diagnosis • Mainstream school • Average IQ • No previous occupational therapy • No behavior problems	*Intervention* • Over a 6-mo period • 16 sessions occupational therapy using SI: — Sessions 1–4 were assessment, — Sessions 5–14 were treatment, and — Sessions 15–16 were reassessment; 1 hr/wk. *Treatment and Equipment* • Well described • Up to 5 activities providing tactile, vestibular, proprioceptive inputs; nondirective treatment; tapped child motivation; encouraged adaptive response; and followed a developmental course • Parent education • School liaison/consult • Home activities *Outcome Measures* BOTMP	4 of 5 participants improved on measures of motor proficiency, especially on the gross motor composite, using standard scores, which accounts for increasing age. Mean average improvement was 10 mo over an average treatment time of 5 mo for 4 of 5 participants. Functional qualitative gains from intervention were based on teacher and parent observation.	Variable of parent understanding was uncontrolled because parents were present in treatment when possible. Treating or assessing therapists were not blinded. No significance testing was done, so results are largely qualitative. Small sample size is a limitation.
Ayres (1972a)	The objective was to determine whether children with LD and SI problems make greater gains with a SI remediation program or academic work.	Level II Non-RCT Matched for type and level of SI dysfunction *Participants* • 2 matched groups, each with 30 participants • Generalized SI dysfunction • 12 with auditory–language disorder • Ages 5–9 *Inclusion:* Participants identified by their school as having LD. Performance on a battery of SI and academic tests fell below a specified level of dysfunction. Resulted in groups of 2 types of SI dysfunction: generalized dysfunction and auditory–language dysfunction.	*Intervention* *Experimental group:* Individualized SI intervention, 25–40 min/session, 5 days/wk, for 5–6 mo *Control group:* Equivalent time of classroom intervention *Outcome Measures* Portions of the SCSIT; ITPA; WRAT, academic test of spelling, reading, and arithmetic; Slosson Oral Reading Test, reading assessment	The experimental group with generalized SI dysfunction demonstrated significant gains in reading on the WRAT and on total WRAT score. The experimental group with auditory–language disorder demonstrated significant gains in WRAT reading and Slosson Oral Reading Test reading. Both experimental groups demonstrated significant gains in change scores in auditory–language skill on the ITPA beyond the $p = .01$ level and on the SCSIT.	The study demonstrates strengths in participant selection on the basis of the type and severity of SI dysfunction, resulting in a homogeneous participant pool specifically selected as appropriate for SI intervention. Testers were blind to group assignment. Groups were matched, but it was not specifically stated whether they were randomly assigned or not. Specific subtests of the SCSIT were not reported, and specific results of some significant statistical analyses were not reported. Small sample size may result in lack of significant results. Type II error (false negative).

(Continued)

Table C4. Summary of the Evidence of the Effectiveness of Occupational Therapy Interventions Using a Sensory Integration Approach for Children and Adolescents (cont.)

Author/Year	Study Objectives	Level/Design/Participants	Intervention and Outcome Measures	Results	Study Limitations
Ayres (1977)	The objective was to evaluate the effectiveness of sensory integrative therapy to improve the eye–hand coordination of children with LD, SI dysfunction, and choreathetosis.	Level II Non-RCT *Participants* • N = 54; 31 choreathetosis, 23 control • Participants were taken from a larger population used in a study on SI treatment to affect academic improvement.	*Interventions* • SI treatment interventions 0.5 hr 5×/wk for 6 mo over a 1-yr period • Control participants equivalent to time in special education classroom • Approximately 130 hr *Outcome Measures* Motor Accuracy Test right and left hand as pretest and posttest measure	There were no differences after the test on the Motor Accuracy Test between participants in the intervention and control groups.	The study needed more power. The small sample size was a limitation.
Baranek (2002)	The objective was to examine the efficacy of sensory and motor interventions with children with autism and to describe implications of findings for education and research.	Level I Systematic review *Inclusion* Remedial intervention targeting specific sensory or motor components; compensatory skills training approaches; task/environmental modifications *Sample* 29 studies: • 3 classical SI • 3 SI-based • 5 sensory stimulation • 9 auditory integration training/auditory • 3 visual • 2 sensory handling • 4 exercise	*Intervention* • SI therapy • Other SI-based approaches • Sensory stimulation techniques • Auditory integration training and related acoustic interventions • Visual therapies • Sensorimotor handling techniques • Physical exercise *Outcome Measures* Varied by study, but included outcomes such as play, language, behaviors, tactile sensitivity, sound sensitivity, developmental/cognitive performance, and physiological measures	*SI therapy:* Results showed improvements in mastery of play, engaged behaviors, increased adult and general social interaction, improved response to movement and affection, and improved approach to new activities. Children with hyperresponsivity to touch and movement had better outcomes than those with hyporesponsivity. No change was reported in peer interactions. *SI-based therapy:* Improvement occurred in various aspects of behavior. Improvement in all areas occurred after treatment and decreased sensory defensiveness. Fine motor activities elicited more speech variety, longer utterances, and decreased autistic speech than did vestibular treatment. *Sensory stimulation:* Decreased tension and anxiety were reported for the treatment group. Response to sounds improved. Stereotypic/self-stimulatory behaviors decreased. Social behavior improved. Vocalizations increased. *Auditory integration training:* Some evidence of improved attention and decreased sound sensitivity or other sensory problems were reported, and a decrease in aberrant behaviors was reported. Control groups often had just as many positive effects.	Limited studies were found on any 1 intervention. Some treatments (e.g., sensorimotor handling) are questionable because of outdated neurological theory. Individual studies were frequently methodologically weak with small sample sizes and lack of control participants. The author stated that the greatest limiting factor is the failure to link changes in the purported dysfunctional mechanism (e.g., auditory, vestibular, or visual dysfunction) to functional changes in behavior. The author also stated that the heterogeneity of the autism population may contribute to mixed results in these studies.

			Some studies reported adverse effects.	The author questioned generalizability and long-term effects of the interventions.
			• *Visual:* Improved body posture, facial expression, and ball catching; decreased aberrant behaviors	
			• *Sensory handling:* Few significant changes; increase in visual competency and mobility; short-term improvement on language and socialization	
			• *Exercise:* Decrease in self-stimulatory behaviors	
Bullock & Watter (1978)	The objective was to examine the effectiveness of an SI treatment program.	Level II Non-RCT 3 and 6 mo posttesting *Inclusion:* • Referral to clinic for learning, behavioral, or clumsiness problems • Normal intelligence • Absence of genetic defects • Presence of areas of abnormal functioning as determined by a neurodevelopmental screening *Participants* Treatment group = 78 children with minimal cerebral dysfunction. Treatment group divided into preschool, school-age, and total group. Control group = 7 children with minimal cerebral dysfunction. Ages: 3–12; 4.7:1 ratio boys to girls.	*Intervention* • Individualized clinic-based program providing sensory inputs addressing postural responses and motor planning • Home programming of daily activities also conducted • Control group received NT *Frequency* 6 mo of clinic/home intervention; undetermined frequency of clinic service *Outcome Measures* Neurodevelopmental assessment developed by authors Assessment examined 10 subtests of gross motor abilities, neurological signs, visual responses, primitive reflexes, orientation, postural reactions, posture relative to position, tactile, proprioception, and vestibular functioning; spatial relations; fears and compensatory actions in motor abilities. Each subtest was rated on a 4-point scale from normal to severe. Reliability and test–retest reliability were reported as highly consistent.	In the treatment group, both school-age and preschool-age children demonstrated marked decreases at 6-mo retest in incidence as reported in total percentage of children scored as "abnormal" (vs. "normal") on all 10 subtests of the Neurodevelopmental Evaluation. There was a decrease of 86% and 75% in total number of abnormalities in school-age and preschool-age groups compared with an increase of 7% and 14% in the control group. No significance tests were conducted. On tests of vestibular reactions, tonic reflexes, postural reactions, tone, touch, and motor planning, initial incidence was 50%–100% and 0%–9% after 6 mo. Severity of dysfunction in each testing category decreased over the 6-mo period. By the end of the period, most children went from moderate/severe dysfunction to mild dysfunction.	Nonblinding of examiner and treatment therapist was a limitation. The same therapist did all assessment and treatment. The specific frequency of intervention both in clinic and at home was not specified. The home program component was not specified and confounds description of program as SI. No significance tests were conducted.

(Continued)

Appendix C. Evidence Tables 163

Table C4. Summary of the Evidence of the Effectiveness of Occupational Therapy Interventions Using a Sensory Integration Approach for Children and Adolescents (cont.)

Author/Year	Study Objectives	Level/Design/Participants	Intervention and Outcome Measures	Results	Study Limitations
Bundy, Shia, Qi, & Miller (2007)	The objective was to examine whether sensory processing disorder interferes with playfulness, how the major manifestations of sensory processing disorder relate to playfulness, and whether OT/SI intervention results in increased playfulness.	Level II Non-RCT *Inclusion:* • Part of a larger sensory processing disorder intervention study • Diagnosis of sensory processing disorder by an experienced therapist • Low scores on Short Sensory Profile • Profile of scores on SIPT (note: only 4 children had low praxis) • Normal IQ *Participants* • $N = 2$ groups of 20 children • *Sensory processing disorder:* 4 girls, 16 boys; ages 4.4–9.8 (mean age = 6.9, $SD = 1.6$) • *Typically developing:* 9 girls, 11 boys; ages 4.7–11.7 (mean age = 7.5, $SD = 1.7$)	*Intervention* SI intervention, 20 1-hr sessions; described in L. J. Miller, Schoen, James, & Schaaf (2007) *Outcome Measures* • ToP, a test of components of playfulness and engagement in play • Short Sensory Profile for sensitivity to sensory information • 6 of the SIPT praxis tests—Bilateral Motor Coordination, Constructional Praxis, Oral Praxis, Postural Praxis, Sequencing Praxis, and Design Copying—for sensory processing disorder group only	Typically developing children demonstrated higher (better) ToP scores. ToP scores correlated significantly ($r = .72$, $p < .0005$) with the total score of the Short Sensory Profile. ToP scores correlated with SIPT scores at –.42. There was no significant difference on ToP scores in children with sensory processing disorder after SI intervention. Post hoc analysis identified that children with sensory processing disorder had relatively normal playfulness scores before therapy, suggesting there was not much room for improvement. Further analysis showed that children with sensory processing disorder engaged in more sedentary vs. active play, and lower ToP scores were found in the area of active play. Children with sensory processing disorder were more likely to engage in active play after SI intervention.	The small convenience sample was a limitation. The study group did not demonstrate much delay in play at the onset, leaving little room for change. The use of an observation-based measure of playfulness vs. a standard play format may have influenced the reliability of the test–retest results.
Candler (2003)	The objective was to examine the effectiveness of a summer camp program on occupational performance in children with SMD.	Level III Pretest–posttest *Participants* $N = 12$ children (8 boys, 4 girls) with SMD: 6 diagnosed with pervasive developmental disorder; 1 diagnosed with Down syndrome; 3 with no diagnosis; 2 diagnosed with ADHD; ages 5–13	*Intervention* Participation in a 1-wk day camp with an SI approach and therapeutic riding program to address occupational performance in school-age children with SMD Occupational therapists provided SI-based intervention, sensory diets, and environmental sensory adaptations. Therapeutic riding instructors provided horse-related activities. *Outcome Measure* Canadian Occupational Performance Measure with a modified interview format	There was a statistically significant improvement in performance or satisfaction for at least 1 of the goals reported by 9 of the 10 families that participated in postintervention interviews.	Results cannot be generalized to other populations because of the small study size, lack of randomization, and lack of a control group. The modifications to the Canadian Occupational Performance Measure influenced families' identification of goals. Almost half of the 116 goals were generated after review of a behavioral outcome list. This approach introduced a risk that the interviewer influenced the responses. The study design did not isolate which aspects of the camp experience contributed to the results.

Carte, Morrison, Sublett, Uemura, & Setrakian (1984)	The objective was to investigate the effects of SI intervention on hyporesponsive nystagmus, perceptual processing dysfunction, and academic performance in LD children with reading deficits.	Level I RCT *Participants* $N = 87$ children (66 boys, 21 girls): • Middle-class hyponystagmus group (treatment $n = 23$, 10 younger, 13 older; control $n = 22$, 15 younger, 7 older) • Ages 6–11 *Inclusion:* SCSIT identified SI deficits in addition to LDs.	*Intervention* 66 sessions ($2-3 \times 45$ min/wk for 9 mo) *SI intervention:* Individualized program emphasizing equalization and integration of tactile-proprioceptive and vestibular systems by stressing linear and rotary movement, improvement of bilateral coordination and motor planning, graduated nonresistive to resistive responses, passive to active participation, and context of child-directed approach. *Control participants:* No program description given. *Outcome Measures* • Gates-MacGintie—reading comprehension • WRAT Reading and Arithmetic Tests • Target Test—visual tracking, attention, and immediate memory • Underlining Test—rapid visual-perceptual analysis	Only hyponystagmus group results were reported. Authors reported that results were the same for total group. Significant increased duration was reported for nystagmus post-treatment for group ($p = .032$) and time ($p = 0$). SI group had significantly more normalized nystagmus ($p = .02$). Group × Time interaction effect was nonsignificant ($p = .102$.) Target test had a significant time effect, with both SI and control groups improving over time. Similar effects were found for reading comprehension and arithmetic.	Results discussed older and younger groups, but no age ranges were given for the groups, nor was a rationale for dividing by age. Very small sample size as a result of dividing by age could contribute to a lack of significant results ($n = 7$ to $n = 15$). Authors concluded that the lack of significant Group × Time interaction effects indicates that SI intervention is not effective in changing vestibular or perceptual processing.
Case-Smith & Bryan (1999)	The objective was to examine the effect of an occupational therapy intervention using an SI approach with preschool children with autism.	Level IV Single-participant AB design: • Nonengagement • Mastery play • Interaction *Participants* • 5 boys with autism; 1 child also had bilateral hearing loss and another had bipolar disorder • 4 boys were age 5 • 1 was age 4 (1 participant discontinued when started Lovass training)	*Interventions* After a 3-wk baseline period, individual occupational therapy with an SI approach was provided for 30 min/wk and weekly teacher consults; study lasted for 10 wk *Outcome Measures* Engagement Checklist Mastery Play rated by author. Videotape segments were viewed out of sequence from dates taped to decrease bias.	4 children decreased the frequency of nonengagement. 3 increased the frequency of mastery (goal-directed play). Improvements in frequency of interaction were minimal. Results supported the use of the Engagement Checklist as an intervention measurement.	Case studies have limited external validity, but because of outcomes rated in the natural environment, the authors feel positively that the changes in purposeful behavior and decrease of nonengagement behaviors are true functional improvements for this group of people. Study lacked a control group.

(Continued)

Table C4. Summary of the Evidence of the Effectiveness of Occupational Therapy Interventions Using a Sensory Integration Approach for Children and Adolescents (cont.)

Author/Year	Study Objectives	Level/Design/Participants	Intervention and Outcome Measures	Results	Study Limitations
Grimwood & Rutherford (1980)	The objective was to assess the effectiveness of SI treatment on children predicted to be "at risk" for reading failure.	Level I RCT Posttesting at 1 and 2 yr after treatment *Participants* • $N = 21$ children (16 boys, 5 girls): treatment group $n = 9$; control group $n = 10$ • Grade 1 students, mean age = 5.7 yr *Inclusion*: Identified as "at risk" for reading failure with the Satz Battery • SI diagnosis from SCSIT, SCPNT, and clinical observations	*Intervention* *SI intervention*: 24 wk, 2×0.5 hr/wk Had individualized treatment plans; provided sensory input, addressed postural mechanisms and bilateral coordination *Control participants*: NT *Outcome Measures* • Iota Word Test, word recognition test • St. Lucia Graded Word Reading Test • Neale Analysis of Reading Ability	SI intervention group had significantly increased reading skills, $p < .05$ on all measures. Final performance results of the SI group were consistent with those of their overall age peers. Results were sustained over a 2-yr period.	Study is not clear about whether evaluators were blind or not. The assessment was done by psychology students. The sample size was small. The control group was "no treatment," so there was a possible Hawthorne effect for the SI group.
Hoehn & Baumeister (1994)	The objective was to determine whether children with learning disabilities differentially exhibit concomitant problems in SI and whether such children are helped in any way by means specific and unique to SI-based therapy.	Level I Systematic review *Study Selection* 7 studies using SI treatment with students with LD published after Ottenbacher's (1982b) meta-analysis. *Inclusion Criteria* Same as Ottenbacher study; limited to only studies of children with LD; 6 studies were Level II non-RCTs, and 1 was a Level IV single-participant design *Sample Characteristics* Ages 5–11 Had LD and SI dysfunction	*Intervention* All studies included SI treatment described generally as "using specific SI therapy principles and techniques designed to provide vestibular, proprioceptive, and tactile stimulation within a meaningful, self-directed activity in order to elicit an adaptive motor response." *Outcome Measures* Outcomes included measures of sensorimotor functioning (e.g., postrotary nystagmus), perceptual processing, motor skills, academic abilities, attention self-concept, and behavior.	*Motor outcomes*: 3 of 7 studies had only time-of-test main effects. Authors concluded that on the basis of this finding, all other motor effects in other studies were caused by maturation, although they reported various significant positive Time × Group interaction effects for vestibular and motor outcomes on the other 4 studies. *Cognitive, language, and academic measures*: Significant time-of-test results were found in several studies, but no significant Time × Group main effects were reported for any study. *Self-esteem/self-concept*: 3 studies included these outcomes. No significant Time × Group main effects were found for any study, although pretest–posttest improvement was found in 2 studies, with the SI groups improving on more measures.	Qualitative analysis frequently focused on postrotary nystagmus outcomes that do not necessarily reflect functional gains. Similarly, critique of changes in nystagmus does not reflect a good understanding of SI theory. The authors equated the simple increase in duration of nystagmus with the effectiveness of SI intervention irrespective of whether the end nystagmus is within average ranges or not. Although inconsistent across studies, positive results were found for gross motor or motor planning outcomes in several studies. In some studies, significant effects were found for pretest–posttest results for these outcomes, but because those studies did not have a reported significant Group × Time interaction effect, the results were dismissed as maturation

Study	Objective	Design/Participants	Intervention/Outcome Measures	Results	Comments
Humphries, Snider, & McDougall (1993)	The objective was to compare SI and PM effectiveness while valuing the therapist's clinical impressions of change as an outcome measure and to specifically examine the effects of interventions on a subgroup with vestibular problems.	Level I RCT Participants • N = 103 participants with LD and SI dysfunction • Ages 58–107 mo • 35 in SI group, 35 in PM group, 33 in NT group	Intervention 72 hr, 3×60 min/wk for SI and PM SI group: Therapeutic application of selected activities that provided tactile and vestibular experiences and proprioceptive input to help the child make an adaptive response PM group: Motor training to remediate specific motor skill weaknesses and warm-ups, gross motor, and fine motor activities Outcome Measures Calculations were made regarding the reduction of number of systems of dysfunction (e.g., vestibular, tactile, dyspraxia, vestibular dyspraxia, tactile and vestibular dysfunction, tactile and vestibular dyspraxia, and generalized dysfunction).	SI and PM were better than NT, but SI was not better than PM to improve motor skills. No greater treatment effects were found for those with vestibular dysfunction than those without; however, there were greater effects for those with mild vs. severe SI dysfunction. NT group showed improvement on SI function, but only SI and PM groups showed improvement on motor skills.	effects. Because the alternate treatment groups in those studies were PM groups, the lack of differences between groups may have reflected problems with differentiating between interventions with adequate fidelity. Description of SI treatment provided in the study suggests the intervention may or may not have adhered to essential characteristics of SI intervention. In addition, a form of fidelity measurement occurred by rating the amount to which each therapist adhered to individual treatment plans, further indicating possible departure from essential characteristics of SI treatment. The NT group did not receive equivalent amounts of one-on-one attention. Only measuring a decrease in symptoms of sensorimotor dysfunction does not address the functional gains children may have made despite retention of their initial diagnostic categories.
Humphries, Wright, McDougall, & Vertes (1990)	The objective was to compare the effect of SI/PM and NT on language, PM, and cognitive function.	Level I RCT Participants N = 30; ages 72–99 mo LD, SI problems (10 per group); 7 girls, 3 boys in each group	Intervention 24 sessions (1×60 min/wk) SI group: Individualized SI therapy PM group: 1:1 perceptual training Control group: NT Outcome Measures BOTMP, SCSIT subtests, SCPNT, WRAT, Test of Language Development	SI group performed significantly better than PM and NT on BOTMP Battery Composite Measure and Gross Motor Composite Measure and the SCSIT Motor Accuracy–Right Measure. No group differences were observed on higher level cognitive, language, or academic performance.	Rating of improvement on clinical observations was rated as only "change or no change," score of 0 or 1, which greatly limited the range and variability in the data. Comparison made to Ayres' (1972a) claims that SI improves academic abilities with no mention that the participants received 5× more treatment before retest (e.g., 5 sessions/wk over 6 mo).

(Continued)

Table C4. Summary of the Evidence of the Effectiveness of Occupational Therapy Interventions Using a Sensory Integration Approach for Children and Adolescents (cont.)

Author/Year	Study Objectives	Level/Design/Participants	Intervention and Outcome Measures	Results	Study Limitations
					Authors noted there was no wait time after treatment ended before posttest; therefore, there was no time for consolidation of gains, which may have diminished the measurement of positive effects that may have occurred.
Humphries, Wright, Snider, & McDougall (1992)	The objective was to confirm the results of a previous study on the effectiveness of SI therapy compared with PM training and NT.	Level I RCT *Participants* • $N = 103$ children, primarily boys, ages 58–107 mo; mean age = 79 mo • Motor coordination problems; LD: SI ($n = 35$), PM ($n = 35$), NT ($n = 33$)	*Intervention* 72 hr 3×60 min/wk over 8 mo: • Intervention was delivered by 8 occupational therapists certified in SI assessment and experienced in SI intervention. • Fidelity to intervention was addressed as therapists identified acceptable activities for each intervention and were observed to determine extent of adherence. Adherence was 85% for SI and 79% for PM. • Outcome examiners were blind. *Outcome Measures* *Motor/sensory outcomes:* SCSIT; SCPNT; BOTMP; Beery-Buktenica Test of Visual–Motor Integration; clinical observations defined by Dunn and divided into categories of motor planning and vestibular dysfunction *Psychoeducational measures:* Wechsler Intelligence Scale for Children, Wechsler Preschool and Primary Scale of Intelligence, Test of Visual–Perceptual Skills, Gestalt closure and number recall tests from Kaufman Assessment Battery for Children; WRAT; handwriting measure; language measures from ITPA; Clinical Evaluation of Language Functions; Durrell Analysis of Reading Difficulty; short form of the Rosner Test	Only motor variables demonstrated significant gains ($p = .04$). Psychoeducational variables did not reach significance. The gross motor composite score of the BOTMP accounted for most of the significance of group differences. *Design copying:* PM group did better than the SI group but not the NT group ($p = .05$). *Balance subtest of BOTMP:* PM group did better than the SI group but not the NT group ($p = .05$). *Bilateral coordination subtest of BOTMP:* PM group did better than the NT group but not the SI group ($p = .05$). Motor planning: SI group did better ($p < .01$) than both the PM and NT groups, with SI group showing superior improvement (but not necessarily significant improvement) in all clinical observations of this area. Better performance of SI group on the tongue-to-lip observation ($p = .02$) accounted for most of the significance of this item. Performance on the motor planning measure for the SI group was also the only measure to significantly correlate ($p < .001$) with handwriting readiness performance.	This study was generally well controlled and rigorous. However, the PM intervention provided in this study was not the same as the previous study, but included more activities focused on postural control, balance, and quality of movement, which may have resulted in improvement in those areas through more direct training of those tasks. The difference between SI and PM interventions may be less clear in this study, as seen by less adherence to the PM fidelity.

Author	Study Objectives	Study Design/Participants	Intervention and Outcome Measures	Results	Study Limitations
Leemrijse, Meijer, Vermeer, Adèr, & Diemel (2000)	The objective was to evaluate the effects of Le Bon Départ treatment and SI treatment on the motor performance of children diagnosed with developmental coordination disorder.	Level IV Single-participant design with multiple baselines and alternating treatments. Treatment order was randomized to control for carryover effects. Length of phases was randomized to control for spontaneous improvement and seasonal effects. Children received special treatment during the baseline phase to control for placebo. The tester was blinded for phase and treatment order to control for measurement bias. *Participants* 6 children (5 boys, 1 girl), ages 6.0–8.1, diagnosed with developmental coordination disorder. Participating families spoke Dutch. Children with marked learning disorders, hyperactivity, or other behavioral disorders were excluded. Exclusion was based not on set criteria but on teacher opinion.	of Auditory Analysis; behavior measure of the Conners' Parent–Teacher Questionnaire; Matching Familiar Figures Test; North York Self-Concept Scale *Intervention* Each participant received baseline treatment, Le Bon Départ, and SI for 12–18 wk each in weekly 1-hr one-on-one sessions. Le Bon Départ and SI were provided by an experienced therapist. *Outcome Measures* Movement Assessment Battery for Children, Rhythm Integrated; 6 praxis subtests from the SIPT; and VAS	*Group Effects* During Le Bon Départ treatment, scores on all measures improved significantly. During SI treatment, scores on all measures improved, but only the VAS scores showed significant improvement. However, when gains made during Le Bon Départ were compared with gains made during SI, only the Rhythm Integrated scores showed a significant difference between interventions. Treatment order did not significantly affect assessment scores. *Individual Effects* After all phases were complete, 5 participants had significant improvement in Movement Assessment Battery for Children scores, 2 showed significant improvement on the praxis subtests, and all 6 showed significant improvement on VAS.	All outcome scores were pooled into a single average to increase responsivity. However, pooling made it impossible to state in detail which aspect of motor performance improved the most. Small study size and lack of randomized groups limit the generalizability of this study. Testers were not blinded to Rhythm Integrated and VAS. The underlying causes of developmental coordination disorder were not addressed. The aspects of the intervention responsible for positive effects were not addressed. Although Le Bon Départ appears to adhere to a protocol that could be referenced, the SI therapy in this study was not manualized, and as such it is not possible to verify that the SI treatment administered held true to SI theory.
Linderman & Stewart (1999)	The objective was to examine the effects of SI-based occupational therapy, provided in an outpatient clinic, on the functional behavior of 2 young children diagnosed with autism when measured at home.	Level IV Single-participant, AB design *Participants* N = 2 boys with autism, ages 3.9 and 3.3	*Intervention* SI 1 hr 1 time/wk for 11 and 7 wk for Participant 1 and Participant 2, respectively. Treatment provided by experienced therapist; separate therapist for observations at baseline and other measurement points to decrease bias *Outcome Measures* Functional Behavioral Assessment for Children with SI Dysfunction Scale expanded from 4 to 10 points to increase sensitivity	Significant improvements in social interaction, approach to new activities, response to holding and hugging, and response to movement were reported. Significant gains did not occur in functional communication during mealtime. The child who more poorly registered sensory input made fewer observable gains.	This was a small study with a short duration. Results may have been confounded by other treatment added during the study. It is preferable to do an ABA design rather than only AB. Making inferences from single-participant design is limited because of the small sample size and lack of control group.

(Continued)

Table C4. Summary of the Evidence of the Effectiveness of Occupational Therapy Interventions Using a Sensory Integration Approach for Children and Adolescents (cont.)

Author/Year	Study Objectives	Level/Design/Participants	Intervention and Outcome Measures	Results	Study Limitations
L. J. Miller, Coll, & Schoen (2007)	The objective was to examine whether OT/SI ameliorates attention, cognitive/social, sensory, or behavioral problems better than an active alternative placebo or NT.	Level I RCT 3 groups: OT/SI, activity, NT *Participants* • $N = 24$ children with SMD (7 = OT/SI, 10 = activity protocol, 7 = NT). • 6 girls, 18 boys; ages 3–11.6, mean age = 6	*Intervention* OT/SI 2×/wk for 10-wk manualized *Intervention:* Manualized intervention based on principles proposed by Ayres (1972a) emphasizing clinical reasoning and using a draft fidelity-to-intervention measure with 6 therapists providing intervention and parent education *Alternate treatment:* Activity protocol provided by educators or raters with a psychology degree and experience with children: • No parent education with this group • No specific intervention related to child's problems • Included engaging in tabletop play activities, games, puzzles, blocks, arts and crafts *NT group:* 10-wk waitlist for OT/SI *Outcome Measures* Leiter Attention and Cognitive/Social subscores; Short Sensory Profile; Vineland Adaptive Behavior Scales; CBCL; Goal Attainment Scales; Electrodermal Response using the Sensory Challenge Protocol Functional behaviors mentioned for each participant varied depending on results of pretest observations and parent interview	OT/SI group demonstrated significantly greater results than NT and alternate treatment on Goal Attainment Scales and Leiter–Attention and Cognitive/Social subscores. The OT/SI group demonstrated greater reduction in the amplitudes of electrodermal reactivity responses than the other groups. There were no significant differences among groups for the Short Sensory Profile or the CBCL internalizing; however, the OT/SI group showed greater gain scores.	This study had blind examiners for the physiological testing but not for the other measures. There was also no reporting of the qualifications of the therapists who did the testing or intervention. The study had low power, potentially resulting in nonsignificant results because of a very small sample size. Length of intervention sessions was not specified. The study did control for therapeutic alliance, statistical regression, maturation, history, and instrumentation. A power analysis was done for future studies. Parent education was indicated as part of the protocol, but no information was given as to how much or in what format.
L. J. Miller, Schoen, James, & Schaaf (2007)	The objective was to conduct a pilot outcome study to inform a future RCT regarding replicable criteria for identification of a homogeneous group with sensory processing disorder, identify sensitive	Level III Pretest–posttest *Inclusion:* Diagnosis by expert occupational therapist of SMD *Exclusion:* IQ <85, other developmental, psychiatric, neural, or orthopedic problems except	*Intervention* OT/SI 2×/wk for 10 wk Intervention based on principles by Ayres emphasizing clinical reasoning with focus on attaining occupational goals. Used pilot intervention manual using the STEP–SI.	Demonstrated significant improvement on the following measures: • Leiter Cognitive/Social Subscale: $d = .50$ • Short Sensory Profile: Total score, $d = 1.62$	Length of intervention sessions was not specified. Number of cancelled intervention sessions was reported but not specified. Staff turnover may have affected service provision.

Study	Objective	Level/Design/Participants	Intervention and Outcome Measures	Results	Study Limitations
	outcome measures, develop a manualization of components of treatment, and develop fidelity to treatment measure.	ADHD, LD, and mild Tourette syndrome. *Participants* 30 children with SMD, ages 3.9–11 (mean age = 6.79, SD = 1.75)	*Outcome Measures* • *Sensory functioning:* Short Sensory Profile • *Attention, impulsivity, and activity:* ADD-H Comprehensive Teacher's Rating Scale (ACTeRS); 3 subscales of the Leiter International Performance Scale; Barkley's Behavior Rating Scale; Barkley's Behavior Rating for ADHD; Swanson Nolan and Pelham (SNAP-IV) • *Anxiety:* Multidimensional Anxiety Scale for Children • *Activities of daily living:* Vineland Adaptive Behavior Scale • *Social and emotional behaviors:* CBCL • *Physiological measures:* electrodermal reactivity using the Sensory Challenge Protocol • *Changes in natural settings:* behavior rating scale based on videotape of treatment • *Individualized Measure of Parent-Perceived Priorities for Change:* Goal Attainment Scales	• Vineland Socialization subscore: $d = 0.82$ • CBCL externalizing subscore: $d = 0.54$ • CBCL internalizing subscore: $d = 0.43$ • Goal Attainment Scales: $d = 2.16$ No differences were seen on the Barkley's Behavior Rating, the SNAP-IV, the Anxiety-Multidimensional Anxiety Scale for Children, and other subsets of the Vineland, CBCL, and Leiter.	Study duration was longer than anticipated. Evaluators were not blinded. There were too many outcome variables for the number of participants and no use of statistical adjustments.
Morrison & Sublett (1986)	The objective was to determine whether nystagmus, equilibrium, and visual–motor skills improve with SI treatment compared with continued enrollment in special education classes only.	Level I RCT *Participants* $N = 47$ children who were homogeneous in terms of degree of reading retardation and hyponystagmus, ≤12 s on total direction scores • Control group: 14 girls, 7 boys; mean age = 104 mo • Treatment group: 18 girls, 8 boys; mean age = 96.8 mo	*Interventions* SI treatment provided after school for 66 sessions 2–3×/wk over 8.5 mo. Both control and SI groups remained in their regular LD classroom throughout the day. Treatment consisted of tactile, proprioceptive, and vestibular treatment, with rotary and linear movements, and used hammocks and platform swings. *Outcome Measures* Intell testing, WRAT, Gates MacGinte, Postrotary Nystagmus Test, Equilibrium, Visual-Motor Integration Test	This research supports earlier research that indicated that there is a subgroup of children who do not adequately comprehend what they read and who also demonstrate vestibular processing problems. However, the results do not indicate that SI treatment is uniquely effective in treating these dysfunctions. There were no significant differences between the treatment and control groups on nystagmus, equilibrium, or visual–motor skills.	The study did not reassess reading and may have selected measures (e.g., nystagmus) that are less likely to change than behavior on other measures. Ayres (1972) has stated that duration of nystagmus may not "normalize" with treatment, but end products (e.g., reading skills) may improve. The study also did not look at ocular control, which would likely be the first area to change.
Ottenbacher (1982a)	The objective was to determine whether duration of postrotary nystagmus changes over the course of SI therapy.	Level IV Single-participant design *Participants* $N = 3$ children with LD	*Interventions* • 5-wk baseline • 50-min SI • 3× a week, passive and active vestibular stimulation • 20 wk of intervention	Visual/statistical analysis was used. 2 participants showed changes in nystagmus; the 1 with low duration of nystagmus increased; the 1 with typical nystagmus showed a decrease caused by hypothesized	Only the duration of the Postrotary Nystagmus Test was measured pretest and posttest, not ocular control or functional areas thought to be related to vestibular function.

(Continued)

Table C4. Summary of the Evidence of the Effectiveness of Occupational Therapy Interventions Using a Sensory Integration Approach for Children and Adolescents (cont.)

Author/Year	Study Objectives	Level/Design/Participants	Intervention and Outcome Measures	Results	Study Limitations
			Outcome Measure Duration of postrotary nystagmus	habituation. 1 did not change appreciably; however, in the last treatment session, the child's nystagmus was at 10-s duration. This last participant did not show other signs of vestibular problems.	Making inferences from single-participant design is limited because of the small sample size and lack of control group.
Ottenbacher (1982b)	The objective was to synthesize existing evidence on the efficacy of SI therapy, as applied to various clinical populations, using meta-analysis.	Level I Meta-analysis *Study Selection* Comprehensive literature search for studies, including computer search and hand searches *Study Criteria* • Investigated the effect of SI intervention. Dependent variable evaluated for academic achievement, motor or reflex integration, or language • At least 2 groups: SI and NT control group; results had to allow quantitative analysis • $N = 8$ studies (317 participants) • 7 studies had some type of random assignment or matching • 1 study had no experimental manipulation Participants ages 4–62 *Diagnosis:* $n = 89$ mental retardation, $n = 191$ LD, $n = 18$ aphasia, and $n = 19$ at risk for learning or reading disorder	*Intervention* All studies used SI therapy using sensory stimulation and adaptive responses involving total body movement and including some combination of vestibular, proprioceptive, or tactile stimulation, excluding studies that provided only tactile or vestibular stimulation. *Outcome Measures* Outcomes included the areas of academic achievement, motor or reflex integration, or language function.	SI therapy had a significant effect on motor, academic, and language outcomes compared with NT control participants. The 3 clinical groups commonly identified as having sensory processing issues (mental retardation, LD, language impaired/aphasic) responded to SI therapy at significant levels compared with their same-diagnosis peers not receiving intervention. The effect size analysis indicated that SI had its greatest effect when the outcome was a motor or reflex outcome and was least effective with language outcomes.	Study included a wide range of diagnoses and ages, including adults. Examined SI only in relation to NT. Levels of individual studies not stated. A strength is that this meta-analysis technique was cutting-edge data analysis at the time of publication of this study.
Ottenbacher, Short, & Watson (1979)	The objective was to strengthen the empirical foundation that duration of postrotary nystagmus of different subgroups of children with LD are differentially affected by SI intervention and that changes are more manifest with increasing therapy.	Level III Pretest–posttest *Participants* $N = 43$ children in 6 groups Short treatment was <6 mo with low, medium, and high nystagmus. Long treatment was >6 mo with low, medium, and high nystagmus. Ages = 51–125 mo	*Intervention* • *Long treatment:* ≥6 mo for 5 hr/mo • *Short treatment:* any not meeting the requirements of long treatment Intervention was described as SI therapy. No other information was given.	Children with low initial nystagmus demonstrated a near doubling of duration after intervention of >6 mo. The authors concluded that longer therapy resulted in greater gains. There was a significant interaction of duration of nystagmus with length of therapy.	Specifics of administration of intervention were not clear. No data were given on therapist qualifications, interventions, etc. This study provides some interesting information on nystagmus processing but lacks any significant rigor or control.

Author/Year	Study Objectives	Level/Design/Participants	Intervention and Outcome Measures	Results	Study Limitations
Polatajko, Kaplan, & Wilson (1992)	The objective was to examine the efficacy of SI intervention on improving academic and motor skills of children with learning disabilities.	**Level I** Systematic review *Study Selection* 7 studies using SI treatment with students with LD published since 1978 *Study Criteria* • Children with LD or at risk for learning problems • SI dysfunction • Individualized SI intervention provided • ≥1 comparison group and random assignment to groups (e.g., 2-group randomized clinical trial) • Evaluation of motor or academic outcomes • Pre–post testing, with 2 using follow-up and 1 midtreatment *Sample Characteristics* 311 children ages 4.8–13 with LD and SI dysfunction	*Intervention* • Individualized SI intervention provided in all studies • 2 studies compared with NT groups • 2 studies used PM training groups • 3 studies used alternative treatment (e.g., tutoring, reading readiness, PM strategies) • 1 study used unspecified activities Intervention frequency varied by study; a minimum of 1 hr/wk was given by all. Frequency ranged from 1–3 sessions, rate from 1–3 hr/wk, total dose from 19.5–76 hr. *Outcome Measures* Academic performance measures for reading and math used in 7 of 7 studies. Other measures used in 6 of 7 studies: Motor, visual–motor, sensory–motor, nystagmus, and language performance	Authors found that SI intervention was not an effective treatment for academic problems of children with LD, was inconclusive as to whether it was more effective than PM approaches, and needs more research to determine whether SI was better than maturation alone. • All studies showed improvement on all variables (except 1 study showed no change on reading and math) from pretesting to posttesting. • Across the 6 outcome variables, SI was more effective than NT in 6 of 15 comparisons. • Across outcome variables, SI was more effective than a placebo in 1 of 3 comparisons. • Across outcomes, SI was more effective than other treatments on 2 of 20 comparisons but as effective in 16 of 20 comparisons.	Authors reported the 7 studies presented small to medium intervention effects with low power, likely contributing to Type II errors. The experimental nature of the interventions provided in the studies may not have reflected the clinical application of the approach, and differences between interventions may not have been sufficient. Outcome measures reported may not have been sensitive enough to capture gains made in interventions and may not reflect the gains that are meaningful to the children and parents.
Polatajko, Law, Miller, Schaffer, & Macnab (1991)	The objective was to assess whether there is a difference between the effects of an occupational therapy program using SI and one using a PM program in improving academic performance, motor performance, or self-esteem in children with SI dysfunction.	**Level I** RCT, with follow-up at 9 mo; SI and PM groups, no nontreatment control *Participants* $N = 67$ children (35 SI, 32 PM); 58 boys, 9 girls; mean age = 7.4 yr (standard deviation = 71–109 mo); LD; identified SI dysfunction	*Intervention* 60 min/wk for 6 mo, 3-mo break from intervention SI program used sensory modalities to elicit an adaptive response, graded activities selected according to child's motor skills, and ability to tolerate sensory stimulation. PM program used activities designed to improve PM function, including table-top activities, fine and gross motor activities, and eye–hand coordination tasks. Did not include any activities used in SI program.	*Academic performance:* Both SI and PM groups demonstrated significant gains on the Woodcock–Johnson in reading, math, and written language compared with the standardization sample norms at both the 6-mo termination of intervention and follow-up at 9 mo. There were no significant differences in performance among the SI and PM groups in academic areas, with the exception that the SI group approached significance in mathematics ($p = .054$ at 6 mo and $p = .058$ at 9 mo using a 2-tailed test; would be significant with 1-tail test).	Although maturation may be a factor in the results, the growth rates of the sample suggest that maturation alone does not account for the gains. Further examination with a control group would be necessary. In this study, authors were unable to recruit a sufficient number of control participants. Low power of the study with greater-than-expected outcome variance made detection of difference

(Some data were obtained by means of a record review.)
Outcome Measures
SCPNT
• Low group: < -1.0 SD
• Medium group: -1.0 to $+1.0$ SD
• High group: $> +1.0$ SD

Children with high nystagmus demonstrated a decrease in nystagmus duration. Maturation was ruled out as a factor in the increase in duration. There were no significant effects of age on nystagmus.

(Continued)

Table C4. Summary of the Evidence of the Effectiveness of Occupational Therapy Interventions Using a Sensory Integration Approach for Children and Adolescents (cont.)

Author/Year	Study Objectives	Level/Design/Participants	Intervention and Outcome Measures	Results	Study Limitations
			A treatment manual was developed at the onset of the study and included activities coded as PM or SI. Therapists were restricted to activities specified in the manual. Fidelity was monitored with an activity recording form and randomized checks by the investigators. *Outcome Measures* BOTMP; Woodcock–Johnson measured reading, math, and written language; Coopersmith Behavioral Assessment of Self-Esteem; and the Personality Inventory for Children	*Motor performance:* No significant changes in performance were noted relative to the standardization sample norms; however, the authors pointed out that the scores are age-adjusted. They suggested that both the PM and SI groups were able to maintain a motor performance growth rate commensurate with the standardization sample (e.g., demonstrating an actual improvement in raw score performance) that they did not appear to demonstrate before. Half of the children improved at a greater rate than the normal rate of development. There were no significant differences in motor performance between SI and PM. *Self-esteem:* The SI group showed significant improvement on the Behavioral Assessment of Self-Esteem at both 6 and 9 mo. The PM group showed no change. However, differences between the SI and PM groups were not significant.	difficult, suggesting that a larger sample is needed. Although this study attempted to manualize the interventions, strict adherence to specific activities is not necessarily conducive to the underlying principles of SI intervention. For example, eye–hand coordination activities may be incorporated into both SI and PM activities. A research assistant who was not an occupational therapist administered study testing and was blinded to group status.
Roberts, King-Thomas, & Boccia (2007)	The objective was to examine behavioral treatment effects of classical SI therapy.	Level IV Single-case participant ABAB design *Participants* N = 1 boy, 3 yr 5 mo, with average nonverbal intellectual skills, delayed communication skills, and SMD	*Intervention* • During intervention phase, SI intervention • 1 hr 3×/wk involving clinic-based services only • No classroom consultation • Treatment provided by a highly trained therapist *Protocol:* • 2 wk NT, 5 wk treatment • 2 wk NT • 2 wk treatment *Outcome Measures* Observational ratings conducted by teacher and teacher aide of behavioral regulation in preschool setting within 3 contexts: circle time, outdoor play, and activity/work time	Results suggest a significant reduction in aggressive acts, mouthing objects, and intensity of teacher input and an increase in engagement associated with treatment phases. Degree of teacher intensity needed to manage the participant's behavior during the first intervention phase and second NT phase was significantly lower than that needed in the first NT phase. The estimates of level of engagement suggest an increase across phases.	Typically, information from single-case studies has limited applicability; however, given the multiple repeated measures taken across the four conditions, this study provides a nice pilot study that might be most easily replicated in clinical and educational settings. Additional single-case studies in this model could add to the body of evidence on the effectiveness of SI intervention, one case at a time, while researchers ready themselves to have all necessary tools to apply for funding for a Level 1 RCT study.

			resulting in 35 days of behavior rating. Raters were blind to the intervention and to treatment phases of the study. 2 raters allowed for comparison of reliability.	
Schroeder (1982)	The objective was to determine whether 1st graders with suspected neurological problems would benefit from Rosner's Perceptual Skills Curriculum, Ayres's SI intervention, or a combination of both.	Level II Non-RCT *Participants* Treatment group: $n = 15$ children from a sample of 87 1st graders evaluated with Bender Visual–Motor Gestalt Test, Wepman Auditory Discrimination Test, and Manual Form Perception Test from SCSIT ($n = 5$ per group). Control group: $n = 5$, no treatment, children remained in regular classroom	*Intervention* • 16-wk remedial program • Group 1: Rosner Curriculum for three 30-min sessions • Group 2: SI for two 45-min sessions • Group 3: Both approaches • Group 4: 5 control participants with no neurological problems *Outcome Measures* Bender, Wepman, SCSIT, WRAT	Group 3, who received both approaches, showed improvement in visual, auditory, and tactile gains. Group 2, who received only SI, showed greater tactile gains. Group 1, who received only Rosner, showed greater auditory gains. Both SI and Rosner were similar on visual improvements. On the WRAT for reading, there was a 6-mo improvement with SI, 1-yr improvement with Rosner, and 9-mo improvement with both SI and Rosner. Children in the SI group demonstrated more improvement in math than the other groups. Spelling achievement was similar for both groups. Progress with both interventions appears similar to or better than control group progress.	This study presents data as graphics only with no statistical analysis. There were no well-defined cutoff criteria for sample inclusion. The authors did not identify number of boys and girls, and the sample sizes were small.
Vargas & Camilli (1999)	The objective was to determine whether existing studies support the efficacy of SI intervention.	Level I Meta-analysis *Study Selection* Comprehensive literature search for studies published from 1972 through 1994, including computer search and hand searches *Study Criteria* • Investigated the effect of SI intervention • At least 2 groups • Reported results in a manner to allow quantitative comparison • Reported outcomes of academic skills, motor function, behavior, language, or sensorimotor function	*Interventions* SI treatment defined as a treatment aimed to enhance development of basic SI processes with activities that provided vestibular, proprioceptive, tactile, or other somatosensory inputs to elicit adaptive body responses. *Variables* Several study variables were examined to determine effects on the intervention outcomes reported. *Study Design Variables* Quality of treatment using SI, total treatment hours, diagnosis, age, design quality, sampling method, number of outcome measures,	SI intervention demonstrated small to moderate effects with psychoeducational and motor outcomes compared with no intervention, but was as effective as alternate interventions with larger effects reported in earlier studies. *SI/NT:* Found significant effects, $d = 0.29$, but larger effects were found with earlier studies that had fewer measurement categories and fewer outcome measures. Significant effects were found for measurement categories of psychoeducational ($d = 0.39$) and motor ($d = 0.40$) measures. SI/alternative treatment: SI and alternate conditions showed equal effects ($d = 0.09$).	The author reported that there was a limited number of studies, which often had poor reporting of pertinent information, such as types of disability, provider qualifications, descriptions of treatment strategies, and the like. Interrater reliability of the coding process was not verified. There were potential coding problems. Results of children with _D were combined with those of children with mental retardation. The criteria of SI intervention were unclear, and it was not clear whether studies were appropriate.

(Continued)

Appendix C. Evidence Tables

Table C4. Summary of the Evidence of the Effectiveness of Occupational Therapy Interventions Using a Sensory Integration Approach for Children and Adolescents (cont.)

Author/Year	Study Objectives	Level/Design/Participants	Intervention and Outcome Measures	Results	Study Limitations
		Study Sample 27 articles representing 24 studies; 18 comparisons for SI/NT; 16 comparisons for SI/alternative treatment *Sample Characteristics* • SI/NT studies: 341 participants in experimental group, 237 in control • SI/alternative treatment studies: 250 participants in experimental group, 191 in control • Ages: 3–adult • Diagnosis: LD, minor brain dysfunction, at risk, motor delay, psychiatric, aphasia, mental retardation	number of measurement categories, professional affiliations of researcher, geographic location, publication year *Outcome Measures* Psychoeducational, motor function, behavior, language, and sensory–perceptual outcomes		Adult studies were included with child studies, which may have diluted results. The question of whether more recent studies have controlled intervention to the point of affecting essential characteristics of SI intervention may be an issue with fidelity to intervention of some studies included in this review.
Werry, Scaletti, & Mills (1990)	The objective was to assess the effectiveness of SI intervention compared with a control group in children with LD.	Level I RCT • SI and untreated control • SI group further divided into early and late-aged groups for data analysis *Inclusion:* Children identified by teachers as having learning difficulties, difficulties paying attention, or clumsiness; SI dysfunction determined by Ayres (1972) *Clinical Observations* *Exclusion:* Children with mental retardation, major neurological disorders, previous SI treatment, on any medication, parents refused inclusion, no SI problems observed, failure to respond to recruitment letter, or considered unlikely to respond to treatment in available time *Participants* Treatment group $n = 39$, control group $n = 35$. Children randomly	*Intervention* Based on Ayres (1972b) SI theory *Frequency* • 11–18 sessions (median = 13), 1-hr sessions over 4–5 mo • Control group received NT *Outcome Measures* Peabody Picture Vocabulary Test to estimate verbal IQ; Burt Word Reading Test to test word recognition; Neale Analysis of Reading Ability to assess reading comprehension; Bankson Language Screening Test for subtests of visual and auditory processing; Unstandardized Handwriting Test; Bruininks–Oseretsky Short Form to measure gross and fine motor skills, including visual–motor; SCSIT for SI assessment of sensory processing and praxis skills. Conners' Teacher Rating Scale is a teacher report of conduct, inattention, anxiety, and hyperactivity.	All groups improved significantly on word recognition, reading, vocabulary, and motor performance. Differences were less significant when the SI group was divided by age. No significant Time × Group effects were found, with the exception of the Bankson Visual Matching test, which found significant improvement in the SI group.	Determination of SI dysfunction was based on minimal assessment. Intervention techniques were not described. The intervention setting was an empty classroom with no mention of suspended equipment or how vestibular input was provided in lieu of suspended equipment. The tester was not blind to the group assignment. Short-term intervention and small sample size were weaknesses. Examination of the mean and standard deviation data indicated that the SI group typically made larger gains and had higher posttest scores than the control group; however, many outcomes had large standard deviations, resulting in nonsignificant results.

		assigned by blinded therapist. Groups matched by school, age, gender, and degree of SI dysfunction. Intervention group divided into early ($n = 16$) and late ($n = 13$) groups.		The intervention provided in this study is highly questionable as to its adherence to the core concepts of SI intervention. In addition, serious methodological flaws and duration of intervention may have contributed to the negative findings.
M. White (1979)	The objective was to examine the effectiveness of SI therapy on children at risk for reading failure.	Level I RCT *Inclusion* Total 1st-grade enrollment from 2 elementary schools screened with Satz and Friel predictive test battery and identified as severe and mild risk *Participants* • Average IQ • Ages 5.2–6.9 • $N = 21$ (2 groups; $n = 11$ treatment, $n = 10$ control) • Sample is same as used in Grimwood & Rutherford (1980) study	*Intervention* SI therapy; individualized intervention programs Therapy was carried out in school hall of 1 school and specially equipped caravan of another, with both having fixed equipment. Therapy was described as organizing sensory information from the environment to make an adaptive response and to address disordered sensory integrative mechanisms lowest on the developmental scale and work upward. Therapy enhanced sensory functioning and provided graded neuromuscular techniques and activities to assist integration of postural reflexes and balance. *Frequency* 2×30 min/wk for 48 sessions *Outcome Measures* Satz Battery to measure alphabet recitation; Peabody Picture Vocabulary, Benton Finger Localization; Recognition–Discrimination, Beery–Buktenica Test of Visual–Motor Integration; Iota Word Test and teacher assessment for reading competency (completed at end of therapy); Lucia Graded Word Reading Test and teacher ratings (1 yr after treatment); Neale Analysis of Reading Ability Accuracy and Comprehension Scales; and Lucia Graded Word Reading Test (2 yr after treatment)	Significant gains in reading skills were found in the treatment group on the Iota Word Test at the end of the treatment period. These word-reading gains were sustained at 1 yr after treatment on the St. Lucia Word Reading Test. Reading accuracy and comprehension at the end of 2 yr after treatment continued to be significantly higher than the control group. In addition, at each testing period, the treatment group members were closer to the scores of their total class peers.	Small sample size is a weakness. The qualifications of students doing testing is questionable. The use of different tests at different measurement points is questionable. Study would have been better if it had used the same test or different versions of the same test.

(Continued)

Appendix C. Evidence Tables

Table C4. Summary of the Evidence of the Effectiveness of Occupational Therapy Interventions Using a Sensory Integration Approach for Children and Adolescents (cont.)

Author/Year	Study Objectives	Level/Design/Participants	Intervention and Outcome Measures	Results	Study Limitations
B. N. Wilson & Kaplan (1994)	This was a follow-up study to assess the long-term effects of SI treatment on the academic skills, motor skills, and behavior of children with LD when compared with tutoring.	Level I RCT *Inclusion:* Participants who participated in initial study (i.e., evidence of deficits in motor coordination, vestibular–proprioceptive functioning, SI, LD, or at risk for LD) *Exclusion:* ADHD, neurological disorder *Participants* 22 of the 29 original participants participated in the follow-up study: 11 participants from the SI group and 11 participants from the tutoring group. Age at follow-up ranged from 8 yr 2 mo to 11 yr 7 mo.	*Intervention* Originally 2 groups: SI and tutoring Authors recorded further instances of therapy that occurred during the follow-up period. 5 of the children from the SI group received further occupational therapy, tutoring, or speech therapy. None of the children who received tutoring had received further treatment. *Outcome Measures* Woodcock–Johnson cognitive index and reading clusters to measure academic skills; BOTMP to evaluate fine and gross motor skills; the Developmental Test of Visual–Motor Integration, Design Copying and Motor Accuracy Tests of the SCSIT to evaluate visual–motor skill; the Abbreviated Symptom Questionnaire to obtain a measure of behavior and hyperactivity	The only statistically significant difference found was on the gross motor composite and upper-limb coordination subtest of the BOTMP. The SI group's mean remained exactly the same, whereas the tutoring group's mean dropped.	*Control group:* The initial study did not include a control group, which affects the strength of the conclusions that can be reached from this treatment efficacy study. *Ceiling effect:* The moderate negative relationship found between how well a child initially responded to treatment and how well those gains were maintained may be indicative of a ceiling effect in the skills being measured or instrument used.
B. N. Wilson, Kaplan, Fellowes, Gruchy, & Faris (1992)	The objective was to compare the effectiveness of SI to tutoring with regard to the effect of improvement on academic, motor, and behavioral measures.	Level I RCT *Participants* $N = 29$; 6 boys, 23 girls; ages 5.2–8.6; 14 in SI; 15 in tutoring condition *Inclusion* • Average intelligence • SI dysfunction • Hyposensitive to vestibular input • Below average on at least 3 vestibular- or proprioceptive-related clinical observations • Below average on at least 1 of 3 Woodcock–Johnson subtests, 1 visual–motor test, and 1 of the coordination subtests of BOTMP	*Interventions* SI: Focusing on the provision of vestibular, proprioceptive, and tactile stimulation within meaningful and self-directed activities Tutoring: Carried out in a quiet room of the child's school *Frequency* Both treatments 50 min, 2×/wk Assess at 40 sessions and again after 75–80 sessions *Outcome Measures* Abbreviated Symptom Questionnaire; Woodcock–Johnson; BOTMP; Motor Accuracy Test–Revised; Behavioral Observation forms of the Miller Assessment for Preschoolers	At 6 mo, no difference was noted between groups on any measures except the behavioral measure (Abbreviated Symptom Questionnaire). The SI group improved to within normal limits; the tutoring group improved slightly. These results were maintained for both groups at 12 mo. The authors stated that both tutoring and SI can be valuable therapies.	No control group was available to truly compare differences between SI/tutoring and maturation. No parent participation or parent or teacher consultation was allowed. These are typically critical components for both treatments, and the ability to have suggestions from therapists and tutors carried over to the classroom and home environments may be critical elements of both programs' success.

Study	Objective	Level/Design/Participants	Intervention and Outcome Measures	Results	Study Limitations
Ziviani, Poulsen, & O'Brien (1982)	The objective was to investigate the effect of neurodevelopment and SI techniques on motor skills and academic performance of children with LD.	Level I RCT • Matched pairs • Alternate treatment control *Participants* N = 8 matched pairs; all boys, ages 5.7–13, mean age = 8.8 yr; LD	*Intervention* • Neurodevelopmental and SI-based occupational therapy program 1.5 hr/wk for 13 wk • Used SCSIT and SCPNT for treatment programming • Control participants participated in remedial activities in class that were not part of regular curriculum. *Outcome Measures* Blind raters; BOTMP; Hull B Word Recognition Test for reading; Schonell Graded Word Spelling Test A for spelling	A discriminant analysis found the experimental group had significantly more improvement in motor skills than control participants ($p = .01$). The experimental group demonstrated significant gains over the control group on all subtests of the BOTMP, with fine motor composite contributing the most discriminant function. There were no significant differences between groups on the Hull Word Recognition Test or the Graded Word Spelling test.	Intervention was not well-defined. Sample size was very small. Quality of treatment was not stated, nor was the specific intervention fully described. Length of treatment sessions was not specified. The use of a reportedly combined intervention confounds the effects of "pure" SI intervention but may better reflect clinical practice.

Note. ADHD = attention deficit hyperactivity disorder; BOTMP = Bruininks–Oseretsky Test of Motor Proficiency; CBCL = Child Behavior Checklist; ITPA = Illinois Test of Psycholinguistic Abilities; LD = learning disabilities; NT = no treatment; OT/SI = occupational therapy/sensory integration; PM = perceptual–motor; RCT = randomized controlled trial; SCPNT = Southern California Post-Rotary Nystagmus Test; SCSIT = Southern California Sensory Integration Tests; SD = standard deviation; SI = sensory integration; SIPT = Sensory Integration and Praxis Tests; SMD = sensory modulation disorder; STEP-SI = STEP-SI Model of Treatment of Sensory Modulation Disorder; ToP = Test of Playfulness; VAS = visual analogue scales; WRAT = Wide Range Achievement Tests.

This table is a product of AOTA's Evidence-Based Practice Project and the *American Journal of Occupational Therapy.* Copyright © 2010 by the American Occupational Therapy Association. May be freely reproduced for personal use in clinical or educational settings as long as the source is cited. All other uses require written permission from the American Occupational Therapy Association. To apply, visit www.copyright.com.

From May-Benson, T. A., & Koomar, J. A. (2010). Systematic review of the research evidence examining the efficacy of interventions using a sensory integrative approach for children (Suppl. Table 1). *American Journal of Occupational Therapy, 64,* 403–414. doi: 10.5014/ajot.2010.09071

Table C5. Summary of the Evidence of the Effectiveness of Occupational Therapy Interventions Other Than the Sensory Integration Approach for Children and Adolescents

Author/Year	Study Objectives	Level/Design/Participants	Intervention and Outcome Measures	Results	Study Limitations
Individual Studies: Consultation					
Dunn (1990)	The objective was to examine the effectiveness of direct and collaborative consultation models of service delivery on the attainment of educationally relevant outcomes.	Level VI RCT 2 groups *Participants* *Inclusion:* Diagnosis: ≥1 yr delay in ≥2 areas on developmental profile; attending special education programs and referred to occupational therapy *Exclusion:* Diagnoses of deafness, blindness, or nonambulatory *Sample:* 12 preschoolers and 2 kindergarteners (6 girls, 8 boys; 35–79 mo old)	*Intervention* Throughout school year; 24 hr, 60 min/wk *Direct service:* Outside the classroom; activities designed by occupational therapists to address gross motor, fine motor, or self-help skills; only neutral, supportive comments to teachers *Consultation:* Verbal and written instructions, demonstrations to teachers *Outcome Measures* • IEP goals • Teacher/occupational therapist rating form	*IEP goals:* Both groups achieved the same percentage of IEP goals. More fine motor and language goals were met by the direct group. More cognitive and gross motor goals were met by the consultation group. *Teacher/occupational therapist form:* Teachers in the consultation group reported that the occupational therapist contributed to the achievement of the goals at a higher percentage and to more positive attitudes.	No statistical analysis was completed to examine between-group differences reported. Generalizability is limited by the small sample size and the fact that the amount of occupational therapist–teacher interaction in the consultation group is unusually high for clinical practice and may have contributed to the more positive perceptions by teachers.
Kemmis & Dunn (1996)	The objective was to examine the success of weekly consultation between therapists and teachers for children identified as having SI dysfunction and learning problems.	Level III 1 group, pretest–posttest *Participants* *Inclusion:* Diagnosis of learning disability, behavior disorder, or developmental delays; deficits in socialization, learning, or communication; poor sensory processing *Exclusion:* Diagnoses of neuromuscular conditions *Sample:* 10 children (7 boys, 3 girls; age range = 5 yr 7 mo–9 yr 7 mo)	*Intervention* 60 min/wk *Consultation:* Each session, the occupational therapist–teacher pair targeted a specific performance problem and developed an intervention strategy for the teacher to use and implement the next week. *Outcome Measures* • Individualized rating scale to rate intervention success; weekly goals were coded as met, unmet, or questionable. • Performance areas and intervention approaches coded.	*Intervention success:* 63% of weekly goals met; "therapist" was the only variable that had a significant effect on success rate. *Performance areas:* Academic goals most frequently chosen (62%) *Intervention approach:* Compensatory approach most frequently chosen (59%)	Interrater reliability on the categorization of performance area and intervention approach was not established, making the consistency in findings unclear. Generalizability is limited because of small sample size and because frequency and type of intervention do not represent prevalent model of service delivery.
Sugden & Chambers (2003)	The objective was to determine the extent to which parents and teachers, with guidance, can assist in the management of children with DCD.	Level II Crossover, 2 groups Assessment (Ax) → No Rx → Ax → A]; B → Ax → B]; A → Ax → No Rx → Follow-up *Participants* *Inclusion:* Diagnosis of movement difficulties identified by teachers	*Intervention* 4 × 20 min/wk for 20 wk (per condition) *Teacher intervention:* A profile of the child was prepared, and priorities were set by teachers and parents. Every week, teachers were given abilities to work on activities and the like. Underlying principles came from a cognitive–motor approach.	Children made gains in their motor performance as a result of treatment. These gains were maintained at follow-up. In Phase 1, the group that received teacher intervention scored significantly better than the group that received parent intervention. This difference was not found in Phase 2.	In the study design, some children received a seemingly adequate amount of intervention but displayed little or no improvement, whereas others who received little intervention made significant progress. A different study design would be needed to further explore the reasons for this variability in response.

		Exclusion: Diagnoses of learning difficulty, medical condition that could explain coordination difficulties *Sample:* 31 children (22 boys, 9 girls; ages 7–9)	*Parent intervention:* Same except conducted by parents *Outcome Measure* M–ABC and checklist	
Direct Service Approaches					
Impairment-Oriented Approaches: Sensory-Based Approaches					
Fertel-Daly, Bedell, & Hinojosa (2001)	The objective was to examine the effect of using a weighted vest on attention to a fine motor task and self-stimulatory behaviors in preschool children with PDD.	Level IV SCED: ABA (A: baseline; B: vest) *Participants* *Inclusion:* Diagnosis of PDD; exhibiting difficulties with attention to task; attending the same self-contained class in a 5-day/wk, 3-hr/day preschool *Exclusion:* Current use of weighted vest *Sample:* 5 children (4 boys, 1 girl; ages 2.5–3.1 yr)	*Intervention* 15 1.5- to 2-hr sessions over 6 wk Children wore a weighted vest while doing fine motor activities. *Outcome Measures* • Behavioral observation at 5-min intervals • Parent and teacher report	*Behavioral observation:* Positive (all children); attention, distractions, and self-stimulatory behaviors. Attention to task decreased when the vest was removed but was longer than baseline. Self-stimulation increased when the vest was removed. *Parent and teacher report:* Positive effects on tantrums, staying seated, aggressive behavior, self-stimulatory behaviors, and seated posture	On the visual graph analysis, there were no guidelines for inspecting single-case data. The data collection was brief; there was a single intervention phase. Interobserver agreement was not performed; thus, there was a lack of control for observer drift. In the study design, some behaviors did not return to baseline after B. Multiple baselines would have addressed this situation. Generalizability is limited by the small sample size.
Hall & Case-Smith (2007)	The objective was to investigate the effects of incorporating a therapeutic listening program with a sensory diet on children with SPD and visual–motor delays.	Level III 1 group, 2 interventions Comparison, AB (A: sensory diet; B: A + therapeutic listening) *Participants* *Inclusion:* Diagnoses of visual–motor delay and SPD; referred to occupational therapy *Exclusion:* Diagnoses of intellectual delays, cerebral palsy, Down syndrome, visual or hearing impairment, severe autism *Sample:* 10 children (9 boys, 1 girl; ages 5 yrs 8 mo–10 yr 11 mo)	*Intervention* 4-wk A followed by 8-wk B Sensory diet: Based on Sensory Profile; activities that provided sensory input (e.g., movement, heavy work, tactile stimulation) Therapeutic listening: Children listened to prescribed music 2×/day for 20 min to 30 min. *Outcome Measures* • Sensory Profile • VMI • ETCH	*Sensory Profile:* 9 of 14 subscales improved (unclear which phases were compared). *VMI:* Mixed results; difference on 1 subtest pre-A and post-B only *ETCH:* Results were mixed. There were differences on 2 subtests (not total score) pre-A and post-B only.	The listening program was administered by parents; thus, the researchers were unable to monitor adherence to treatment protocol. Generalizability is limited by the small sample size.

(Continued)

Table C5. Summary of the Evidence of the Effectiveness of Occupational Therapy Interventions Other Than the Sensory Integration Approach for Children and Adolescents (cont.)

Author/Year	Study Objectives	Level/Design/Participants	Intervention and Outcome Measures	Results	Study Limitations
VandenBerg (2001)	The objective was to examine the effect of weighted vests on visual attention for fine motor activities in children with ADHD.	Level IV SCED: AB (A: baseline; B: vest) *Participants* *Inclusion:* Diagnosis of ADHD; sensory modulation problem and difficulty writing identified by occupational therapy *Exclusion:* None reported *Sample:* 4 children (2 boys and 2 girls; range = 5 yr 9 mo–6 yr 10 mo)	*Intervention* Six 15-min observations were conducted within a 15-day period for each condition during an activity. Vests with weights about the shoulder girdle area were 5% of the child's body weight. Children were allowed to wear the vest when not being observed. *Outcome Measure* Time on task	All 4 students demonstrated an increase (54%–64% to 79%–82%) in time on task during a fine motor activity while wearing the weighted vests compared with baseline without the vest.	With regard to the study design, an ABA design would have been preferable to strengthen validity of study. Generalizability is limited by the small sample size.
\multicolumn{6}{l}{*Impairment-Oriented Approaches: Sensory–Motor Approaches*}
Candler (2003)	The objective was to examine the effectiveness of a summer camp program on occupational performance in children with SPD.	Level III 1 group, pretest–posttest *Participants* *Inclusion:* Diagnosis of sensory modulation disorder *Exclusion:* None mentioned *Sample:* 12 children (8 boys, 4 girls)	*Intervention* Weekday camp with an SI-based approach (by occupational therapist; sensory diets, etc.) and therapeutic riding program (by riding instructors) *Outcome Measure* COPM, modified interview	Significant improvement occurred in performance and satisfaction scores at follow-up.	Generalizability is limited by the small sample size.
Chia & Chua (2002)	The objective was to investigate the effects of PT on sensory-motor function, academic scores, learning behavior, and social–emotional status of school-age children with DCD and learning difficulties.	Level I RCT 2 groups *Participants* *Inclusion:* Diagnosis of sensorimotor difficulties; in school's learning support program *Exclusion:* Diagnoses of medical conditions that may interfere with PT; previous PT or occupational therapy intervention *Sample:* 14 boys (ages 6–9)	*Intervention* PT group: 12 wk 2×/wk (8 wk 1:1 and 4 wk of group); provide normal sensory stimuli while facilitating normal responses; address muscle tightness, weakness, postural misalignment Control group: No therapy *Outcome Measures* • Modified NSMDA to evaluate neuromotor function • Academic performance • Teacher survey (learning behavior, social responses)	*Neuromotor function:* PT demonstrated the greatest mean improvement. *Academic performance:* There was no significant difference between groups. *Teacher survey:* There was no significant difference between groups.	There appears to be large within-group variability on outcome measures. Sample size of only 14 participants (7 per group) may have reduced the power of the statistical analysis.
Hartshorn et al. (2001)	The objective was to assess the effect of movement therapy on social skills and on-task behavior in children with autism.	Level I RCT: 2 groups *Participants* *Inclusion:* Diagnosis of autism; attending a school for children with autism	*Intervention* 30 min 2×/wk for 8 wk *Movement therapy:* Warm-up (greetings while clapping), activities (e.g., obstacle course), cool down (song and movement)	Improvements were found compared with the control group in time spent wandering in the classroom, time spent negatively responding to touch, time spent resisting teachers, and time spent doing on-task passive behaviors.	Teachers and therapists were not blinded to group assignment. Outcome behaviors were assessed only during the movement sessions.

			Exclusion: None mentioned *Sample:* 2 groups of 38 children (ages 3–7)	*Control group:* No intervention; observed during 2 movement sessions at 8-wk intervals *Outcome Measure* Behavioral observation for 6 1-min periods during first 18 min of pre-post session	
Inder & Sullivan (2005)	The objective was to examine the effect of selected Edu–K techniques on the postural responses of children with DCD.	Level IV SCED Multiple baselines, AB with follow-up *Participants* *Inclusion:* Diagnosis of motor coordination below age level affecting academic achievement or ADLs; attendance at a Movement Development Clinic *Exclusion:* No other medical, neurological, or mental disorder *Sample:* 4 children (2 boys, 2 girls; ages 9–11)	*Intervention* 6 weekly sessions Home programming including PACE, 4 activities (drinking water, brain buttons, cross crawls, Cooks Hook Up) to ensure learning readiness, and Dennison Laterality Repatterning, a 5-step balance process that simulates stages of laterality, infancy to walking *Outcome Measure* Dynamic posturography: SOT to quantify postural stability; various sensory conditions	Improved performance for 2 of 4 children at follow-up. The number of falls decreased significantly for all children.	Study constraints prevented the establishment of stable patterns at baseline. There was no monitoring of adherence to the intervention program. Illness and holidays compromised consistency of the intervention. With regard to the outcome measure, the authors noted that a learning effect is possible on the SOT.
Schilling & Schwartz (2004)	The objective was to investigate the effect of use of therapy balls as seating on engagement and in-seat behavior of children with autism.	Level IV SCED ABAB (A: baseline, natural setting; B: therapy ball) *Participants* *Inclusion:* Diagnosis of autism; attending a specific integrated preschool program; difficulties with in-seat, on-task behaviors reported by teacher *Exclusion:* None noted *Sample:* 4 boys (range = 3 yr 11 mo–4 yr 2 mo)	*Intervention* Variable but minimum 2 wk; data collected for 5–10 min 3×/wk *Natural setting:* Art activities, seated reciprocal play, small group table activities, circle time *Therapy balls:* Balls with molded feet fitted to the child replaced standard seating chairs during the intervention phase *Outcome Measures* • Seating behavior • Engagement on task • Opposition behavior (1 child)	*Seating behavior:* 3 of 4 children demonstrated an increase during the intervention phases with a return to baseline on withdrawal. *Engagement on task:* 4 of 4 children demonstrated an increase during intervention phases with a return to baseline on withdrawal. *Oppositional behavior:* Oppositional behavior was absent during intervention with a return to baseline on withdrawal.	The heterogeneity of the diagnoses/problems and the variability of the intervention settings introduce variability into the results, potentially limiting confidence in the findings. Variability in the length of time of intervention is a significant confound. Generalizability is limited by the small sample size.
			Performance-Oriented Approaches: Direct Skills Teaching		
Hodge, Murata, & Porretta (1999)	The objective was to determine the effect of preparatory activities on the fundamental motor skill performance of elementary-age children	Level I RCT: 3 groups *Participants* *Inclusion:* Diagnoses of learning disabilities with attention deficits; in special education programs	*Intervention* TS: Preliminary practice period in which the participants performed the selected motor skills to be assessed several times	The only significant difference found between groups was for throwing accuracy. The mental preparation group performed significantly better than the TS and control group.	There are potentially confounding differences between the groups. Although MP observed the motor skills to be assessed, TS practiced the skill without

(Continued)

Appendix C. Evidence Tables

Table C5. Summary of the Evidence of the Effectiveness of Occupational Therapy Interventions Other Than the Sensory Integration Approach for Children and Adolescents (cont.)

Author/Year	Study Objectives	Level/Design/Participants	Intervention and Outcome Measures	Results	Study Limitations
	with learning disabilities and attention deficits.	Exclusion: None mentioned Sample: 46 children (36 boys, 10 girls; ages 9–11)	MP: Preliminary practice period involving mental imagery and verbal directions after a demonstration of the selected motor skills to be assessed Control group: No activities Outcome Measure Selected items from the Adapted Physical Education Assessment Scale		demonstration. An element of teaching was thus present in MP but not in TS. Children in TS practiced their own movement (correct or not), whereas children in MP were shown an appropriate movement for completing the skill.
P. H. Wilson, Thomas, & Maruff (2002)	The objective was to explore the efficacy of a computer-based, motor/kinesthetic, imagery-based intervention program compared with a conventional perceptual–motor intervention and a control group.	Level I RCT 3 groups Participants Inclusion: Identified by school specialists as having motor coordination difficulties; <50th percentile on M–ABC Exclusion: Diagnosis of neurological disorders, ADHD Sample: 54 children divided into 3 groups of 18; M–ABC score of 11 per group <15th percentile	Intervention Five 1-hr/wk sessions Imagery training: On computer, increasing complexity: (1) visual imagery exercises predictive timing, (2) relaxation and MP, (3) visual modeling of motor skills, (4) mental rehearsal from an external/internal perspective, (5) practice Perceptual–motor training: Gross and fine motor and perceptual–motor activities. Control group: No treatment Outcome Measure M–ABC	M–ABC scores improved in the imagery group and the perceptual–motor group but not in the control group.	Because 11 of 18 per group obtained M–ABC scores <15th percentile, the results from this study may not be comparable with others that typically use <15th percentile as an inclusion criterion. With regard to the outcome measure, the impact of the intervention on motor imagery abilities was not assessed.
		Performance Oriented Approaches: Cognitive-Based Approaches			
Martini & Polatajko (1998)	The objective was to demonstrate generalizability across therapists of positive outcomes obtained by the CO–OP intervention approach.	Level IV SCED replication AB-post Participants Inclusion: Diagnosis of motor deficit Exclusion: Diagnoses of neurological disorder or a physical/sensory deficit causing the motor problem Sample: 4 children (3 boys and 1 girl)	Intervention CO–OP (see L. T. Miller et al., 2001) Outcome Measures • COPM • Behavioral observations to measure use/understanding of global cognitive strategy • Performance Quality Rating Scale to assess performance of chosen goals	COPM: Significant improvement for all Behavioral observations: All demonstrated use and understanding of the global cognitive strategy. Performance Quality Rating Scale: Participants' performance improved in their chosen activities.	Visual graph analysis was chosen to analyze data. There are no formal guidelines for visually inspecting single case data and determining the effects of an intervention.

Author/Year	Study Objectives	Level/Design/Participants	Intervention and Outcome Measures	Results	Study Limitations
L. T. Miller, Polatajko, Missiuna, Mandich, & Macnab (2001)	The objective was to pilot the procedures and measures for a full-scale RCT that will evaluate the efficacy of the CO–OP approach in improving the functioning of children with DCD.	Level I Pilot RCT 2 groups *Participants* *Inclusion:* Diagnosis of motor deficits characteristic of DCD; recruited from university clinic *Exclusion:* Diagnoses of neurological disorder or a physical or sensory deficit affecting motor skills; IQ < 85 *Sample:* 20 children (10 per group; 14 boys, 6 girls; ages 7–13)	*Intervention* 10 50-min sessions, 2 to 3×/wk *CO–OP:* Children were taught to apply cognitive strategy to solve their motor problems and learned to perform 3 chosen goals. Guidance was used by occupational therapists to enable children to discover strategies to help them learn their goals. Generalization and transfer were promoted. *Current treatment approach:* Multisensory, neuromuscular, and biomechanical. Therapists set goals, instruct participants how to perform tasks and provide skill instructions. *Outcome Measures* • COPM • VABS • Bruininks–Oseretsky Test of Motor Proficiency • VMI • SPPC • Follow-up interview	*COPM:* Both groups improved, but larger gains were made by the CO–OP group. *VABS:* Improvements were made by CO–OP participants. *Bruininks–Oseretsky Test of Motor Proficiency:* Improvements were made by both groups. *VMI and SPPC:* No significant change in either group. *Follow-up:* All parents of CO–OP and 71% of current treatment approach parents reported improvements in their child's confidence during motor tasks. All parents of CO–OP indicated that acquired motor skills had been maintained, whereas 3 of 7 current treatment approach reported that the goals had been maintained. 2 reported that some aspect of the goals had been maintained, and 2 reported that goals had not been maintained.	Because there was no control group in this pilot study, it is unclear whether for those outcomes where equal improvements were seen in both groups, the results were caused by treatment or some other factor, such as maturation. The current treatment approach intervention was an eclectic mix of treatments and was not manualized. As a result, it is not possible to assess which aspects of the current treatment approach treatment resulted in positive outcomes or replicate the study.
Polatajko, Mandich, Miller, & Macnab (2001)	The objective was to provide a summary of the evidence for CO–OP, including 2 intervention studies not published elsewhere: a SCED series (Study 1) to evaluate the effect of CO–OP as an approach to help children with DCD meet functional goals and a retrospective chart audit (Study 2) to determine whether the effects reported in experimental studies are replicable in a clinic by different therapists with different children.	*Study 1* Level IV 1 SCED (AB, posttest, follow-up) with 9 replications Level III 1 group comparison, pre-post/follow-up test *Study 2* Level III 1 group comparison, pre-post *Participants* *Inclusion:* Diagnosis of motor difficulties characteristic of DCD *Exclusion:* Diagnoses of neurological disorder or a physical or sensory deficit affecting motor skills *Sample:* Study 1 = 10 children; Study 2 = charts of 25 children	*Study 1: Intervention* CO–OP (see L. T. Miller et al., 2001) SCED *Outcome Measures* • SCED • Behavioral observations of performance on 3 goals per child at baseline, throughout the intervention, posttest, and at 12-wk follow-up • 1 group comparison • COPM • VABS • VMI • Test of Motor Impairment • Child Behavior Checklist • Eyberg Child Behavior Inventory *Study 2: Intervention* CO–OP (see L. T. Miller et al., 2001) *Outcome Measures* • COPM • VABS • M–ABC • VMI	*Study 1* *SCED:* Child 1 improved performance from baseline on all 3 skills and maintained that improvement at posttest and the 12-wk follow-up. These results were replicated in 9 more SCEDs for 26 of the 27 additional goals. Group data showed significant improvement relative to pretest at posttest and follow-up on COPM and VABS. The other measures did not achieve significance. *Study 2* *COPM:* Improvement *VABS:* Improvement in motor performance and communication *M–ABC:* Improvement in ball skills *VMI:* Improvement Improvements noted on VABS, M–ABC, and VMI indicate that the skills learned were generalized and transferred to other areas.	The Study 1 SCED design had good internal validity but poor external validity, making for weak generalizability. The 1-group design did not account for placebo effect. Study 2 had missing data, which resulted in a relatively (N = 25) small sample size.

(Continued)

Table C5. Summary of the Evidence of the Effectiveness of Occupational Therapy Interventions Other Than the Sensory Integration Approach for Children and Adolescents (cont.)

Author/Year	Study Objectives	Level/Design/Participants	Intervention and Outcome Measures	Results	Study Limitations
			Meta-Analyses and Systematic Reviews		
Baranek (2002)	The objective was to examine the efficacy of sensory and motor interventions with children with autism.	Level I Systematic review *Studies* *Inclusion:* Remedial intervention targeting specific sensory or motor components; compensatory skills training approaches; task/environmental modifications *Exclusion:* Traditional behavioral interventions; pharmacological interventions; comprehensive educational models (e.g., TEACHH) *Sample:* 29 studies	*Intervention* (no. of studies) • SI therapy (3) • SI-based approaches (3) • Sensory stimulation (5) • AIT and acoustic interventions (9) • Visual therapies (3) • Sensorimotor techniques (2) • Physical exercise (4) *Variables* Varied by study; the author described the outcomes of each study.	*SI and SI-based:* Despite positive outcomes documented, the author questioned the results of the studies given the numerous study limitations. *Sensory stimulation:* Some positive results were found from studies using touch pressure. *AIT and related acoustic:* Mixed results. Numerous outcomes were difficult to interpret. *Visual therapies:* Inconsistencies in findings were reported. *Sensorimotor handling:* Mixed results were obtained. No study found dramatic improvement on any measure. *Physical exercise:* All studies found some beneficial, albeit short-lived, effects of exercise for decreasing self-stimulatory behaviors and mixed findings for improving other simple cognitive/play tasks.	Studies included were often methodologically weak, with small sample sizes and lack of control participants. In addition, the heterogeneity of the autism population was not considered in the inclusion criteria, which may explain some of the mixed results obtained. In general, there were a limited number of studies found for any 1 intervention, preventing the author from reaching definite conclusions.
Kavale & Mattson (1983)	The objective was to assess the efficacy of perceptual–motor training.	Level I Meta-analysis *Studies* *Inclusion:* Perceptual–motor training; presence of a control group *Sample:* 180 studies	*Intervention* Perceptual–motor training (including Barsch, Cratty, Delacato, Frostig, Getman, Kephart, Combination, and others) *Variables* • Outcomes • Interventions • Designs • Participants	ES was 0.082, which indicates that perceptual–motor training is no better than no treatment. *Outcomes:* The only area revealing a modest gain was adaptive behavior (ES = 0.267). *Interventions:* All revealed small or negative ES, and no single intervention revealed any advantage. *Designs:* Studies categorized as "low validity" revealed the largest ES (0.198), whereas studies categorized as "high" revealed a negative ES (−0.119). Both ESs were small. *Participants:* Small ESs were found for all subject groups and at all grade levels.	Nolan (2004) completed a critical analysis of Kavale and Mattson's (1983) meta-analysis and uncovered methodological flaws concerning study selection, completeness of data, and analysis value. These flaws bring uncertainty about the results reported by Kavale and Mattson. However, Nolan did not redo the statistical calculations necessary for a meta-analysis, and accordingly, it is unknown at this time whether the results obtained by Kavale and Mattson would have been different if a more rigorous methodology were followed.

Author/Year	Study Objectives	Level/Design/Participants	Intervention and Outcome Measures	Results	Study Limitations
Pless & Carlsson (2000)	The objective was to evaluate the effectiveness of motor skill interventions for children with DCD.	Level I Meta-analysis and systematic review *Studies* *Inclusion*: Investigating the effects of a motor skill intervention using an experimental design with >1 control group or single-subject design; diagnosis of DCD or motor problems consistent with DCD; ages 3–13; 1970–1996 *Key terms*: Not reported but included physically awkward, motor impaired, DCD, clumsy, sensory integrative deficit *Sample*: 21 studies included in the review; 13 studies included in the meta-analysis	*Intervention* GA: Consists mainly of facilitation of balance and other physical abilities and training of specific perceptual and motor tasks SI: Consists of provision of proprioceptive, tactile, and vestibular stimulation through activities requiring full body movement and training in specific perceptual and motor skills SS: Consists of a combination of correctly performed practice of functional skills, appropriate repetition, and sufficient guidance and time to facilitate skill retention and generalization *Variables* • Intervention • Age of children • Intervention setting • Intervention length • Intervention frequency	*Intervention*: SS intervention was the most effective (ES = 1.46), followed by GA (ES = 0.71) and SI (ES = 0.21). *Age of children*: Interventions with children ages 6–13 were more effective (ES = 0.77) compared with interventions with younger children (ES = 0.14). *Intervention setting*: Home programs (ES = 1.41) were more effective than group (ES = 0.96) or one-on-one interventions (0.45). *Intervention length*: Shorter interventions—less than 3 mo (ES = 0.72)—were as effective as longer interventions—more than 3 mo (ES = 0.69). *Intervention frequency*: Similar outcomes occurred when conducted less than 3×/wk (ES = 0.60) and more than 3–5×/wk (ES = 0.86).	24 outcome measures were used to evaluate intervention outcomes in the various studies included in this meta-analysis. In their statistical analysis, the authors averaged the ESs from the different measures without assessing the statistical heterogeneity of the data, which might have been inappropriate. A comparison of the 3 intervention categories identified by the authors was not the primary objective of the studies included in the meta-analysis. Accordingly, the authors' conclusions about the relative effectiveness of the different intervention categories should be interpreted with care.
Sinha, Silove, Wheeler, & Williams (2006)	The objective was to identify, evaluate, and combine any clinical trial-based evidence of the effects of sound therapy in people with ASD.	Level I Systematic review *Studies* *Inclusion*: RCT that assessed the effectiveness of sound therapies to treat people with ASD; years of studies to 2002 *Sample*: 6 studies	*Intervention* Sound therapies: Involve listening to filtered and modulated music Control: Compared with no sound therapy (control conditions in all trials involved listening to unmodified music) *Variables* Outcomes	3 studies did not demonstrate beneficial effects, and 3 studies reported improvements at 3 mo (although the authors question the validity of the outcome measure used).	Few studies met the RCT criteria. Studies that did qualify were judged to have inadequate allocation concealment and used a wide variety of outcome measures and statistical methods, and the data were presented in forms that did not lend themselves to statistical comparison software.

Note. ADHD = attention deficit hyperactivity disorder; ADLs = activities of daily living; AIT = auditory integration training; ASD = autism spectrum disorders (ASD); CO-OP = Cognitive Orientation to daily Occupational Performance; COPM = Canadian Occupational Performance Measure; DCD = developmental coordination disorder; Edu-K = Education Kinesiology; ES = effect size; ETCH = Evaluation Tool of Children's Handwriting; GA = general ability; IEP = individualized education plan; M–ABC = Movement Assessment Battery for Children; MP = mental preparation; NSMDA = Neuro-Sensory Motor Development Assessment; PACE = Positive, Active, Clear, Energetic; PDD = pervasive developmental disorders; PT = physiotherapy; RCT = randomized controlled trial; SCED = single case experimental design; SI = sensory integration; SOT = Sensory Organization Test; SPD = sensory processing disorder; SPPC = Self-Perception Profile for Children; SS = specific skills; TEACHH = Treatment and Education of Autistic and related Communication–Handicapped cHildren; TS = task-specific warm-up; VABS = Vineland Adaptive Behavior Scales; VMI = Developmental Test of Visual–Motor Integration.

This table is a product of AOTA's Evidence-Based Practice Project and the *American Journal of Occupational Therapy*. Copyright © 2010 by the American Occupational Therapy Association. May be freely reproduced for personal use in clinical or educational settings as long as the source is cited. All other uses require written permission from the American Occupational Therapy Association. To apply, visit www.copyright.com.

From Polatajko, H. J., & Cantin, N. (2010). Exploring the effectiveness of occupational therapy interventions, other than the sensory integration approach, with children and adolescents experiencing difficulty processing and integrating sensory information (Suppl. Table 1). *American Journal of Occupational Therapy, 64*, 415–429. doi: 10.5014/ajot.2010.09072

Appendix C. Evidence Tables

Appendix D. History and Occupational Profile

HISTORY AND OCCUPATIONAL PROFILE
(This form is intended to be completed by the child's parents or primary caregivers)

FAMILY INFORMATION
Child's Name: _____ Date _____
Birth date: _____ Age: _____ Phone Number: _____
Parent's Name: _____
Address: _____

With whom does child live most of the time?
    Biological Parent: Mother [ ] Father [ ] Step-parent: Mother [ ] Father [ ]
    Adoptive Parents   [ ] Adopted at what age: _____ Other [ ] Specify: _____
    Siblings – how many? [ ] Grandparents [ ] Other _____

REFERRING INFORMATION
Who referred this child for an evaluation? _____
Reason for referral: _____
_____
What are your primary concerns/goals regarding your child? _____
_____
When did you first have those concerns? _____
_____
What do you see as your child's strengths? _____
_____
In one sentence, how would you describe your child? _____
_____
Do you have any additional information that will help to better understand your child?
_____

SCHOOL HISTORY:
Hand preference: _____ Current school placement: _____
Present grade: _____ Have any grades been repeated? _____
Is your child in a special class or receiving any support services (specify)?
_____
What does the teacher say about your child?
_____

INTERVENTION HISTORY: Please check any of the following with whom you have contacted concerning your child and include name and contact information if possible.

[ ] Occupational Therapist _____
[ ] Physical Therapist _____
[ ] Speech and Language Pathologist _____
[ ] Developmental Pediatrician _____
[ ] Developmental Optometrist _____
[ ] Behaviorist _____
[ ] Orthopedist _____
[ ] Psychologist _____
[ ] Counseling _____
[ ] Others (please specify) _____

From *Sensory Integration: Applying Clinical Reasoning to Practice with Diverse Populations*, by R. C. Schaaf and S. Smith Roley, 2006, Austin, TX: Pro-Ed. Reprinted with permission.

MEDICAL HISTORY

Any difficulties during pregnancy or delivery? (Specify)_____

Length of pregnancy: _____ Length of labor: _____
Birth was: Normal [ ]   Caesarian [ ]   Breech [ ]   Twins or more [ ]
Birth Weight: _____ Did baby require assistance in starting to breathe?   Yes [ ]   No [ ]
Remarks: _____
Were there any complications/problems in early infancy? Yes [ ]   No [ ]   (please specify)

_____

Were there any feeding difficulties in early infancy?   Yes [ ]   No [ ]   (please specify)

_____

Who is your child's present physician? _____
Does your child have a diagnosis? _____
Diagnosed by whom? _____ Date: _____
Does your child have now or in the past had significant health problems?
Surgery? Explain _____ Hospitalization? Explain _____
Respiratory, lung, or bronchial difficulties? _____ Cardiac Problems? _____
Seizures (when and how often) _____
Allergies? _____ Ear Infections? _____
Is your child currently on any medications?   Yes [ ]   No [ ]
(If yes, please give a list and state reasons)

_____
Previously tried medications _____

Does your child use any specialized equipment? (Explain)

Has your child had a hearing evaluation?   Yes [ ]   No [ ]
By whom: _____ Date: _____
Has your child had a vision evaluation?   Yes [ ]   No [ ]
By whom: _____ Date: _____
Has your child had a psychological evaluation?   Yes [ ]   No [ ]
By whom: _____ Date: _____
Has your child had a neurological evaluation?   Yes [ ]   No [ ]
By whom: _____ Date: _____

From *Sensory Integration: Applying Clinical Reasoning to Practice with Diverse Populations*, by R. C. Schaaf and S. Smith Roley, 2006, Austin, TX: Pro-Ed. Reprinted with permission.

DEVELOPMENTAL HISTORY

List the age at which your child accomplished each activity.
Indicate "not yet" if they have not yet accomplished it.

Motor:
Head control
Roll over both ways _____ Reaching for objects _____
Sitting alone _____ Finger feeding _____
Creeping on all fours
Pulling to stand _____ Eating with spoon _____
Walking _____ Drawing a circle _____
Jumping _____ Cutting with scissors _____
Hopping on one-foot _____ Using knife for cutting _____
Riding bike _____
Does your child have difficulty learning new motor skills? _____

Language:
Said first word _____ Pointing to simple pictures _____
Combined words _____ Following one-step commands _____
Spoke sentences _____ Following several-step commands _____
Looking when called _____ Looks in direction that others point _____

Self-Help:

Dressing   **Grooming**
Put on shirt independently _____ Bathing independently _____
Button independently _____ Combing hair _____
Zips independently _____ Toilet trained
                                                Bowel
                                                Bladder _____
Snaps independently _____ Toileting independently _____
Dress self independently _____ Ties shoes _____

Describe your child as an infant:	YES	NO	SOMETIMES
A. Cried a lot, fussy, irritable			
B. Non-demanding			
C. Alert			
D. Quiet			
E. Passive			
F. Active			
G. Liked being held			
H. Resisted being held			
I. Floppy when held			
J. Tense when held			
K. Good sleep patterns			
L. Irregular sleep patterns			

From *Sensory Integration: Applying Clinical Reasoning to Practice with Diverse Populations*, by R. C. Schaaf and S. Smith Roley, 2006, Austin, TX: Pro-Ed. Reprinted with permission.

Describe your child at present:	YES	NO	SOMETIMES
A. Mostly quiet			
B. Overly active			
C. Tires easily			
D. Talks constantly			
E. Too impulsive			
F. Restless			
G. Stubborn			
H. Resistant to changes			
I. Fights frequently			
J. Usually happy			
K. Exhibits frequent temper tantrums			
L. Clumsy			
M. Difficulty separating from primary caretaker			
N. Nervous habits or tics			
O. Falls often			
P. Wets bed			
Q. Wets or soils pants (how often)			
R. Has poor attention span			
S. Frustrated easily			
T. Has unusual fears			
U. Rocks self frequently			
Comments:			

From *Sensory Integration: Applying Clinical Reasoning to Practice with Diverse Populations*, by R. C. Schaaf and S. Smith Roley, 2006, Austin, TX: Pro-Ed. Reprinted with permission.

OCCUPATIONAL HISTORY
Copyright Susanne Smith Roley, 2003.

Please answer the following questions. Note if participation was more difficult when you or your child was younger. Include comments as appropriate. Feel free to use the other side of the paper.

	Often	Sometimes	Rarely	Often	Sometimes	Rarely
Socially	Does your child:			Do you or others in your family:		
Socialize with extended family and close friends?						
Communicate needs, wants, and interests effectively?						
Find it hard to make friends among age-related peers?						
Prefer to stay home rather than going with the group.						
Join in community activities?						
Seek out friends and companions?						
Need or desire a companion or caregiver in close contact during the day or at night?						
Comments						
While at Play	Does your child:			Do you or others in your family:		
Tend to play or interact with others that are younger or require caregiving?						
Have fun with other children in the neighborhood, at school or other social situations?						
Enjoy toys and games that are developmentally appropriate?						
Enjoy time alone entertained by hobbies and interests?						
Comments						
In the Community	Is your child comfortable:			Is it difficult for you or others in your family when:		
Running errands?						
Going shopping for groceries, supplies or clothes?						
Eating in restaurants?						
Attending birthday parties?						

From *Sensory Integration: Applying Clinical Reasoning to Practice with Diverse Populations*, by R. C. Schaaf and S. Smith Roley, 2006, Austin, TX: Pro-Ed. Reprinted with permission.

Attending family gatherings (e.g. holidays, birthdays, etc.)						
Going on outings with the family?						
Comments:						

During Daily Routines	Does your child accept and respond well when:			Is it difficult for you or others in your family when:		
Preparing to leave the house?						
Putting on clothes in the morning?						
Bathing and grooming?						
Preparing meals and cleaning up?						
Going to bed and during bedtime routines?						
Putting their things away to do something else?						
When moving from one activity and place to another (transitions)?						
There are changes in routine?						
Comments:						

Describe a typical day for your child from waking till bedtime including whether it is different for your child to get to sleep at night and stay asleep. (Use back of page if necessary) _____

_____
_____
_____
_____
_____
_____
_____
_____
_____
_____
_____
_____
_____
_____
_____
_____
_____
_____

From *Sensory Integration: Applying Clinical Reasoning to Practice with Diverse Populations*, by R. C. Schaaf and S. Smith Roley, 2006, Austin, TX: Pro-Ed. Reprinted with permission.

Appendix E. Selected *CPT*™ Coding for Occupational Therapy Evaluations and Interventions

The following chart can assist with selecting the most clinically appropriate *CPT* code to describe occupational therapy evaluation and intervention for children and adolescents with challenges in sensory processing and sensory integration. Occupational therapy practitioners should use the most relevant code from the current *CPT* book based on specific services provided, individual patient goals, payer policy, and common usage.

Examples of Occupational Therapy Evaluation and Intervention	Suggested *CPT* Code(s)
Evaluation	
Evaluate/assess functional performance in areas such as: • Sensory processing, integration and praxis necessary for motor planning and occupational performance • Cognitive, communication, and social skills • Emotion regulation • Activities of daily living (ADLs) and instrumental activities of daily living (IADLs), play and school activities	**97003**—Occupational therapy evaluation **97004**—Occupational therapy reevaluation
Administer and analyze results of standardized assessments such as: • Sensory Integration and Praxis Tests (Ayres, 1989), the Sensory Processing Measure (SPM; Miller Kuhaneck, Henry, Glennon, 2007), and the Sensory Processing Measure–Preschool (SPM–P; Ecker & Parham, 2010; Miller Kuhaneck, Glennon, & Henry, 2010) as part of the sensory processing and integration assessment • Peabody Developmental Motor Scales, 2nd ed. (PDMS–2; Folio & Fewell, 2000) or Bruininks–Oseretsky Test of Motor Proficiency, 2nd ed. (BOT–2; Bruininks & Bruininks, 2005) as part of the motor assessment • Pediatric Evaluation of Disability Inventory (PEDI; Haley, Coster, Ludlow, Haltiwanger, & Andrellos, 1992), Vineland (Sparrow, Cicchetti, & Balla, 2005) or Scales of Independent Behavior, Revised (SIB–R; Bruininks, Woodcock, Weatherman, & Hill, 1997) as part of the adaptive assessment	**96111**—Developmental testing extended (includes assessment of motor, language, social, adaptive, and/or cognitive functioning by standardized developmental instruments) with interpretation and report
Administer and analyze results of standardized cognitive assessments such as: • Behavior Rating Inventory of Executive Function (Gioia, Guy, & Kenworthy, 2000) • School Function Assessment (Coster, Deeney, Haltiwanger, & Haley, 1998) • School Assessment of Motor and Process Skills (Fisher, Bryze, Hume, & Griswold, 2005)	**96125**—Standardized cognitive performance testing (e.g., Ross Information Processing Assessment [Ross-Swain, 1996]) per hour of a qualified health care professional's time, both face-to-face time administering tests to the patient and time interpreting these test results and preparing the report
• Participate in a team conference as part of a diagnostic team in which the team conveys evaluation findings, diagnoses, and recommendations to a client's family • Participate in a team conference to review results of a retest (such as the SPM or SPM–P) to determine the results of intervention and progress noted	**99366**—Medical team conference with an interdisciplinary team of health care professionals, face-to-face with patient and/or family, 30 minutes or more, participation by non-physician qualified health care professional

(continued)

Examples of Occupational Therapy Evaluation and Intervention	Suggested *CPT* Code(s)
Evaluation *(cont.)*	
Participate in a team conference as part of a diagnostic team in which the team reviews evaluation findings and clarifies diagnostic considerations and recommendations prior to meeting with a client's family	**99368**—Medical team conference with an interdisciplinary team of health care professionals, patient and/or family not present, 30 minutes or more, participation by nonphysician qualified health care professional
Intervention	
Design and implement occupational therapy interventions using sensory integrative techniques to facilitate adaptive responding and optimal arousal to allow for enhanced participation in play, school, and adaptive occupations	**97533**—Sensory integrative techniques to enhance sensory processing and promote adaptive responses to environmental demands, direct one-on-one patient contact by the provider, each 15 minutes
Design and implement graded activities to increase coordination, balance, and sensory awareness to enhance participation in daily occupations	**97112**—Neuromuscular reeducation of movement, balance, coordination, kinesthetic sense, posture, and/or proprioception for sitting and/or standing activities
Design and lead therapeutic social-skill groups with a sensory integrative emphasis for individuals with restricted interpersonal skills and/or lack of engagement due to poor sensory processing and integration	**97150**—Therapeutic procedure(s), group (2 or more individuals; report 97150 for each member of group); group therapy procedures involve constant attendance of the physician or therapist, but by definition do not require one-on-one patient contact by the physician or therapist
Design and implement a variety of individual therapeutic play activities to facilitate participation and performance on the playground, in the classroom, and at home	**97530**—Therapeutic activities, direct one-on-one patient contact by the provider (use of dynamic activities to improve functional performance), each 15 minutes
• Provide instruction and compensatory training to improve participation and performance in adaptive/self-care activities • May include interventions such as training in a sensory diet designed to support self-regulation in order to successfully perform self-care activities	**97535**—Self-care home management training (e.g., activities of daily living and compensatory training, meal preparation, safety procedures, instruction in use of assistive technology devices/adaptive equipment), direct one-on-one contact by the provider, each 15 minutes
Provide exercises to increase range of motion, strength, and mobility to enhance ability to participate in daily activities	**97110**—Therapeutic procedure, one or more areas, each 15 minutes; therapeutic exercises to develop strength and endurance, range of motion, and flexibility **97113**—Aquatic therapy with therapeutic exercises

Note. The *CPT*™ 2011 codes referenced in this document do not represent all of the possible codes that may be used in occupational therapy evaluation and intervention. Not all payers will reimburse for all codes. *CPT* codes are updated annually and become effective January 1. Always refer to annual updated *CPT* publication for most current codes.

CPT™ is a trademark of the American Medical Association (AMA). *CPT* five-digit codes, nomenclature, and other data are Copyright ©2010 by the American Medical Association. All Rights Reserved. Reprinted with permission. No fee schedules, basic units, relative values, or related listings are included in *CPT*. The AMA assumes no liability for the data contained herein.

Adapted from *CPT 2011*, by American Medical Association, 2010, Chicago: Author. Adapted with permission.

Appendix F. Data Collection Forms

Sensory Input and Written Production

Child's Name _____ Date _____
Location _____ Time _____
Therapist _____ Period/Subject _____

Time sensory input provided _____
Type of sensory input _____

Of times they stood up/out of seat _____ (tally) Comment: _____

Re-direction Verbal _____ (tally) Comment: _____
              Physical _____ (tally) Comment: _____

Postural adjustment _____ Leaning on desk Comment: _____
                     _____ Head on desk
                     _____ Other _____

Non-engagement _____ Fidgets w/ objects or put in mouth Comment: _____
                _____ Looks away from task   Comment: _____
                _____ Touches others or other's work   Comment: _____
                _____ Other _____   Comment: _____

Purposeful engagement   _____ (mins) _____ (mins) _____ (mins) Comment: _____
(Time on task/doing individual work)
Frequency/duration   _____ (mins) _____ (mins) _____ (mins)
                                   _____ (mins) _____ (mins) _____ (mins)

Completed assignment? Y/N (circle one)
                       # Of lines written/produce _____ Comment: _____
                       Picture completion? Y/N (circle one)

Printed with permission from Dora Sarkodie, MS, OTR/L

Sensory-Based Intervention Data Collection Sheet

Client/Student:

Date of PreTests (Initial Observation and Baseline): Pre Test 1: _____ Pre Test 2: _____
Date of PostTest (Observation after Intervention and Follow Up): Post Test 1: _____ Post Test 2: _____
Time of Day of Observation: Pre 1 _____ Pre 2 _____ Post 1 _____ Post 2 _____

Goal of Intervention-Targeted Outcomes:

Intervention Used Between Pre and Post Observation:

"Dosage" (How many days, how often during the day):

Who did the intervention? (Child, parent, teacher, aide):

Protocol for Intervention (Include any modifications to the intervention):

Client/Student Assessment and Feedback on Intervention:

Frequency Codes for _____ (record the number of occurrences of behaviors the sensory-based intervention is trying to address)	Pre Test 1 Observation Activity:	Pre Test 2 Observation Activity:	Post Test 1 Observation Activity:	Post Test 2 Observation Activity:
a.				
b.				
c.				

Reprinted with permission from ©Kristie Patten Koenig, PhD, OTR, FAOTA.

Sensory-Based Intervention Data Collection Sheet

Client/Student:

Date of PreTests (Initial Observation and Baseline): Pre Test 1: _____ **Pre Test 2:** _____
Date of PostTest (Observation after Intervention and Follow Up): Post Test 1: _____ **Post Test 2:** _____
Time of Day of Observation: Pre 1 _____ **Pre 2** _____ **Post 1** _____ **Post 2** _____

Goal of Intervention-Targeted Outcomes:

Intervention Used Between Pre and Post Observation:

"Dosage" (How many days, how often during the day):

Who did the intervention? (Child, parent, teacher, aide):

Protocol for Intervention (Include any modifications to the intervention):

Client/Student Assessment and Feedback on Intervention:

Duration Codes for _____ (record the amount of time that the desired behavior is occurring during a designated observation period)	Pre Test 1 Observation Activity:	Pre Test 2 Observation Activity:	Post Test 1 Observation Activity:	Post Test 2 Observation Activity:
a.				
b.				
c.				

Reprinted with permission from ©Kristie Patten Koenig, PhD, OTR, FAOTA.

Appendix G. Application to Adults With Mental Health Concerns

As Dunn (2001) described, response to sensation and patterns of responsivity may change with exposure, intervention, and environment but are surprisingly consistent and enduring across the life span. Children who have challenges in processing and integrating sensory information may have received direct intervention and learned coping strategies, but as they transition to young adulthood and adulthood they may find that these issues continue to affect their daily lives. Relationships between sensory processing abnormalities and anxiety and depression (Kinnealey, Koenig, & Smith, in press; Pfeiffer & Kinnealey, 2006) and obsessive–compulsive disorder (Rieke & Anderson, 2009) are found in the literature. Occupational therapy using a sensory integration approach and sensory-based interventions is used with adults with difficulty processing and integrating sensory information (Heller, 2002; Kinnealey, Oliver, & Wilbarger, 1995; Pfeiffer & Kinnealey, 2006), as well as adults with mental health diagnoses (Champagne, 2005; Champagne & Stromberg, 2004). Pfeiffer and Kinnealey (2006) implemented a treatment protocol for adults with sensory defensiveness without a mental health diagnosis that included insight into the sensory issues and regular and daily sensory input that provided primarily proprioceptive, vestibular, and tactile input. This intervention model advocated self-treatment after a session with a trained occupational therapist to provide an evaluation and interpretation and allowed the subjects to choose activities that they felt met their sensory needs. After a month of intervention, sensory defensiveness and secondary anxiety decreased (Pfeiffer & Kinnealey, 2006). Champagne and her colleagues (Champagne, 2005; Champagne & Stromberg, 2004; Mullen, Champagne, Krishnamurty, Dickson, & Gao, 2008) used sensory-based strategies such as deep pressure stimulation (e.g., weighted blankets) in acute inpatient psychiatric settings and found that deep pressure stimulation produced calming and reduced anxiety in a sample of typical adults and may be an alternative to restraints and seclusion used in mental health settings (Champagne & Stromberg, 2004). Mollo, Schaaf, and Benevides (2008) reported on the use of Kripalu yoga in occupational therapy to help adults with sensory sensitivity and anxiety. These direct intervention and consultation models now are used to assist adults who continue to encounter challenges in sensory processing and sensory integration. Continued study with rigorous research design and implementation is needed to assess the efficacy of sensory-based treatments in these additional populations.

Appendix H. Glossary

Adaptive response: "Purposeful, goal-directed actions" that are "more effective than that which [an individual] has been able to demonstrate previously" (Ayres, 1972b, p. 126).

Auditory processing: The ability to take in and make sense of individuals' speech sounds rapidly and efficiently enough to comprehend spoken language. A brain processing function in which the individual has the ability to recognize and interpret sounds (National Institute on Deafness and Other Communication Disorders, 2004).

Auditory system: The sensory system for hearing. Consists of a series of structures by which sounds are received from the environment and conveyed as signals to the central nervous system; it consists of the outer, middle, and inner ear and the tracts in the auditory pathways (Free Dictionary, n.d.-a).

Body scheme: An unconscious mechanism underlying spatial motor coordination that provides the central nervous system with information about the relationship of the body and its parts to environmental space (Bundy, Lane, & Murray, 2002). "Ayres believed that the ability to process and integrate sensation formed the basis for the development of body scheme, sometimes referred to as *body percept*" (Bundy et al., 2002, p. 71).

Cognitive approaches: Intervention "approaches that use cognitive strategies to support the specific training on the activities of interest" (Polatajko & Cantin, 2010, p. 417).

Consultation: A type of intervention in which occupational therapy practitioners use their knowledge and expertise to collaborate with a client. The collaborative process involves identifying the problem, creating possible solutions, trying solutions, and altering them as necessary for greater effectiveness. When providing consultation, the practitioner is not directly responsible for the outcome of the intervention (Dunn, 2000, p. 113).

Developmental dyspraxia: A disorder of motor organization in children not attributed to an overt, known neurological cause. Historically, it was referred to as "clumsy child syndrome." In a sensory integration frame of reference, it is conceived as primarily a developmental deficit in motor-planning skills. In psychological and neuropsychological fields, however, it may have a specific meaning as a deficit in gesture use (May-Benson, personal communication, January 28, 2011).

Direct service: Traditional model of practice in which "the therapist engages a child in an activity with the goal of promoting the child's skill acquisition and minimizing the consequences of a disability" (Jaffe, Humphrey, & Case-Smith, 2010, p. 127).

Dunn's model: Sensory thresholds and patterns of responding. This model explains an interaction between the nervous system and behavior in relation to sensory stimulation. Specifically, the model explicates the interaction between the amount of sensory stimulation needed for the nervous system to respond and behaviors exhibited in response to sensory stimuli. Four sensory processing patterns are described: sensory seeking, sensory avoiding, sensory sensitivity, and low registration (Dunn, 2001).

Dyspraxia: A disorder of integrating tactile, vestibular, and proprioceptive sensory information resulting in interference with the ability to plan and execute skilled or nonhabitual motor plans (Ayres, 1972b). Dyspraxia can be observed in an individual's inaccurate or ineffective movements, despite the person's best efforts.

Emotion regulation: "A complex process involving physiological, cognitive, and behavioral responses to internal and external factors in an attempt to maintain homeostasis of the body and engage effectively in context" (Watling & Miller Kuhanek, 2010, p. 116).

Exteroception: Sensations arising from stimuli that are external to the body (Kandel, Schwartz, & Jessell, 2000), including visual, auditory, and tactile sensations.

Feedforward: Signals sent ahead of a movement to prepare for an upcoming motor command or to ready the system for the receipt of some kind of feedback information (Bundy et al., 2002).

Gravitational insecurity: Excessive fear of ordinary movement, being out of an upright position, or having one's feet off the ground. Children with this fear are uncomfortable with gravity, and their reactions are out of proportion to any real danger that exists or to any postural deficits the child may have (North Shore Pediatric Therapy, 2009).

Habituation: The gradual adaptation to a stimulus or to the environment, with a decreasing response (The Free Dictionary, n.d.-b).

Integration: "The interaction and coordination of two or more functions or processes" (Ayres, 1972b, p. 26).

Interoception: Sensations that arise from within the body and are used primarily for survival (Kandel et al., 2000).

Motor planning: Ability to plan and execute voluntary actions. Organizing a plan for action that involves movement.

Neuroplasticity: Ability of the human brain to change as a result of one's experience (Babylon Free Dictionary, n.d.).

Perceptual–motor approaches: Intervention that includes activities that require both movement and perception skills (Kephart, 1971; Sherrill, 1998).

Practic: Pertaining to the ability to plan and execute coordinated movement.

Praxis: "The ability to plan and carry out an unfamiliar action" (Ayres, 1979, p. 87). "Primarily pertains to the planning aspect of a motor act; it is a process that requires knowledge of actions and of objects, motivation, and intention on the part of the person" (Bundy et al., 2002, p. 71).

Proprioception: "The sense of position and movement of one's own limbs and body without using vision" (Kandel et al., 2000, p. 443). Proprioceptive sensations are "information arising from the body, especially from muscles, joints, ligaments, and receptors associated with bones" (Ayres, 1972b, p. 66). Proprioceptive information plays a critical role in sensory integration influencing motor actions and modulating emotional state (Ayres, 1972b).

Self-regulation: An organized behavioral state whereby the individual is able to successfully adapt to the demands of his or her environment (Boekoerts & Pintrich, 2005). More specifically, self-regulation has been defined as "the ability to monitor and modulate cognition, emotion, and behavior to accomplish one's goal and/or to adapt to the cognitive and social demands of specific situations" (Berger, Kofman, Livneh, & Henik, 2007, p. 257).

Sensation: A perception associated with stimulation of a sense organ or with a specific body condition; the faculty to feel or perceive (Free Dictionary, n.d.-c).

Sensorimotor approaches: Intervention approaches that "provide a variety of motor activities with an inherent variety of sensory stimuli (e.g., therapeutic riding, movement therapy, therapy balls)" (Polatajko & Cantin, 2010, p. 417).

Sensory diet: A strategy for developing individualized home programs that are practical, carefully scheduled, and based on the concept that controlled sensory input can affect functional abilities (Bundy et al., 2002; J. Wilbarger & Wilbarger, 2002).

Sensory discrimination: The ability to take in information from the physical environment and perceive qualities of stimuli such as spatial or temporal features.

Sensory integration: "The neurological process that organizes sensation from one's own body and from the environment and makes it possible to use the body effectively within the environment" (Ayres 1972b, p. 11).

Sensory integrative dysfunction: A condition in which "the brain is not processing or organizing the flow of sensory impulses in a manner that gives the individual good, precise sensory input well . . . [and] is not directing behavior effectively" (Ayres, 1979, p. 51).

Sensory-based approaches: Intervention approaches that provide "specific sensory stimulation" (Polatajko & Cantin, 2010, p. 417).

Sensory modulation: Enhancement or dampening of sensory input; "the capacity to regulate and organize the degree, intensity, and nature of responses to sensory input in a graded and adaptive manner so that persons can maintain an optimal range of performance and adapt to challenges" (Lane, Miller, & Hanft, 2000, p. 2); the active process by which central nervous system mechanisms adjust or otherwise adapt to incoming information (Lane, 2002).

Sensory processing: Functions related to sensation occurring in the central nervous system (Bundy et al., 2002).

Sensory registration: Detection of sensation and the initial point of perception; a response to change or novelty in the sensory environment.

Sensory stories: An adaptation of Social Stories™. Sensory stories depict situations in which the individual experiences difficulties in sensory processing or integration and subsequently implements sensory strategies to support coping and engagement. Sensory stories are designed to help children learn about situations when challenges in sensory processing and integration may interfere with engagement and how to implement strategies to enable successful participation in everyday activities at school, home, and in the community (Therapro, 2009).

Social Stories™: Stories used to describe a situation, skill, or concept in terms of relevant social cues, perspectives, and common responses in a specifically defined style and format. Social Stories often are customized so that the individual with whom the story is being used is the main character. The goal of a Social Story is to share accurate social information in a patient and reassuring manner that is easily understood and instructive in helping the individual to understand and develop appropriate and effective social skills. Originally developed for use with children with autism, Social Stories have now been extended to many additional domains (Gray Center for Social Learning and Understanding, n.d.).

Vestibular–proprioceptive integration: The integration of vestibular and proprioceptive sensations for perception of the body's position in space, the body's parts in relation to one another, and the dynamic movement of the body through space, providing the basis for a variety of functional skills, including postural control, balance, coordination, bilateral integration, and sequencing (Ayres, 1979; Koomar & Bundy, 2002).

Vestibular/vestibular system: The vestibular system is responsible for maintaining balance, posture, and the body's orientation in space. The vestibular system consists of the semicircular canals, the utricle and saccule, the vestibular portion of the vestibulococochlear nerve, and the central nervous system structures that interpret and respond to the information derived from these structures.

Visual perception: Registration and integration of visual information for perception. The ability to perceive or understand what is being seen; the integration of an image with an idea of what it represents (Encyclopedia.com, n.d.).

References

Achenbach, T. M. (2009). *The Achenbach System of Empirically Based Assessment (ASEBA): Development, findings, theory, and applications.* Burlington: University of Vermont Research Center for Children, Youth, and Families.

Agency for Healthcare Research and Quality. (2009). *Standard recommendation language.* Retrieved February 14, 2009, from http://www.ahrq.gov/clinic/uspstf/standard.htm

Ahn, R. R., Miller, L. J., Milberger, S., & McIntosh, D. N. (2004). Prevalence of parents' perceptions of sensory processing disorders among kindergarten children. *American Journal of Occupational Therapy, 58,* 287–302.

Allen, S., & Donald, M. (1995). The effect of occupational therapy on the motor proficiency of children with motor/learning difficulties. *British Journal of Occupational Therapy, 58*(9), 385–391.

Allik, H., Larsson, J., & Smedje, H. (2006). Sleep patterns of school-age children with Asperger syndrome or high-functioning autism. *Journal of Autism and Developmental Disorders, 36,* 585–595.

Ameratunga, D., Johnston, L., & Burns, Y. (2004). Goal-directed upper-limb movements by children with and without DCD: A window into the perceptuo–motor dysfunction. *Physiotherapy Research International, 9,* 1–12. doi: 10.1002/prt.295

American Medical Association. (1997). *Physician's current procedural terminology (CPT).* Chicago: Author.

American Medical Association. (2010). *CPT 2011.* Chicago: Author.

American Occupational Therapy Association. (1979). *Occupational therapy product output reporting system and uniform terminology for reporting occupational therapy services.* (Available from American Occupational Therapy Association, 4720 Montgomery Lane, PO Box 31220, Bethesda, MD 20824-1220)

American Occupational Therapy Association. (1989). *Uniform terminology for occupational therapy* (2nd ed.). (Available from American Occupational Therapy Association, 4720 Montgomery Lane, PO Box 31220, Bethesda, MD 20824-1220)

American Occupational Therapy Association. (1994). Uniform terminology for occupational therapy (3rd ed.). *American Journal of Occupational Therapy, 48,* 1047–1054.

American Occupational Therapy Association. (2002). Occupational therapy practice framework: Domain and process. *American Journal of Occupational Therapy, 56,* 609–639.

American Occupational Therapy Association. (2006). Policy 1.44: Categories of occupational therapy personnel. In *Policy manual* (2009 ed., 33–34). Bethesda, MD: Author.

American Occupational Therapy Association. (2007a). Accreditation standards for a doctoral-degree-level educational program for the occupational therapist. *American Journal of Occupational Therapy, 61,* 641–651.

American Occupational Therapy Association. (2007b). Accreditation standards for a master's-degree-level educational program for the occupational therapist. *American Journal of Occupational Therapy, 61,* 652–661.

American Occupational Therapy Association. (2007c). Accreditation standards for an educational program for the occupational therapy assistant. *American Journal of Occupational Therapy, 61,* 662–671.

American Occupational Therapy Association. (2008a). Guidelines for documentation of occupational therapy. *American Journal of Occupational Therapy, 62,* 684–690.

American Occupational Therapy Association. (2008b). Occupational therapy practice framework: Domain and process (2nd ed.). *American Journal of Occupational Therapy, 62,* 625–683.

American Occupational Therapy Association. (2009a). Guidelines for supervision, roles, and responsibilities during the delivery of occupational therapy services. *American Journal of Occupational Therapy, 63,* 779–803.

American Occupational Therapy Association. (2009b). Providing occupational therapy using sensory integration theory in school-based practice. *American Journal of Occupational Therapy, 63,* 823–842.

American Occupational Therapy Association. (2010). Standards of practice for occupational therapy. *American Journal of Occupational Therapy, 64*(Suppl.), S106–S111.

Amundson, M. (1995). *Evaluation Tool of Children's Handwriting.* Homer, AK: OT Kids.

Antrop, I., Roeyers, H., Van Oost, P., & Buysse, A. (2000). Stimulation seeking and hyperactivity in children with ADHD. *Journal of Child Psychology and Psychiatry and Allied Disciplines, 41,* 225–231. doi: 10.1017/S0021963099005302

Ayres, A. J. (1964). Tactile functions: Their relation to hyperactive and perceptual–motor behavior. *American Journal of Occupational Therapy, 18,* 6–11.

Ayres, A. J. (1965). Patterns of perceptual–motor dysfunction in children: A factor analytic study. *Perceptual and Motor Skills, 20,* 335–368.

Ayres, A. J. (1972a). Improving academic scores through sensory integration. *Journal of Learning Disabilities, 5,* 338–343.

Ayres, A. J. (1972b). *Sensory integration and learning disorders.* Los Angeles: Western Psychological Services.

Ayres, A. J. (1972c). *Southern California Sensory Integration Tests.* Los Angeles: Western Psychological Services.

Ayres, A. J. (1977). Effect of sensory integrative therapy on the coordination of children with choreoathetoid movements. *American Journal of Occupational Therapy, 31,* 291–293.

Ayres, A. J. (1979). *Sensory integration and the child.* Los Angeles: Western Psychological Services.

Ayres, A. J. (1980). *Southern California Tests of Sensory Integration Tests Manual: Revised.* Los Angeles: Western Psychological Services.

Ayres, A. J. (1989). *Sensory Integration and Praxis Tests.* Los Angeles: Western Psychological Services.

Babylon Free Dictionary. (n.d.) *Neuroplasticity.* Retrieved January 20, 2011, from http://dictionary.babylon.com/neuroplasticity/

Bach-y-Rita, P. (2004). Tactile sensory substitution studies. *Annals of the New York Academy of Sciences, 1013,* 83–91.

Bangert, M., & Altenmüller, E. (2003). Mapping perception to action in piano practice: A longitudinal DC–EEG study. *BMC Neuroscience, 4,* 26. Available from http://www.biomedcentral.com/1471-2202/4/26

Bar-Shalita, T., Vatine, J., & Parush, S. (2008). Sensory modulation disorder: A risk factor for participation in daily life activities. *Developmental Medicine and Child Neurology, 50,* 932–937.

Baranek, G. T. (1999). Autism during infancy: A retrospective video analysis of sensory–motor and social behaviors at 9–12 months of age. *Journal of Autism and Developmental Disorders, 29,* 213–224.

Baranek, G. (2002). Efficacy of sensory and motor interventions for children with autism. *Journal of Autism and Developmental Disorders, 32,* 397–422.

Baranek, G. T., Chin, Y. H., Hess, L. M., Yankee, J. G., Hatton, D. D., & Hooper, S. R. (2002). Sensory processing correlates of occupational performance in children with fragile X syndrome: Preliminary findings. *American Journal of Occupational Therapy, 56,* 538–546.

Baranek, G. T., David, F. J., Poe, M. D., Stone, W. L., & Watson, L. R. (2006). Sensory Experiences Questionnaire: Discriminating sensory features in young children with autism, developmental delays, and typical development. *Journal of Child Psychology and Psychiatry and Allied Disciplines, 47,* 591–601.

Baum, C. M., & Edwards, D. (2008). *Activity Card Sort* (2nd ed.). Bethesda, MD: AOTA Press.

Bavelier, D., Brozinsky, C., Tomann, A., Mitchell, T., Neville, H., & Liu, G. (2001). Impact of early deafness and early exposure to sign language on the cerebral organization for motion processing. *Journal of Neuroscience, 21,* 8931–8942.

Bayley, N. (2005). *Bayley Scales of Infant and Toddler Development* (3rd ed.). San Antonio, TX: Psychological Corporation.

Beery, K. E., Buktenica, N. A., & Beery, N. A. (2004). *Beery–Buktenica Developmental Test of Visual–Motor Integration (VMI)* (5th ed.). Parsippany, NJ: Modern Curriculum Press.

Bennett, E. L., Diamond, M. C., Krech, D., & Rosenzweig, M. R. (1964). Chemical and anatomical plasticity of brain. *Science, 146,* 610–619.

Bennett, E. L., Diamond, M. C., Krech, D., & Rosenzweig, M. R. (1996). Chemical and anatomical plasticity of brain. *Journal of Neuropsychiatry and Clinical Neurosciences, 8,* 459–470.

Bennett, E. L., Rosenzweig, M. R., Diamond, M. C., Morimoto, H. M., & Hebert, M. (1974). Effects of successive environments on brain measures. *Physiology and Behavior, 12*(4), 621–631.

Berg, C., & LaVesser, P. (2006). The Preschool Activity Card Sort. *OTJR: Occupation, Participation and Health, 26*(4), 143–151.

Berger, A., Kofman, O., Livneh, U., & Henik, A. (2007). Multidisciplinary perspectives on attention and the development of self-regulation. *Progress in Neurobiology, 82,* 256–286.

Berk, R., & DeGangi, G. (1983). *DeGangi–Berk Test of Sensory Integration.* Los Angeles: Western Psychological Services.

Bieberich, A. A., & Morgan, S. B. (2004). Self-regulation and affective expression during play in children with autism or Down syndrome: A short-term longitudinal study. *Journal of Autism and Developmental Disorders, 34,* 439–448.

Blanche, E. (2002). *Observations based on sensory integration theory.* Los Angeles: Western Psychological Corporation.

Blanche, E. (2010). *Observations based on sensory integration theory* [video and book]. Torrence, CA: Pediatric Therapy Network.

Blanche, E., & Schaaf, R. (2001). Proprioception: A cornerstone of sensory integration intervention. In S. S. Roley, E. Blanche, & R. Schaaf (Eds.), *Understanding the nature of sensory integration with diverse populations* (pp. 109–124). San Antonio, TX: Therapy Skill Builders.

Boekoerts, M., & Pintrich, P. R. (2005). *Handbook of self-regulation.* Burlington, MA: Elsevier Academic Press.

Braun, C., Heinz, U., Schweizer, R., Wiech, K., Nirbaumer, N., & Topka, H. (2001). Dynamic organization of the somatosensory cortex induced by motor activity. *Brain, 124,* 2259–2267.

Brown, C., & Dunn, W. (2002). *Adolescent/Adult Sensory Profile, user's manual.* San Antonio, TX: Psychological Corporation.

Brown, C., Tollefson, N., Dunn, W., Cromwell, R., & Filion, D. (2001). The Adult Sensory Profile: Measuring patterns of sensory processing. *American Journal of Occupational Therapy, 55,* 75–82.

Brown, J., Cooper-Kuhn, C. M., Kempermann, G., Van Praag, H., Winkler, J., Gage, F. H., et al. (2003). Enriched environment and physical activity stimulate hippocampal but not olfactory bulb neurogenesis. *European Journal of Neuroscience, 17,* 2042–2046.

Bruininks, R. H., & Bruininks, B. D. (2005). *Bruininks–Oseretsky Test of Motor Proficiency* (2nd ed.). Circle Pines, MN: AGS.

Bruininks, R. H., Woodcock, R. W., Weatherman, R. F., & Hill, B. K. (1997). *Scales of Independent Behavior–Revised.* Itasca, IL: Riverside.

Bryan, L. C., & Gast, D. L. (2000). Teaching on-task and on-schedule behaviors to high-functioning children with autism via picture activity schedules. *Journal of Autism and Developmental Disorders, 30,* 553–567.

Bullock, M. I., & Watter, P. (1978). A study of the effectiveness of physiotherapy in the management of young children with minimal cerebral dysfunction. *Australian Journal of Physiotherapy, 24,* 111–119.

Bundy, A. C. (2002). Using sensory integration theory in schools: Sensory integration and consultation. In A. C. Bundy, S. J. Lane, & E. A. Murray (Eds.), *Sensory integration: Theory and practice* (2nd ed., pp. 3–33). Philadelphia: F. A. Davis.

Bundy, A. C., Lane, S. J., & Murray, E. A. (2002). *Sensory integration: Theory and practice* (2nd ed.). Philadelphia: F. A. Davis.

Bundy, A. C., & Murray, E. A. (2002). Sensory integration: A. Jean Ayres' theory revisited. In A. C. Bundy, S. J. Lane, & E. A. Murray (Eds.), *Sensory integration: Theory and practice* (2nd ed., pp. 3–33). Philadelphia: F. A. Davis.

Bundy, A. C., Shia, S., Qi, L., & Miller, L. J. (2007). How does sensory processing dysfunction affect play? *American Journal of Occupational Therapy, 61,* 201–208.

Cairney, J., Hay, J., Faught, B., Wade, T., Corna, L., & Flouris, A. (2005). Developmental coordination disorder, generalized self-efficacy toward physical activity, and participation in organized and free play activities. *Journal of Pediatrics, 147,* 515–520. doi:10.1016/j.jpeds.2005.05.013

Candler, C. (2003). Sensory integration and therapeutic riding at summer camp: Occupational performance outcomes. *Physical and Occupational Therapy in Pediatrics, 23,* 51–64. doi:10.1300/J006v23n03_04

Carte, E., Morrison, D., Sublett, Uemura, A., & Setrakian, W. (1984). Sensory integration therapy: A trial of a specific neurodevelopmental therapy for the remediation of learning disabilities. *Developmental and Behavioral Pediatrics, 54,* 189–194.

Case-Smith, J. (1995). The relationships among sensorimotor components, fine motor skill, and functional performance in preschool children. *American Journal of Occupational Therapy, 49,* 645–652.

Case-Smith, J. (2010). An overview of occupational therapy for children. In J. Case-Smith & J. C. O'Brien (Eds.), *Occupational therapy for children* (6th ed., pp. 1–21). Maryland Heights, MI: Mosby.

Case-Smith, J., & Bryan, T. (1999). The effects of occupational therapy with sensory integration emphasis on preschool-age children with autism. *American Journal of Occupational Therapy, 53,* 489–497.

Case-Smith, J., & O'Brien, J. C. (2010). *Occupational therapy for children* (6th ed.). Maryland Heights, MI: Mosby.

Ceponiene, R., Lepistö, T., Shestakova, A., Vanhala, R., Alku, P., Naatanen, R., et al. (2003). Speech–sound–selective auditory impairment in children with autism: They can perceive but do not attend. *Proceedings of the National Academy of Sciences of the United States of America, 100,* 5567–5572.

Cermak, S. (2009). Deprivation and sensor processing in institutionalized and postinstitutionalized children: Part II. *Sensory Integration Special Interest Section Quarterly, 32*(3), 1–4.

Champagne, T. (2005). Expanding the role of sensory approaches in acute psychiatric settings. *Mental Health Special Interest Section Quarterly, 28*(1), 1–4.

Champagne, T., & Stromberg, N. (2004). Sensory approaches in inpatient psychiatric settings: Innovative alternatives to seclusion and restraint. *Journal of Psychosocial Nursing, 42*(9), 35–44.

Channon, S., Charman, T., Heap, J., Crawford, S., & Rios, P. (2001). Real-life-type problem-solving in Asperger's syndrome. *Journal of Autism and Developmental Disorders, 31,* 461–469.

Chia, L. C., & Chua, L. W. (2002). Effects of physiotherapy on school-aged children with developmental coordination disorder and learning difficulties: A pilot study. *Physiotherapy Singapore, 5,* 75–80.

Cohn, E. S., & Cermak, S. A. (1998). Including the family perspective in sensory integration outcomes research. *American Journal of Occupational Therapy, 52,* 540–546.

Colarusso, R. P., & Hammill, D. D. (2003). *Motor-Free Visual Perception Test* (3rd ed., MVPT–3). Novato, CA: Academic Therapy Publications.

Coleman, R., Piek, J. P., & Livesey, D. J. (2001). A longitudinal study of motor ability and kinaesthetic acuity in young children at risk of developmental coordination disorder. *Human Movement Science, 20,* 95–110.

Constantino, J. N., & Gruber, C. P. (2005). *The Social Responsiveness Scale.* Los Angeles: Psychological Corporation.

Coster, W. (1998). Occupation-centered assessment for children. *American Journal of Occupational Therapy, 52,* 337–344.

Coster, W., Deeney, T., Haltiwanger, J., & Haley, S. (1998). *The School Function Assessment.* San Antonio, TX: Psychological Corporation.

Cummins, A., Piek, J. P., & Dyck, M. J. (2005). Motor coordination, empathy, and social behaviour in schoolaged children. *Developmental Medicine and Child Neurology, 47,* 437–442. doi:10.1017/S001216220500085X

Dawson, G., & Watling, R. L. (2000). Interventions to facilitate auditory, visual, and motor integration in autism: A review of the evidence. *Journal of Autism and Developmental Disorders, 30,* 415–421.

Davies, P. L., & Tucker, R. (2010). Evidence review to investigate the support for subtypes of children with difficulty processing and integrating sensory information. *American Journal of Occupational Therapy, 64,* 391–402.

Davis, R. A. O., Bockbrader, M. A., Murphy, R. R., Hetrick, W. P., & O'Donnell, B. F. (2006). Subjective perceptual distortions and visual dysfunction in children with autism. *Journal of Autism and Developmental Disorders, 36,* 199–210.

DeGangi, G. (2000). *Pediatric disorders of regulation in affect and behavior.* San Diego, CA: Academic Press.

DeGangi, G. A., & Greenspan, S. I. (1989). *Test of Sensory Functions in Infants manual.* Los Angeles: Western Psychological Services

Dettmer, S., Simpson, R. L., Myles, B. S., & Ganz, J. B. (2000). The use of visual supports to facilitate transitions of students with autism. *Focus on Autism and Other Developmental Disabilities, 15,* 163–169.

Dewey, D., Kaplan, B. J., Crawford, S. G., & Wilson, B. N. (2002). Developmental coordination disorder: Associated problems in attention, learning, and psychosocial adjustment. *Human Movement Science, 21,* 905–918.

Diamond, M. C., Rosenzweig, M. R., Bennett, E. L., Lindner, B., & Lyon, L. (1972). Effects of environmental enrichment and impoverishment on rat cerebral cortex. *Journal of Neurobiology, 3*(1), 47–64.

Dooley, P., Wilczenski, F. L., & Torem, C. (2001). Using an activity schedule to smooth school transitions. *Journal of Positive Behavior Interventions, 3,* 57–61.

Doucet, M. E., Guillemot, J. P., Lassonde, M., Gagné, J. P., Leclerc, C., & Lepore, F. (2005). Blind subjects process auditory spectral cues more efficiently than sighted individuals. *Experimental Brain Research, 160,* 194–202.

Downs, A., & Smith, T. (2004). Emotional understanding, cooperation, and social behavior in high-functioning children with autism. *Journal of Autism and Developmental Disorders, 34,* 625–635.

Dunbar, S. B. (1999). A child's occupational performance: Considerations of sensory processing and family context. *American Journal of Occupational Therapy, 53,* 231–235.

Dunn, W. (1990). A comparison of service provision models in school-based occupational therapy services: A pilot study. *OTJR: Occupation, Participation and Health, 10,* 300–320.

Dunn, W. (1997). The impact of sensory processing abilities on the daily lives of young children and their families: A conceptual model. *Infants and Young Children, 9,* 23–35.

Dunn, W. (1999). *The Sensory Profile: User's manual.* San Antonio, TX: Psychological Corporation.

Dunn, W. (2000). *Best practice in occupational therapy in community service with children and families.* Thorofare, NJ: Slack.

Dunn, W. (2001). The sensations of everyday life: Empirical, theoretical and pragmatic concerns. *American Journal of Occupational Therapy, 55,* 608–620.

Dunn, W. (2002). *Infant/Toddler Sensory Profile manual.* San Antonio, TX: Psychological Corporation.

Dunn, W. (2006). *Sensory Profile School Companion.* San Antonio, TX: Psychological Corporation.

Dunn, W., & Bennett, D. (2002). Patterns of sensory processing in children with attention deficit hyperactivity disorder. *Occupational Therapy Journal of Research, 22,* 4–15.

Dunn, W., & Brown, C. (1997). Factor analysis on the Sensory Profile from a national sample of children without disabilities. *American Journal of Occupational Therapy, 51,* 490–495.

Dunn, W., & Daniels, D. (2001). Initial development of the Infant/Toddler Sensory Profile. *Journal of Early Intervention, 25*(1), 27–41.

Dunn, W., Myles, B. B., & Orr, S. (2002). Sensory-processing issues associated with Asperger's syndrome: A preliminary investigation. *American Journal of Occupational Therapy, 56,* 97–102.

Dziuk, M. A., Gidley Larson, J. C., Apostu, A., Mahone, E. M., Denckla, M. B., & Mostofsky, S. H. (2007). Dyspraxia in autism: Association with motor, social, and communicative deficits. *Developmental Medicine and Child Neurology, 49,* 734–739.

Ecker, C., & Parham, D. (2010). *Sensory Processing Measure–Preschool (SPM–P), Home Form.* Los Angeles: Western Psychological Services.

Encyclopedia.com. (n.d.). *Beery–Buktenica Test.* Retrieved January 24, 2011, from www.encyclopedia.com/doc/1G2-3447200079.html

Ermer, J., & Dunn, W. (1998). The Sensory Profile: A discriminant analysis of children with and without disabilities. *American Journal of Occupational Therapy, 52,* 283–290.

Fertel-Daly, D., Bedell, G., & Hinojosa, J. (2001). Effects of a weighted vest on attention to task and self-stimulatory behaviors in preschoolers with pervasive developmental disorders. *American Journal of Occupational Therapy, 55,* 629–640.

Fisher, A. G., Bryze, K., Hume, V., & Griswold, L. A. (2005). *School AMPS: School Version of the Assessment of Motor and Process Skills* (2nd ed.). Fort Collins, CO: Three Star Press.

Fisher, A., & Murray, E. (1991). Introduction to sensory integration theory. In A. Fisher, E. Murray, & A. C. Bundy (Eds.), *Sensory integration theory and practice* (pp. 3–26). Philadelphia: F. A. Davis.

Folio, R., & Fewell, R. (2000). *Peabody Developmental Motor Scales* (2nd ed.). Austin, TX: Pro-Ed.

Forseth, A. K., & Sigmundsson, H. (2003). Static balance in children with hand–eye coordination problems. *Child: Care, Health, and Development, 29,* 569–579.

Free Dictionary. (n.d.-a). *Auditory system.* Retrieved February 1, 2011, from http://medical-dictionary.thefreedictionary.com/auditory+system

Free Dictionary. (n.d.-b). *Habituation.* Retrieved January 22, 2011, from http://medical-dictionary.thefreedictionary.com/habituation

Free Dictionary. (n.d.-c). *Sensation.* Retrieved February 1, 2011, from http://www.thefreedictionary.com/sensation

Frick, S. M., & Hacker, C. (2001). *Listening with the whole body.* Madison, WI: Vital Links.

Gal, E., Cermak, S. A., & Ben-Sasson, A. (2007). Sensory processing disorders in children with autism: Nature, assessment, and intervention. In R. Gabriels & D. Hill (Eds.), *Growing with autism: Working with school-age children and adolescents* (pp. 95–123). New York: Guilford Press.

Gardner, M. F. (1992). *Test of Visual–Motor Skills–Upper Level (TVMS–UL).* Novato, CA: Academic Therapy Publications.

Gardner, M. F. (1995). *Test of Visual–Motor Skills–Revised (TVMS–R).* Los Angeles: Western Psychological Services.

Gardner, M. F. (1997). *Test of Visual–Perceptual Skills–Upper Level (TVPS–UL).* Los Angeles: Western Psychological Services.

Gardner, M. F. (1998). *Test of Handwriting Skills.* Los Angeles, CA: Western Psychological Services.

Geuze, R. H. (2003). Static balance and development coordination disorder. *Human Movement Science, 22,* 527–548.

Geuze, R. H. (2005). Postural control in children with developmental coordination disorder. *Neural Plasticity, 12,* 183–196.

Gioia, G. A., Espy, K. A., & Isquith, P. K. (2003). *Behavior Rating Inventory of Executive Function–Preschool Version.* Odessa, FL: Psychological Assessment Resources.

Gioia, G. A., Isquith, P. K., Guy, S. C., & Kenworthy, L. (2000). *The Behavior Rating Inventory of Executive Function.* Lutz, FL: Psychological Assessment Resources.

Gomez, R., & Condon, M. (1999). Central auditory processing ability in children with ADHD with and without learning disabilities. *Journal of Learning Disabilities, 32,* 150–158.

Gómez-Pinilla, F., Ying, Z., Roy, R. R., Molteni, R., & Edgerton, V. R. (2002). Voluntary exercise induces a BDNF-mediated mechanism that promotes neuroplasticity. *Journal of Neurophysiology, 88,* 2187–2195.

Gordon, J. A., & Stryker, M. P. (1996). Experience-dependent plasticity of binocular responses in the primary visual cortex of the mouse. *Journal of Neuroscience, 16,* 3274–3286.

Graetz, J. E., & Spampinato, K. (2008, Winter). Asperger's syndrome and the voyage through high school: Not the final frontier. *Journal of College Admission, 1,* 19–24.

Graven, S. N., & Browne, J. V. (2008a). Auditory development in the fetus and infant. *Newborn and Infant Nursing Reviews, 8,* 187–193.

Graven, S. N., & Browne, J. V. (2008b). Visual development in the human fetus, infant, and young child. *Newborn and Infant Nursing Reviews, 8,* 194–201.

Gray Center for Social Learning and Understanding. (n.d.) *What are Social Stories™?* Retrieved February 1, 2011, from http://www.thegraycenter.org/social-stories/what-are-social-stories

Gresham, F. M., & Elliott, S. N. (2008). *Social Skills Improvement System—Rating Scales.* Minneapolis, MN: Pearson.

Grimwood, L. M., & Rutherford, E. M. (1980). Sensory integrative therapy as an intervention procedure with Grade One "at risk" readers: A 3-year study. *International Journal of Disability, Development, and Education, 27,* 52–61.

Grüsser, S. M., Mühlnickel, W., Schaefer, M., Villringer, K., Christmann, C., Koeppe, C., et al. (2004). Remote activation of referred phantom sensation and cortical reorganization in human upper-extremity amputees. *Experimental Brain Research, 154,* 97–102.

Guest, S., & Spence, C. (2003). What role does multisensory integration play in the visuotactile perception of texture? *International Journal of Psychophysiology, 50,* 63–80.

Halder, P., Sterr, A., Brem, S., Bucher, K., Kollias, S., & Brandeis, D. (2005). Electrophysiological evidence for cortical plasticity with movement repetition. *European Journal of Neuroscience, 21,* 2271–2277.

Haley, S. M., Coster, W. J., Ludlow, L. H., Haltiwanger, J. T., & Andrellos, P. J. (1992). *Pediatric Evaluation of Disability Inventory: Development, standardization, and administration manual, version 1.0.* Boston: Trustees of Boston University, Health and Disability Research Institute.

Hall, L., & Case-Smith, J. (2007). The effect of sound-based intervention on children with sensory-processing disorders and visual–motor delays. *American Journal of Occupational Therapy, 61,* 209–215.

Hammill, D. D., Pearson, N. A., & Voress, J. K. (1993). *Developmental Test of Visual Perception* (2nd ed.; DTVP–2). Austin, TX: Pro-Ed.

Hanft, B., & Shepherd, J. (2008). Introduction. In B. Hanft & J. Shepherd, *Collaborating for student success* (pp. xix–xxiii). Bethesda, MD: AOTA Press.

Harlow, H. (1958). The nature of love. *American Psychologist, 13,* 673–685.

Harlow, H. F., Harlow, M. K., & Suomi, S. J. (1971). From thought to therapy: Lessons from a primate laboratory. *American Scientist, 59*(5), 538–549.

Harrison, P. L., & Oakland, T. (2003). *Adaptive Behavior Assessment System—2nd edition: Manual.* San Antonio, TX: Psychological Corporation.

Hartshorn, K., Olds, L., Field, T., Delage, J., Cullen, C., & Escalona, A. (2001). Creative movement therapy benefits children with autism. *Early Child Development and Care, 166,* 1–5.

Hauck, J. A., & Dewey, D. (2001). Hand preference and motor functioning in children with autism. *Journal of Autism and Developmental Disorders, 31,* 265–277.

Heller, S. (2002). *Too loud, too bright, too fast, too tight.* New York: Harper Collins.

Hilton, C., Graver, K., & LaVesser, P. (2007). Relationship between social competence and sensory processing in children with high functioning autism spectrum disorders. *Research in Autism Spectrum Disorders, 1,* 164–173. doi: 10.1016/j.rasd.2006.10.002

Hinojosa, J., & Foto, M. (2004). Occupational therapy for documentation for reimbursement: Sensory integration. *Sensory Integration Special Interest Section Quarterly, 27*(4), 1–3.

Hodge, S. R., Murata, N. M., & Porretta, D. L. (1999). Enhancing motor performance through various preparatory activities involving children with learning disabilities. *Clinical Kinesiology, 53,* 76–82.

Hodzic, A., Veit, R., Karim, A. A., Erb, M., & Godde, B. (2004). Improvement and decline in tactile discrimination behavior after cortical plasticity induced by passive tactile coactivation. *Journal of Neuroscience, 24,* 442–446.

Hoehn, T. P., & Baumeister, A. A. (1994). A critique of the application of sensory integration therapy to children with learning disabilities. *Journal of Learning Disabilities, 27,* 338–350.

Honomichl, R. D., Goodlin-Jones, B. L., Burnham, M., Gaylor, E., & Anders, T. F. (2002). Sleep patterns of children with pervasive developmental disorders. *Journal of Autism and Developmental Disorders, 32,* 553–561.

Hubel, D. H., & Wiesel, T. N. (1964). *Binocular interaction in striate cortex of kittens reared with artificial squint.* Boston: Neurophysiology Laboratory, Department of Pharmacology, Harvard Medical School.

Humphries, T., Krekewich, K., & Snider, L. (1996). Evidence of nonverbal learning disability among learning disabled boys with sensory integrative dysfunction. *Perceptual and Motor Skills, 82*(3, Part 1), 979–987.

Humphries, T. W., Snider, L., & McDougall, B. (1993). Clinical evaluation of the effectiveness of sensory integrative and perceptual–motor therapy in improving sensory integrative function in children with learning disabilities. *Occupational Therapy Journal of Research, 13,* 163–182.

Humphries, T., Wright, M., McDougall, B., & Vertes, J. (1990). The efficacy of sensory integration therapy for children with learning disabilities. *Physical and Occupational Therapy in Pediatrics, 10,* 1–17.

Humphries, T., Wright, M., Snider, L., & McDougall, B. (1992). A comparison of the effectiveness of sensory integrative therapy and perceptual–motor training in treating children with learning disabilities. *Developmental and Behavioral Pediatrics, 13,* 31–40.

Inder, J. M., & Sullivan, S. (2004). Does an educational kinesiology intervention alter postural control in children with a developmental coordination disorder? *Clinical Kinesiology, 58,* 9–26.

Inder, J. M., & Sullivan, S. J. (2005). Motor and postural response profiles of four children with developmental coordination disorder. *Pediatric Physical Therapy 17,* 18–29.

Iwanaga, R., Ozawa, H., Kawasaki, C., & Tsuchida, R. (2006). Characteristics of the sensory–motor, verbal, and cognitive abilities of preschool boys with attention deficit/hyperactivity disorder combined type. *Psychiatry and Clinical Neurosciences, 60*(1), 37–45.

Jackson, C. T., Fein, D., Wolf, J., Jones, G., Hauck, M., Waterhouse, L., et al. (2003). Responses and sustained interactions in children with mental retardation and autism. *Journal of Autism and Developmental Disorders, 33,* 115–121.

Jacobs, S. E., & Schneider, M. L. (2001). Neuroplasticity and the environment: Implications for sensory integration. In S. S. Roley, E. I. Blanche, & R. C. Schaaf (Eds.), *Understanding the nature of sensory integration with diverse populations* (pp. 29–42). San Antonio, TX: Therapy Skill Builders.

Jaffe, E. G., & Epstein, C. F. (1992). *Occupational therapy consultation: Theory, principles, and practice.* St. Louis, MO: Mosby.

Jaffe, L., Humphry, R., & Case-Smith, J. (2010). Working with families. In J. Case-Smith & J. O'Brien (Eds.), *Occupational therapy for children* (6th ed., pp. 108–140). Maryland Heights, MO: Mosby.

Jansiewicz, E. M., Goldberg, M. C., Newschaffer, C. J., Denckla, M. B., Landa, R., & Mostofsky, S. H. (2006). Motor signs distinguish children with high functioning autism and Asperger's syndrome from controls. *Journal of Autism and Developmental Disorders, 36,* 613–621.

Jarrold, C., Gilchrist, I. D., & Bender, A. (2005). Embedded figures detection in autism and typical development: Preliminary evidence of a double dissociation in relationships with visual search. *Developmental Science, 8,* 344–351.

Johnson-Ecker, C. L., & Parham, L. D. (2000). The evaluation of sensory processing: A validity study using contrasting groups. *American Journal of Occupational Therapy, 54,* 494–503.

Kagerer, F. A., Bo, J., Contreras-Vidal, J. L., & Clark, J. E. (2004). Visuomotor adaptation in children with developmental coordination disorder. *Motor Control, 8,* 450–460.

Kandel, E. R., Schwartz, J. H., & Jessell, T. M. (2000). *Principles of neural science.* New York: McGraw-Hill.

Kaplan, B. J., Wilson, B. N., Dewey, D., & Crawford, S. G. (1998). DCD may not be a discrete disorder. *Human Movement Science, 17,* 471–490.

Kavale, K., & Mattson, P. D. (1983). "One jumped off the balance beam": Meta-analysis of perceptual–motor training. *Journal of Learning Disabilities, 16,* 165–173.

Kemmis, B. L., & Dunn, W. (1996). Collaborative consultation: The efficacy of remedial and compensatory interventions in school contexts. *American Journal of Occupational Therapy, 50,* 709–717.

Kempermann, G., & Gage, F. H. (1999). Experience-dependent regulation of adult hippocampal neurogenesis: Effects of long-term stimulation and stimulus withdrawal. *Hippocampus, 9,* 321–332.

Kempermann, G., Kuhn, H. G., & Gage, F. H. (1998). Experience-induced neurogenesis in the senescent dentate gyrus. *Journal of Neuroscience, 18*(9), 3206–3212.

Kephart, N. C. (1971). *The slow learner in the classroom* (2nd ed.). Columbus, OH: Merrill.

Kern, J. K., Trivedi, M. H., Garver, C. R., Grannemann, B. D., Andrews, A. A., Savla, J. S., et al. (2006). The pattern of sensory processing abnormalities in autism. *Autism, 10,* 480–494.

Kielhofner, G. (2006). Developing and evaluating quantitative data collection instruments. In G. Kielhofner (Ed.), *Research in occupational therapy: Methods of inquiry for enhancing practice* (pp. 155–176). Philadelphia: F. A. Davis.

Kielhofner, G., & Fossey, E. (2006). The range of research. In G. Kielhofner (Ed.), *Research in occupational therapy: Methods of inquiry for enhancing practice* (pp. 20–35). Philadelphia: F. A. Davis.

Kientz, M. A., & Dunn, W. (1997). A comparison of the performance of children with and without autism on the Sensory Profile. *American Journal of Occupational Therapy, 51,* 530–537.

King, G., Law, M., King, S., Hurley, P., Rosenbaum, P., Hanna, S., et al. (2005). *Children's Assessment of Participation and Enjoyment (CAPE) and Preferences for Activities of Children (PAC).* San Antonio, TX: Harcourt.

Kinnealey, M., Koenig, K. P., & Smith, S. (in press). The relationship among sensory processing, health related quality of life, and social supports in adults. *American Journal of Occupational Therapy.*

Kinnealey, M., Oliver, B., & Wilbarger, P. (1995). A phenomenological study of sensory defensiveness in adults. *American Journal of Occupational Therapy, 49,* 444–451.

Kinsbourne, M. (1991). Overfocusing: An apparent subtype of attention deficit hyperactivity disorder. In N. Amir, I. Rapin, & D. Branski (Eds.), *Pediatric neurology: Behavior and cognition of the child with brain dysfunction* (Vol. 1, pp. 18–35). Basel, Switzerland: Karger.

Knox, S. (2008). Development and current use of the Knox Preschool Play Scale. In L. Parham & L. Fazio (Eds.), *Play in occupational therapy for children* (pp. 55–70). St. Louis, MO: Mosby.

Koenig, K. P., & Rudney, S. G. (2010). Performance challenges for children and adolescents with difficulty processing and integrating sensory information: A systematic review. *American Journal of Occupational Therapy, 64,* 434–447.

Koomar, J., & Bundy, A. (2002). Creating intervention from theory. In A. C. Bundy, S. J. Lane, A. G. Fisher, & E. A. Murray (Eds.), *Sensory integration theory and practice* (2nd ed., pp. 261–308). Philadelphia: F. A. Davis.

Kourtzi, Z., Betts, L. R., Sarkheil, P., & Welchman, A. E. (2005). Distributed neural plasticity for shape learning in the human visual cortex. *PLoS Biology, 3,* e204.

Kujala, A., Huotilainen, M., Uther, M., Shtyrov, Y., Monto, S., Ilmoniemi, R. J., et al. (2003). Plastic cortical changes induced by learning to communicate with non-speech sounds. *NeuroReport, 14,* 1683–1687.

Lacourse, M. G., Turner, J. A., Randolph-Orr, E., Schandler, S. L., & Cohen, M. J. (2004). Cerebral and cerebellar sensorimotor plasticity following motor imagery-based mental practice of a sequential movement. *Journal of Rehabilitation Research and Development, 41,* 505–524.

Lane, S. (2002). Sensory modulation. In A. C. Bundy, S. J. Lane, & E. A. Murray (Eds.), *Sensory integration: Theory and practice* (2nd ed., pp. 101–122). Philadelphia: F. A. Davis.

Lane, S. J., Miller, L. J., & Hanft, B. E. (2000). Toward a consensus in terminology in sensory integration theory and practice: Part 2. Sensory integration patterns of function and dysfunction. *Sensory Integration Special Interest Section Quarterly, 23*(2), 1–3.

Lane, S. J., & Schaaf, R. C. (2010). Examining the neuroscience evidence for sensory-driven neuroplasticity: Implications for sensory-based occupational therapy for children and adolescents with difficulty processing and integrating sensory information. *American Journal of Occupational Therapy, 64,* 375–390.

Law, M., Baptiste, S., Carswell, A., McColl, M. A., Polatajko, H., & Pollock, N. (2005). *Canadian Occupational Performance Measure* (4th ed.). Ottawa, ON: CAOT Publications.

Law, M., & Baum, C. (1998). Evidence-based occupational therapy. *Canadian Journal of Occupational Therapy, 65,* 131–135.

Leemrijse, C., Meijer, O. G., Vermeer, A., Adèr, H. J., & Diemel, S. (2000). The efficacy of Le Bon Départ and sensory integration. *Clinical Rehabilitation, 14,* 147–259.

Lieberman, D., & Scheer, J. (2002). AOTA's evidence-based literature review project: An overview. *American Journal of Occupational Therapy, 56,* 344–349.

Lin, S. H., Cermak, S., Coster, W. J., & Miller, L. (2005). The relation between length of institutionalization and sensory integration in children adopted from Eastern Europe. *American Journal of Occupational Therapy, 59,* 139–147.

Linder, T. W. (2008). *Transdisciplinary Play-Based Assessment: A functional approach to working with young children* (2nd ed.). Baltimore: Paul H. Brookes.

Linderman, T. M., & Stewart, K. B. (1999). Sensory integrative–based occupational therapy and functional outcomes in young children with pervasive developmental disorders: A single-subject study. *American Journal of Occupational Therapy, 53,* 207–213.

Liss, M., Saulnier, C., Fein, D., & Kinsbourne, M. (2006). Sensory and attention abnormalities in autistic spectrum disorders. *Autism, 10,* 155–172. doi:10.1177/1362361306062021

Lloyd, M., Reid, G., & Bouffard, M. (2006). Self-regulation of sport-specific and educational problem-solving tasks by boys with and without DCD. *Adapted Physical Activity Quarterly, 23,* 370–389.

MacDermid, J. C. (2004). An introduction to evidence-based practice for hand therapists. *Journal of Hand Therapy, 17,* 103–104.

Macintosh, K., & Dissanayake, C. (2006). Social skills and problem behaviors in school-aged children with high-functioning autism and Asperger's disorder. *Journal of Autism and Developmental Disorders, 36,* 1056–1076.

Mailloux, Z., May-Benson, T. A., Summers, C. A., Miller, L. J., Brett-Green, B., Burke, J. P., et al. (2007). Goal attainment scaling as a measure of meaningful outcome for children with sensory integration disorders. *American Journal of Occupational Therapy, 61,* 254–259.

Mailloux, Z., Mulligan, S., Smith Roley, S., Blanche, E., Cermak, S., Coleman, G. G., et al. (in press). Verification and clarification of patterns of sensory integrative dysfunction. *American Journal of Occupational Therapy.*

Mandich, A. D., Polatajko, H. J., & Rodger, S. (2003). Rites of passage: Understanding participation of children with developmental coordination disorder. *Human Movement Science, 22,* 583–595.

Marr, D., & Nackley, V. (2009). *Sensory stories: Manual & instructions.* Natick, MA: Theraproducts.

Martin, N. A. (2006). *Test of Visual–Perceptual Skills–3 (TVPS–3).* Los Angeles: Western Psychological Services.

Martin, N. A. (2010). *Test of Visual–Motor Skills–3 (TVMS–3).* Novato, CA: Academic Therapy Publications.

Martini, R., & Polatajko, H. J. (1998). Verbal self-guidance as a treatment approach for children with developmental coordination disorder: A systematic replication study. *OTJR: Occupation, Participation and Health, 18,* 157–181.

Martinussen, R., Hayden, J., Hogg-Johnson, S., & Tannock, R. (2005). A meta-analysis of working memory impairments in children with attention-deficit/hyperactivity disorder. *Journal of the American Academy of Child and Adolescent Psychiatry, 44,* 377–384.

Maurer, D., & Maurer, C. (1988). *The world of the newborn.* New York: Basic Books.

May-Benson, T. A. (2010). Play and praxis in children with an ASD. In H. Miller Kuhaneck & R. Watling (Eds.), *Autism: A comprehensive occupational therapy approach* (pp. 383–426). Bethesda, MD: AOTA Press.

May-Benson, T. A., & Cermak, S. A. (2007). Development of an assessment for ideational praxis. *American Journal of Occupational Therapy, 61,* 148–153.

May-Benson, T. A., & Koomar, J. (2010). Systematic review of the research evidence examining the effectiveness of interventions using a sensory integrative approach for children. *American Journal of Occupational Therapy, 64,* 403–414.

McIntosh, D. N., Miller, L. J., Shyu, V., & Dunn, W. (1999). Overview of the Short Sensory Profile (SSP). In W. Dunn (Ed.), *The Sensory Profile: Examiner's manual* (pp. 59–73). San Antonio, TX: Psychological Corporation.

McIntosh, D. N., Miller, L. J., Shyu, V., & Hagerman, R. (1999). Sensory-modulation disruption, electrodermal responses, and functional behaviors. *Developmental Medicine and Child Neurology, 41,* 608–615.

McWilliam, R. A. (1991). *Children's Engagement Questionnaire.* Nashville, TN: Author, Vanderbilt Center for Child Development.

Mercado, E., Bao, S., Orduña, I., Gluck, M. A., & Merzenich, M. M. (2001). Basal forebrain stimulation changes cortical sensitivities to complex sound. *Neuroreport, 12,* 2283–2287.

Merzenich, M. M., Recanzone, G. H., Jenkins, W. M., & Grajski, K. A. (1990). Adaptive mechanisms in cortical networks underlying cortical contributions to learning and nondeclarative memory. *Cold Spring Harbor Symposia on Quantitative Biology, 55,* 873–887.

Miller, L. J. (1988). *Miller Assessment for Preschoolers.* San Antonio, TX: Psychological Corporation.

Miller, L. J. (2006). *Miller Function and Participation Scales.* San Antonio, TX: Psychological Corporation.

Miller, L. J., Anzalone, M. E., Lane, S. J., Cermak, S. A., & Osten, E. T. (2007). Concept evolution in sensory integration: A proposed nosology for diagnosis. *American Journal of Occupational Therapy, 61,* 135–140.

Miller, L. J., Coll, J. R., & Schoen, S. A. (2007). A randomized controlled pilot study of the effectiveness of occupational therapy for children with sensory modulation disorder. *American Journal of Occupational Therapy, 61,* 228–238.

Miller, L. J., McIntosh, D., McGrath, J., Shuy, V., Lampe, M., Taylor, A., et al. (1998). Electrodermal responses to sensory stimuli in individuals with fragile X syndrome: A preliminary report. *American Journal of Medical Genetics, 83*(4), 268–279.

Miller, L. J., Reisman, J. E., McIntosh, D. N., & Simon, J. (2001). An ecological model of sensory modulation: Performance of children with fragile X syndrome, autistic disorder, attention-deficit/hyperactivity disorder, and sensory modulation dysfunction. In S. S. Roley, E. I. Blanche, & R. C. Schaaf (Eds.), *Understanding the nature of sensory integration with diverse populations* (pp. 57–88). San Antonio, TX: Therapy Skill Builders.

Miller, L. J., Schoen, S., Coll, J. R., Schaaf, R. C., James, K., & Benzel, J. (2007). Part 1: Lessons learned: A pilot study on occupational therapy effectiveness for children with sensory modulation disorder. *American Journal of Occupational Therapy, 61,* 161–169.

Miller, L. J., Schoen, S., James, K., & Schaaf, R. C. (2007). Lessons learned: A pilot study on occupational therapy effectiveness for children with sensory modulation disorder. *American Journal of Occupational Therapy, 61,* 161–169.

Miller, L. J., & Summers, C. (2001). Clinical applications in sensory modulation dysfunction. In S. S. Roley, E. I. Blanche, & R. C. Schaaf (Eds.), *Understanding the nature of sensory integration in diverse populations* (pp. 247–274). San Antonio, TX: Therapy Skill Builders.

Miller, L. T., Polatajko, H. J., Missiuna, C., Mandich, A. D., & Macnab, J. J. (2001). A pilot trial of a cognitive treatment for children with developmental coordination disorder. *Human Movement Science, 20,* 183–210.

Miller Kuhaneck, H., Henry, D., & Glennon, T. (2007). *Sensory Processing Measure (SPM): Main classroom and school environment forms.* Los Angeles, CA: Western Psychological Services.

Miller Kuhaneck, H., Henry, D., & Glennon, T. (2010). *Sensory Processing Measure–Preschool (SPM–P), school form.* Los Angeles, CA: Western Psychological Services.

Minshew, N. J., Sung, K., Jones, B. L., & Furman, J. M. (2004). Underdevelopment of the postural control system in autism. *Neurology, 63,* 2056–2061.

Missiuna, C., Pollock, N., & Law, M. (2004). *Perceived Efficacy and Goal Setting System (PEGS).* Oxford, UK: Harcourt Assessment.

Mollo, K., Schaaf, R., & Benevides, T. (2008). The use of Kripalu yoga to decrease sensory overresponsivity: A pilot study. *Sensory Integration Special Interest Section Quarterly, 31*(3), 14.

Molloy, C. A., Dietrich, K. N., & Bhattacharya, A. (2003). Postural stability in children with autism spectrum disorder. *Journal of Autism and Developmental Disorders, 33,* 643–652.

Morrison, D., & Sublett, J. (1986). The effect of sensory integrative therapy on nystagmus duration, equilibrium reactions, and visual motor integration in reading retarded children. *Child: Care, Health and Development, 12,* 99–110.

Moses, S. N., Martin, T., Houck, J. M., Ilmoniemi, R. J., & Tesche, C. D. (2005). The C50m response: Conditioned magnetocerebral activity recorded from the human brain. *NeuroImage, 27,* 778–788.

Moyers, P., & Dale, L. (2007). *The guide to occupational therapy practice* (2nd ed.). Bethesda, MD: AOTA Press.

Mullen, B., Champagne, T., Krishnamurty, S., Dickson, D., & Gao, R. X. (2008). Exploring the safety and therapeutic effects of deep pressure stimulation using a weighted blanket. *Occupational Therapy in Mental Health, 24,* 65–89.

Mulligan, S. (1998). Patterns of sensory integration dysfunction: A confirmatory factor analysis. *American Journal of Occupational Therapy, 52,* 819–828.

Mulligan, S. (2000). Cluster analysis of scores of children on the Sensory Integration and Praxis Tests. *OTJR: Occupation, Participation and Health, 20,* 258–270.

Mulligan, S. (2003a). Examination of the evidence for occupational therapy using a sensory integration framework with children: Part 2. *Sensory Integration Special Interest Section Quarterly, 26*(2), 1–5.

Mulligan, S. E. (2003b). *Occupational therapy evaluation for children.* Philadelphia: Lippincott Williams & Wilkins.

Murray, E. A., Cermak, S. A., & O'Brien, V. (1990). The relationship between form and space perception, constructional abilities, and clumsiness in children. *American Journal of Occupational Therapy, 44,* 623–628.

Nakahara, H., Zhang, L. I., & Merzenich, M. M. (2004). Specialization of primary auditory cortex processing by sound exposure in the "critical period." *Proceedings of the National Academy of Sciences of the United States of America, 101,* 7170–7174.

National Institute on Deafness and Other Communication Disorders. (2004). *Auditory processing disorder in children.* Retrieved February 1, 2011, from http://www.nidcd.nih.gov/health/voice/auditory.html

Newborg, J. (2004). *Battelle Developmental Inventory—Second Edition manual.* Rolling Meadows, IL: Riverside.

Nolan, J. E. (2004). Analysis of Kavale and Mattson's "balance beam" study (1983): Criteria for selection of articles. *Perceptual and Motor Skills, 99,* 63–82.

North Shore Pediatric Therapy. (2009). *Gravitational insecurity.* Retrieved January 22, 2011, from http://nspt4kids.com/health-topics-conditions/gravitational-insecurity/

O'Brien, V., Cermak, S. A., & Murray, E. (1988). The relationship between visual–perceptual–motor abilities and clumsiness in children with and without learning disabilities. *American Journal of Occupational Therapy, 42,* 359–363.

Orduña, I., Mercado, E., Gluck, M. A., & Merzenich, M. M. (2005). Cortical responses in rats predict perceptual sensitivities to complex sounds. *Behavioral Neuroscience, 119*(1), 256–264.

O'Riordan, M., & Passetti, F. (2006). Discrimination in autism within different sensory modalities. *Journal of Autism and Developmental Disorders, 36,* 665–675.

Orsmond, G. I., Krauss, M. W., & Seltzer, M. M. (2004). Peer relationships and social and recreational activities among adolescents and adults with autism. *Journal of Autism and Developmental Disorders, 34,* 245–256.

Ottenbacher, K. (1982a). Patterns of postrotary nystagmus in three learning disabled children. *American Journal of Occupational Therapy, 36,* 657–663.

Ottenbacher, K. (1982b). Sensory integration therapy: Affect or effect. *American Journal of Occupational Therapy, 36,* 571–578.

Ottenbacher, K., Short, M. A., & Watson, P. J. (1979). Nystagmus duration changes of learning disabled children during sensory integrative therapy. *Perceptual and Motor Skills, 48,* 1159–1164.

Pantev, C., Ross, B., Fujioka, T., Trainer, L. J., Schulte, M., & Shulz, M. (2003). Music and learning induced cortical plasticity. *Annals of the New York Academy of Science, 999,* 438–450.

Parham, L. D. (1998). The relationship of sensory integrative development to achievement in elementary students: Four-year longitudinal patterns. *OTJR: Occupation, Participation and Health, 18,* 105–127.

Parham, L. D., Cohn, E. S., Spitzer, S., Koomar, J. A., Miller, L. J., Burke, J. P., et al. (2007). Fidelity in sensory integration research. *American Journal of Occupational Therapy, 61,* 216–227.

Parham, L. D., & Ecker, C. (2007). *Sensory Processing Measure (SPM): Home form.* Los Angeles: Western Psychological Services.

Parham, L. D., Ecker, C., Miller Kuhaneck, H., Henry, D. A., & Glennon, T. J. (2007). *Sensory Processing Measure (SPM): Manual.* Los Angeles: Western Psychological Services.

Parham, L. D., & Mailloux, Z. (2010). Sensory integration. In J. Case-Smith & J. C. O'Brien (Eds.), *Occupational therapy for children* (6th ed., pp. 325–372). St. Louis, MO: Mosby/Elsevier.

Parham, L. D., Smith Roley, S., Koomar, J., May-Benson, T., Brett-Green, B., Burke, J. P., et al. (2011). Development of a fidelity measure for research on effectiveness of Ayres Sensory Integration.® *American Journal of Occupational Therapy, 65,* 133–142.

Parush, S., Sohmer, H., Steinberg, A., & Kaitz, M. (1997). Somatosensory functioning in children with attention deficit hyperactivity disorder. *Developmental Medicine and Child Neurology, 39,* 464–468.

Pfeiffer, B., & Kinnealey, M. (2006). Treatment of sensory defensiveness in adults. *Occupational Therapy International, 10,* 175–184.

Pfeiffer, B., Kinnealey, M., Reed, C., & Herzberg, G. (2005). Sensory modulation and affective disorders in children and adolescents with Asperger's disorders. *American Journal of Occupational Therapy, 59,* 335–345.

Piek, J. P., Dyck, M. J., Nieman, A., Anderson, M., Hay, D., Smith, L. M., et al. (2004). The relationship between motor coordination, executive functioning, and attention in school-aged children. *Archives of Clinical Neuropsychology, 19,* 1063–1076.

Pless, M., & Carlsson, M. (2000). Effects of motor skill intervention on developmental coordination disorder: A meta-analysis. *Adapted Physical Activity Quarterly, 17,* 381–401.

Polatajko, H. J., & Cantin, N. (2010). Exploring the effectiveness of occupational therapy interventions, other than the sensory integration approach, with children and adolescents experiencing difficulty processing and integrating sensory information. *American Journal of Occupational Therapy, 64,* 415–429.

Polatajko, H. J., Kaplan, B. J., & Wilson, B. N. (1992). Sensory integration treatment for children with learning disabilities: Its status 20 years later. *OTJR: Occupation, Participation and Health, 12,* 323–341.

Polatajko, H. J., Law, M., Miller, J., Schaffer, R., & MacNab, J. J. (1991). The effect of a sensory integration program on academic achievement, motor performance, and self-esteem in children identified as learning disabled: Results of a clinical trial. *Occupational Therapy Journal of Research, 11,* 155–176.

Polatajko, H. J., Mandich, A. D., Miller, L. T., & Macnab, J. J. (2001). Cognitive Orientation to Daily Occupational Performance (CO-OP): Part II—The evidence. *Physical and Occupational Therapy in Pediatrics, 20,* 83–106. doi:10.1300/J006v20n02_06

Polcyn, P., & Bissell, J. (2005). Flexible models of service using the sensory integration framework in school settings. *Sensory Integration Special Interest Section Quarterly, 28*(1), 1–4.

Porges, S. W. (1995). Cardiac vagal tone: A physiological index of stress. *Neuroscience and Biobehavioral Reviews, 19,* 225–233.

Poulsen, A. A., Ziviani, J. M., Cuskelly, M., & Smith, R. (2007). Boys with developmental coordination disorder: Loneliness and team sports participation. *American Journal of Occupational Therapy, 61,* 451–462.

Ptito, M., Moesgaard, S. M., Gjedde, A., & Kupers, R. (2005). Crossmodal plasticity revealed by electrotactile stimulation of the tongue in the congenitally blind. *Brain, 128,* 606–614.

Ragert, R., Schmidt, A., Altenmuller, E., & Dinse, H. R. (2004). Superior tactile performance and learning in professional pianists: Evidence for meta-plasticity in musicians. *European Journal of Neuroscience, 19,* 473–478.

Recanzone, G. H., Schreiner, C. E., & Merzenich, M. M. (1993). Plasticity in the frequency representation of primary auditory cortex following discrimination training in adult owl monkeys. *Journal of Neuroscience, 13*(1), 87–103.

Reeves, G. D. (1998). Case report of a child with sensory integration dysfunction. *Occupational Therapy International, 5,* 304–316. doi:10.1002/oti.84

Reisman, J. E. (1999). *The Minnesota Handwriting Test user's manual*. San Antonio, TX: Psychological Corporation.

Reisman, J. E., & Hanschu, B. (1992). *Sensory Integration Inventory—Revised for individuals with developmental disabilities: User's guide*. Hugo, MN: PDP Press.

Renier, L., Collignon, O., Poirier, C., Tranduy, D., Vanlierde, A., Bol, A., et al. (2005). Crossmodal activation of visual cortex during depth perception using auditory substitution of vision. *NeuroImage, 26,* 573–580.

Reynolds, C. R., & Kamphaus, R. W. (2006). *BASC–2: Behavior Assessment System for Children* (2nd ed.). Upper Saddle River, NJ: Pearson Education.

Reynolds, C. R., Pearson, N. A., & Voress, J. K. (2002). *Developmental Test of Visual Perception—Adolescent and Adult (DTVP–A)*. Lutz, FL: Psychological Assessment Resources.

Reynolds, S., & Lane, S. J. (2008). Diagnostic validity of sensory overresponsivity: A review of the literature and case reports. *Journal of Autism and*

Developmental Disorders, 38, 516–529. doi:10.1007/s10803–007–0418–9

Reynolds, S., Lane, S. J., & Gennings, C. (2010). The moderating role of sensory overresponsivity in HPA activity: A pilot study with children diagnosed with ADHD. *Journal of Attention Disorders, 13*(5), 468–478.

Reynolds, S., Watling, R., Zapletal, A., & May-Benson, T. A. (2010). *Sensory integration in entry-level occupational therapy education.* Manuscript submitted for publication.

Richardson, P. (2010). Use of standardized tests in pediatric practice. In J. Case-Smith & J. C. O'Brien (Eds.), *Occupational therapy for children* (6th ed., pp. 216–243). Maryland Heights, MI: Mosby.

Rieke, E. F., & Anderson, D. (2009). Adolescent/Adult Sensory Profile and obsessive–compulsive disorder. *American Journal of Occupational Therapy, 63,* 138–145.

Rinehart, N. J., Bellgrove, M. A., Tonge, B. J., Brereton, A. V., Howells-Rankin, D., & Bradshaw, J. L. (2006). An examination of movement kinematics in young people with high-functioning autism and Asperger's disorder: Further evidence for a motor planning deficit. *Journal of Autism and Developmental Disorders, 36,* 757–767.

Roberts, J. E., King-Thomas, L., & Boccia, M. L. (2007). Behavioral indexes of the efficacy of sensory integration therapy. *American Journal of Occupational Therapy, 61,* 555–562.

Röder, B., Rösler, F., & Neville, H. J. (2000). Event-related potentials during auditory language processing in congenitally blind and sighted people. *Neuropsychologia, 38,* 1482–1502.

Rodger, S., Ziviani, J., Watter, P., Ozanne, A., Woodyatt, G., & Springfield, E. (2003). Motor and functional skills of children with developmental coordination disorder: A pilot investigation of measurement issues. *Human Movement Science, 22,* 461–478.

Rogers, S. J., Hepburn, S., & Wehner, E. (2003). Parent reports of sensory symptoms in toddlers with autism and those with other developmental disorders. *Journal of Autism and Developmental Disorders, 33,* 631–642.

Rosenzweig, M. R., & Bennett, E. L. (1972). Cerebral changes in rats exposed individually to an enriched environment. *Journal of Comparative and Physiological Psychology, 80*(2), 304–313.

Rosenzweig, M. R., Bennett, E. L., Diamond, M. C., Wu, S.-Y., Slagle, R. W., & Saffran, E. (1969). Influences of environmental complexity and visual stimulation of development of occipital cortex in rat. *Brain Research, 14,* 427–445.

Ross-Swain, D. (1996). *Ross Information Processing Assessment* (2nd ed.). San Antonio, TX: Pearson.

Royeen, C. B. (1987). TIP–Touch Inventory for Preschoolers: A pilot study. *Physical and Occupational Therapy in Pediatrics, 7,* 29–40.

Royeen, C. B., & Fortune, J. C. (1990). Touch Inventory for Elementary-School-Aged Children. *American Journal of Occupational Therapy, 44,* 155–159.

Rubia, K., Taylor, A., Taylor, E., & Sergeant, J. A. (1999). Synchronization, anticipation, and consistency in motor timing of children with dimensionally defined attention deficit hyperactivity behavior. *Perceptual and Motor Skills, 89,* 1237–1258.

Russo, N. M., Nicol, T. G., Zecker, S. G., Hayes, E. A., & Kraus, N. (2005). Research report: Auditory training improves neural timing in the human brainstem. *Behavioural Brain Research, 156,* 95–103.

Sackett, D. L., Rosenberg, W. M., Gray, J. A., Haynes, R. B., & Richardson, W. S. (1996). Evidence-based medicine: What it is and what it isn't. *British Medical Journal, 312,* 71–72.

Salihagic-Kadic, A., Kurjak, A., Medic, M., Andonotopo, W., & Azumendi, G. (2005). New data about embryonic and fetal neurodevelopment and behavior obtained by 3D and 4D sonography. *Journal of Perinatal Medicine, 33,* 478–490.

Schaaf, R., & Davies, P. L. (2010). From the desk of the editor—The evolution of the sensory integration frame of reference. *American Journal of Occupational Therapy, 64,* 363–367.

Schaaf, R. C., Miller, L. J., Seawell, D., & O'Keefe, S. (2003). Children with disturbances in sensory processing: A pilot study examining the role of the parasympathetic nervous system. *American Journal of Occupational Therapy, 57,* 442–449.

Schaaf, R. C., & Nightlinger, K. M. (2007). Occupational therapy using a sensory integrative approach: A case study of effectiveness. *American Journal of Occupational Therapy, 61,* 239–246.

Schaaf, R. C., Schoen, S., Lane, S. J., Smith Roley, S., & May-Benson, T. (2009). The sensory integration frame of reference. In P. Kramer & J. Hinojosa (Eds.), *Frames of reference in pediatric occupational therapy*. Philadelphia: Lippincott Williams & Wilkins.

Schaaf, R. C., Schoen, S. A., Roley, S. S., Lane, S. J., Koomar, J., & May-Benson, T. A. (2010). A frame of reference for sensory integration. In P. Kramer & J. Hinojosa (Eds.), *Frames of reference for pediatric occupational therapy* (pp. 99–186). Philadelphia: Lippincott Williams & Wilkins.

Schaaf, R. C., & Smith Roley, S. (2006). *Sensory integration: Applying clinical reasoning to practice with diverse populations.* Austin, TX: Pro-Ed.

Schaefer, M., Heinze, H., & Rotte, M. (2005). Task-relevant modulation of primary somatosensory cortex suggests a prefrontal–cortical sensory gating system. *NeuroImage, 27,* 130–135.

Schapiro, S., & Vukovich, K. (1970). Early experience effects upon cortical dendrites: A proposed model for development. *Science, 167,* 292–294.

Schell, B. A. B. (2009). Professional reasoning in practice. In E. B. Crepeau, E. S. Cohn, & B.A.B. Schell (Eds.), *Willard and Spackman's occupational therapy* (10th ed., pp. 314–332). Philadelphia: Lippincott Williams & Wilkins.

Schilling, D. L., & Schwartz, I. S. (2004). Alternative seating for young children with autism spectrum disorder: Effects on classroom behavior. *Journal of Autism and Developmental Disorders, 34,* 423–432.

Schreck, K. A., Williams, K., & Smith, A. F. (2004). A comparison of eating behaviors between children with and without autism. *Journal of Autism and Developmental Disorders, 34,* 433–438.

Schroeder, R. J. (1982). Improvement in academic achievement through enhancement of perceptual and sensory integrative functioning. *School Psychology International, 3,* 97–104.

Sherrill, C. (1998). *Adapted physical activity, recreation and sport: Crossdiciplinary and lifespan* (5th ed.). Boston: WCB McGraw-Hill.

Shochat, T., Tzischinsky, O., & Engel-Yeger, B. (2009). Sensory hypersensitivity as a contributing factor in the relation between sleep and behavioral disorders in normal schoolchildren. *Behavioral Sleep Medicine, 7,* 53–62.

Shoener, R. F., Kinnealey, M., & Koenig, K. P. (2008). You can know me now if you listen: Sensory, motor, and communication issues in a non-verbal individual with autism. *American Journal of Occupational Therapy, 62,* 547–553.

Sigmundsson, H., Hansen, P. C., & Talcott, J. B. (2003). Do "clumsy" children have visual deficits? *Behavioral Brain Research, 139,* 123–129.

Sigmundsson H., & Hopkins, B. (2005). Do "clumsy" children have visual recognition deficits? *Child: Care, Health, and Development, 31,* 155–158.

Sinha, H., Silove, N., Wheeler, D., & Williams, K. (2006). Auditory integration training and other sound therapies for autism spectrum disorders: A systematic review. *Archives of Disease in Childhood, 91,* 1018–1022.

Skard, G., & Bundy, A. (2008). Test of Playfulness. In D. Parham & L. Fazio (Eds.), *Play in occupational therapy for children* (2nd ed., pp. 71–94). St. Louis, MO: Mosby.

Smith Roley, S. (with Schaaf, R. C.). (2006a). Evaluating sensory integration function and dysfunction. In R. C. Schaaf & S. Smith Roley (Eds.), *Sensory integration: Applying clinical reasoning to practice with diverse populations* (pp. 15–36). Austin, TX: Pro-Ed.

Smith Roley, S. (2006b). Sensory integration theory revisited. In R. C. Schaaf & S. Smith Roley (Eds.), *Sensory integration*: *Applying clinical reasoning to practice with diverse populations* (pp. 1–13). Austin, TX: Pro-Ed.

Smith Roley, S., Blanche, E. I., & Schaaf, R. C. (2001). *Understanding the nature of sensory integration with diverse populations.* San Antonio, TX: Therapy Skill Builders.

Smith Roley, S., & Jacobs, S. E. (2008). Sensory integration. In E. B Crepeau, E. S. Cohn, & B. A. B. Schell (Eds). *Willard & Spackman's occupational therapy* (11th ed., pp. 792–817). Philadelphia: Lippincott Williams & Wilkins,

Smith Roley, S., Mailloux, Z., Miller Kuhaneck, H, & Glennon, T. (2007). Understanding Ayres Sensory Integration.® *OT Practice, 12*(17), CE1–CE8.

Smits-Engelsman, B. C. M., Wilson, P. H., Westenberg, Y., & Duysens, J. (2003). Fine motor deficiencies in children with developmental coordination disorder and learning disabilities: An underlying open-loop control deficit. *Human Movement Science, 22,* 495–513.

Smyth, M., & Anderson, H. (2000). Coping with clumsiness in the school playground: Social and physical play in children with coordination impairments. *British Journal of Developmental Psychology, 18,* 389–413.

Snow, J. H., Blondis, T. A., Accardo, P. J., & Cunningham, K. J. (1993). Longitudinal assessment of motor and sensory skills in academically disabled and control children. *Archives of Clinical Neuropsychology, 8*(1), 55–68.

Sober, S. J., & Sabes, P. N. (2005). Flexible strategies for sensory integration during motor planning. *Nature Neuroscience 8*(4), 490–497.

Sparrow, S., Balla, E., & Cicchetti, D. (1984). *Vineland Adaptive Behavior Scales.* Circle Pines, MN: American Guidance Service.

Sparrow, S. S., Cicchetti, D. V., & Balla, D. A. (2005). *Vineland Adaptive Behavior Scales* (2nd ed.). San Antonio, TX: Pearson.

Spitzer, S. L. (1999). Dynamic systems theory: Relevance to the theory of sensory integration and the study of occupation. *Sensory Integration Special Interest Section Quarterly, 22*(2), 1–4.

Spitzer, S., & Roley, S. S. (2001). Sensory integration revisited: A philosophy of practice. In S. S. Roley, E. I. Blanche, & R. C. Schaaf (Eds.), *Understanding the nature of sensory integration with diverse populations* (pp. 3–27). San Antonio, TX: Therapy Skill Builders.

Stoeckel, M. C., Pollok, B., Schnitzler, A., Witte, O. W., & Seitz, R. J. (2004). Use-dependent cortical plasticity in thalidomide-induced upper extremity dysplasia: Evidence from somaesthesia and neuroimaging. *Experimental Brain Research, 156,* 333–341.

Stoodley, C. J., Fawcett, A. J., Nicolson, R. I., & Stein, J. F. (2005). Impaired balancing ability in dyslexic children. *Experimental Brain Research, 167,* 370–380.

Stryker, M. P., & Sherk, H. (1975). Modification of cortical orientation selectivity in the cat by restricted visual experience: A reexamination. *Science, 190,* 904–906.

Sugden, D. A., & Chambers, M. E. (2003). Intervention in children with developmental coordination disorder: The role of parents and teachers. *British Journal of Educational Psychology, 73,* 545–561. doi:10.1348/000709903322591235

Tecchio, F., Benassi, F., Zappasodi, F., Gialloreti, L. E., Palermo, M., Seri, S., et al. (2003). Auditory sensory processing in autism: A magnetoencephalographic study. *Biological Psychiatry, 54,* 647–654.

Tervo, R. C., Azuma, S., Fogas, B., & Fiechtner, H. (2002). Children with ADHD and motor dysfunction compared with children with ADHD only. *Developmental Medicine and Child Neurology, 44,*

383–390. [*44, 622*. Correction of dosage error in abstract].

Therapro. (2009). *Sensory stories.* Retrieved February 1, 2011, from http://www.therapro.com/Sensory-Stories-C307930.aspx

Tomchek, S. D., & Case-Smith, J. (2009). *Occupational therapy practice guidelines for children and adolescents with autism.* Bethesda, MD: AOTA Press.

Tomchek, S. D., & Dunn, W. (2007). Sensory processing in children with and without autism: A comparative study using the Short Sensory Profile. *American Journal of Occupational Therapy, 61,* 190–200.

Toplak, M. E., & Tannock, R. (2005). Time perception: Modality and duration effects in attention-deficit/hyperactivity disorder (ADHD). *Journal of Abnormal Child Psychology, 33,* 639–654.

Trachtenberg, J. T., & Stryker, M. P. (2001). Rapid anatomical plasticity of horizontal connections in the developing visual cortex. *Journal of Neuroscience, 21,* 3476–3482.

Trombly, C. (1995). Occupation: Purposefulness and meaningfulness as therapeutic mechanisms. *American Journal of Occupational Therapy, 49,* 960–972.

Urbina, S. (2004). *Essentials of psychological testing.* Hoboken, NJ: Wiley.

U.S. National Center for Health Statistics (Vols. 1–2), & Health Care Financing Administration (Vol. 3). (1997). *International classification of diseases, 9th revision, clinical modification (ICD-9-CM).* Dover, DE: American Medical Association.

U.S. Office of Special Education Programs. (2006). *Monitoring, technical assistance and enforcement.* 20 U.S.C. §§1416 and 1442.

VandenBerg, N. L. (2001). The use of a weighted vest to increase on-task behavior in children with attention difficulties. *American Journal of Occupational Therapy, 55,* 621–628.

van Praag, H., Kempermann, G., & Gage, F. H. (1999). Running increases cell proliferation and neurogenesis in the adult mouse dentate gyrus. *Nature Neuroscience, 2*(3), 266–270.

Van Waelvelde, H., De Weerdt, W., De Cock, P., Janssens, H., Feys, H., & Smits Engelsman, B. C. (2006). Parameterization of movement execution in children with developmental coordination disorder. *Brain and Cognition, 60,* 20–31.

Van Waelvelde, H., De Weerdt, W., De Cock, P., & Smits-Engelsman, B. C. M. (2004). Association between visual–perceptual deficits and motor deficits in children with developmental coordination disorder. *Developmental Medicine and Child Neurology, 46,* 661–666.

Vargas, S., & Camilli, G. (1999). A meta-analysis of research on sensory integration treatment. *American Journal of Occupational Therapy, 53,* 189–198.

Vernazza-Martin, S., Martin, N., Vernazza, A., Lepellec-Muller, A., Rufo, M., Massion, J., & Assaiante, C. (2005). Goal directed locomotion and balance control in autistic children. *Journal of Autism and Developmental Disorders, 35,* 91–102.

Vickers, J. N., Rodrigues, S. T., & Brown, L. N. (2002). Gaze pursuit and arm control of adolescent males diagnosed with attention deficit hyperactivity disorder (ADHD) and normal controls: Evidence of a dissociation in processing visual information of short and long duration. *Journal of Sports Sciences, 20,* 201–216.

Volkmar, F. R., & Greenough, W. T. (1972). Rearing complexity affects branching of dendrites in the visual cortex of the rat. *Science, 176,* 1445–1447.

Walsh, R. N., Cummins, R. A., & Budtz-Olsen, O. E. (1973). Environmentally induced changes in the dimensions of the rat cerebrum: A replication and extension. *Developmental Psychobiology, 6*(1), 3–7.

Watling, R., Bodison, S., Henry, D. A., & Miller-Kuhaneck, H. (2006). Sensory integration: It's not just for children. *Sensory Integration Special Interest Section Quarterly, 29*(4), 1–4.

Watling, R. L., Deitz, J. C., & White, O. (2001). Comparison of the Sensory Profile scores of young children with and without autism spectrum disorders. *American Journal of Occupational Therapy, 55,* 416–423.

Watling, R., & Miller Kuhaneck, H. (with Audet, L.). (2010). Emotion regulation in the autism spectrum disorders. In H. Miller Kuhaneck & R. Watling (Eds.), *Autism: A comprehensive occupational therapy approach* (pp. 115–134). Bethesda, MD: AOTA Press.

Werry, J. S., Scaletti, R., & Mills, F. (1990). Sensory integration and teacher judged learning problems: A controlled intervention trial. *Journal of Paediatrics and Child Health, 26,* 31–35.

West, R. W., & Greenough, W. T. (1972). Effect of environmental complexity on cortical synapses of rats: Preliminary results. *Behavioral Biology, 7,* 279–284.

Wetherby, A. M., & Prizant, B. M. (2002). *Communication and Symbolic Behavior Scales—Developmental Profile.* Baltimore: Brookes.

White, B. P., Mulligan, S., Merrill, K., & Wright, J. (2007). An examination of the relationships between motor and process skills and scores on the Sensory Profile. *American Journal of Occupational Therapy, 61,* 154–160.

White, M. (1979). A first-grade intervention program for children at risk for reading failure. *Journal of Learning Disabilities, 12,* 26–32.

Wiesel, T. N., & Hubel, D. H. (1965). Extent of recovery from the effects of visual deprivation in kittens. *Neurophysiology, 28,* 1060–1072.

Wiesel, T. N., & Hubel, D. H. (1974). Ordered arrangement of orientation columns in monkeys lacking visual experience. *Journal of Comparative Neurology, 158,* 307–318.

Wilbarger, J., & Wilbarger, P. (2002). Alternative and complementary programs for intervention: Clinical application of the sensory diet. In A. C. Bundy, S. J. Lane, A. G. Fisher, & E. A. Murray (Eds.), *Sensory integration theory and practice* (2nd ed., pp. 339–341). Philadelphia: F. A. Davis.

Wilbarger, P., & Wilbarger, J. L. (1991). *Sensory defensiveness in children ages 2–12: An intervention guide for parents and other caretakers.* Santa Barbara, CA: Avanti Educational Programs.

Williams, E., Reddy, V., & Costall, A. (2001). Taking a closer look at functional play in children with autism. *Journal of Autism and Developmental Disorders, 31,* 67–77.

Williams, M. S., & Shellenberger, S. (1994). *How does your engine run? A leader's guide to the Alert Program for Self-Regulation.* Albuquerque, NM: Therapy Works.

Williamson, G. G., Anzalone, M. E., & Hanft, B. E. (2000). Assessment of sensory processing, praxis, and motor performance. In S. I. Greenspan (Ed.), *Clinical practice guidelines: Redefining the standards of care for infants, children and families with special needs* (pp. 155–184). Bethesda, MD: Interdisciplinary Council on Developmental and Learning Disorders.

Wilson, B. N., & Kaplan, B. J. (1994). Follow-up assessment of children receiving sensory integration treatment. *Occupational Therapy Journal of Research, 14,* 244–267.

Wilson, B. N., Kaplan, B. J., Fellowes, S., Gruchy, C., & Faris, P. (1992). The effect of sensory integration treatment compared to tutoring. *Physical and Occupational Therapy in Pediatrics, 12,* 1–36.

Wilson, P. H., Maruff, P., Ives, S., & Currie, J. (2001). Abnormalities of motor and praxis imagery in children with DCD. *Human Movement Science, 20,* 135–159.

Wilson, P. H., & McKenzie, B. E. (1998). Information processing deficits associated with developmental coordination disorder: A meta-analysis of research findings. *Journal of Child Psychology and Psychiatry and Allied Disciplines, 39,* 829–840.

Wilson, P. H., Thomas, P. R., & Maruff, P. (2002). Motor imagery training ameliorates motor clumsiness in children. *Journal of Child Neurology, 17,* 491–498. doi:10.1177/088307380201700704

Windsor, M. M., Smith Roley, S., & Szklut, S. (2001). Assessment of sensory integration and praxis. In S. Smith Roley, E. I. Blanche, & R. C. Schaaf

(Eds.), *Understanding the nature of sensory integration with diverse populations* (pp. 215–245). San Antonio, TX: Therapy Skill Builders.

Wolfberg, P. J. (1995). Enhancing children's play (Appendix: Play Preference Inventory). In K. A. Quill (Ed.), *Teaching children with autism: Strategies to enhance communication and socialization* (p. 217). Independence, KY: Thomson Delmar Learning.

World Health Organization. (2001). *International classification of functioning, disability and health*. Geneva, Switzerland: Author.

Wu, C. W.-H., van Gelderen, P., Hanakawa, T., Yaseen, Z., & Cohen, L. G. (2005). Enduring representational plasticity after somatosensory stimulation. *NeuroImage 27,* 872–884.

Yochman, A., Ornoy, A., & Parush, S. (2006). Co-occurrence of developmental delays among preschool children with attention-deficit-hyperactivity disorder. *Developmental Medicine and Child Neurology, 48,* 483–488.

Yochman, A., Parush, S., & Ornoy, A. (2004). Responses of preschool children with and without ADHD to sensory events in daily life. *American Journal of Occupational Therapy, 58,* 294–302.

You, S. H., Jang, S. H., Kim, Y. H., Kwon, Y. H., Barrow, I., & Hallett, M. (2005). Cortical reorganization induced by virtual reality therapy in a child with hemiparetic cerebral palsy. *Developmental Medicine and Child Neurology, 47,* 628–635.

Zeitlin, S. (1985). *Coping Inventory*. Bensenville, IL: Scholastic Testing Service.

Zeitlin, S., Williamson, G. G., & Szczepanski, M. (1988). *Early Coping Inventory*. Bensenville, IL: Scholastic Testing Service.

Zhang, L. I., Bao, S., & Merzenich, M. M. (2001). Persistent and specific influences of early acoustic environments on primary auditory cortex. *Nature Neuroscience, 4,* 1123–1130.

Zimmerman, B. J. (2000). Attaining self-regulation: A social cognitive perspective. In M. Boekaerts, P. R. Pintrich, & M. Zeidner (Eds.)., *Handbook of self-regulation* (pp. 13–40). Maryland Heights, MI: Academic Press.

Ziviani, J., Poulsen, A., & O'Brien, A. (1982). Effect of a sensory integrative/neurodevelopmental programme on motor and academic performance of children with learning disabilities. *Australian Occupational Therapy Journal, 29,* 27–33.

Zoia, S., Pelamatti, G., Cuttini, M., Casotto, V., & Scabar, A. (2002). Performance of gesture in children with and without DCD: Effects of sensory input modalities. *Developmental Medicine and Child Neurology, 44,* 699–705.